ELITE PHYSIQUE

The New Science of Building a Better Body

Chad Waterbury, PT, DPT, MS

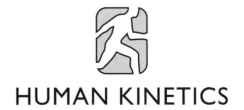

HUMAN KINETICS

Library of Congress Cataloging-in-Publication Data

Names: Waterbury, Chad author.
Title: Elite physique : the new science of building a better body / Chad
  Waterbury.
Description: Champaign, IL : Human Kinetics, 2022. | Includes
  bibliographical references.
Identifiers: LCCN 2021017929 (print) | LCCN 2021017930 (ebook) | ISBN
  9781718203785 (paperback) | ISBN 9781718203792 (epub) | ISBN
  9781718203808 (pdf)
Subjects: LCSH: Bodybuilding. | Muscle strength. | Weight training.
Classification: LCC GV546.5 .W37 2022 (print) | LCC GV546.5 (ebook) | DDC
  613.7/13--dc23
LC record available at https://lccn.loc.gov/2021017929
LC ebook record available at https://lccn.loc.gov/2021017930

ISBN: 978-1-7182-0378-5 (print)

This publication is written and published to provide accurate and authoritative information relevant to the subject matter presented. It is published and sold with the understanding that the author and publisher are not engaged in rendering legal, medical, or other professional services by reason of their authorship or publication of this work. If medical or other expert assistance is required, the services of a competent professional person should be sought.

The web addresses cited in this text were current as of June 2021, unless otherwise noted.

Acquisitions Editor: Michael Mejia; **Developmental Editor:** Laura Pulliam; **Managing Editor:** Shawn Donnelly; **Copyeditor:** Patricia L. MacDonald; **Permissions Manager:** Martha Gullo; **Graphic Designer:** Julie L. Denzer; **Cover Designer:** Keri Evans; **Cover Design Specialist:** Susan Rothermel Allen; **Photographer (cover):** MRBIG Photography/iStock/Getty Images; **Photographer (interior):** Chad Waterbury; **Photo Production Manager:** Jason Allen; **Senior Art Manager:** Kelly Hendren; **Illustrations:** © Human Kinetics; **Printer:** Walsworth

We thank The Prehab Guys in Los Angeles, California, for providing the location for the photo shoot for this book.

Human Kinetics books are available at special discounts for bulk purchase. Special editions or book excerpts can also be created to specification. For details, contact the Special Sales Manager at Human Kinetics.

Printed in the United States of America   10 9 8 7 6 5 4 3 2 1

The paper in this book was manufactured using responsible forestry methods.

Human Kinetics
1607 N. Market Street
Champaign, IL 61820
USA

United States and International
Website: **US.HumanKinetics.com**
Email: info@hkusa.com
Phone: 1-800-747-4457

Canada
Website: **Canada.HumanKinetics.com**
Email: info@hkcanada.com

E8315

Tell us what you think!
Human Kinetics would love to hear what we can do to improve the customer experience. Use this QR code to take our brief survey.

This book is dedicated to all the good teachers, nurses, paramedics, doctors, soldiers, Marines, firefighters, and police officers out there.

CONTENTS

PART I   PLAN FOR MUSCLE

PART II   MUSCLE METHODOLOGY

EXERCISE FINDER

● = online video is available

Chapter 7 Upper Body Training

ACCESSING THE ONLINE VIDEO

This book includes access to online video that contains more than 30 clips demonstrating upper body, lower body, and core exercises. Throughout the book, exercises marked with this play button icon indicate where the content is enhanced by online video clips: ◐

Take the following steps to access the video. If you need help at any point in the process, you can contact us via email at HKPropelCustSer@hkusa.com.
If it's your first time using HK*Propel*:

1. Visit HKPropel.HumanKinetics.com.
2. Click the "New user? Register here" link on the opening screen.
3. Follow the onscreen prompts to create your HK*Propel* account.
4. Enter the access code exactly as shown below, including hyphens. You will not need to re-enter this access code on subsequent visits.
5. After your first visit, simply log in to HKPropel.HumanKinetics.com to access your digital product.

If you already have an HK*Propel* account:

1. Visit HKPropel.HumanKinetics.com and log in with your username (email address) and password.
2. Once you are logged in, navigate to Account in the top right corner.
3. Under "Add Access Code" enter the access code exactly as shown below, including hyphens.

Access code: WATERBURY1E-YHTY-BPUP-CMTX

Once your code is redeemed, navigate to your Dashboard, then select the **Online Video** from the Library. You'll then see an Online Video page with links to two video playlists. Clicking a link will open a video player; each video player contains multiple video clips.

In the player, the clips will appear vertically along the right side. Select the video you would like to watch and view it in the main player window. You can use the buttons at the bottom of the main player window to view the video full screen, to turn captioning on and off, and to pause, fast-forward, or reverse the clip.

Your license to this online video will expire 7 years after the date you redeem the access code. You can check the expiration dates of all your HK*Propel* products at any time in My Account.

For technical support, contact us via email at HKPropelCustSer@hkusa.com.
Helpful tip: You may reset your password from the log in screen at any time if you forget it.

ACKNOWLEDGMENTS

I would like to thank the following people:

John Berardi
Mark Cheng
Justin Dean
Joe DeFranco
Jay and Jen Ferruggia
David Garfinkle
Chris Hitchko
Arash Maghsoodi
Stuart McGill
Stuart McMillan
Michael Mejia
Jason Park

Peter Park
Chris Powers
Wolfgang Puck
John Rusin
Don Saladino
Brad Schoenfeld
Todd Schroeder
Lou Schuler
Susan Sigward
Pavel Tsatsouline
Charlie Weingroff
Fabio Zonin

INTRODUCTION

For most of my life, I've been trying to figure out the mysteries of the human body. Specifically, I've studied how to make it as big, strong, lean, fast, and athletic as possible without using drugs or inflicting the kind of damage that would leave me in pain for the rest of my life.

You could say it was ambitious. It also seemed odd to friends and even some colleagues. What was left to learn? Was there any way to improve the human physique—any exercises, training systems, or diets—that hadn't already been discovered by weightlifters, bodybuilders, and athletes over the past hundred years?

They had a point. Every great physique, from Sandow to Schwarzenegger, was built by manipulating the same basic variables:

- Volume
- Intensity (load)
- Exercise selection
- Frequency
- Recovery

Still, as I saw it, there *was* something left to learn, something we couldn't pick up from following the routines of elite athletes who sometimes trained for three or four hours a day: How could my clients and readers achieve the best possible results in three or four hours *a week*? That led me to decades of experimentation—first in my own workouts, then with my clients, and then with thousands of readers in articles and books.

Here's what I'll share in the following chapters:

- The many ways to build muscle, including some even the most knowledgeable and experienced lifters haven't yet seen or tried
- How to use those systems effectively with whatever equipment you have available
- How to achieve the results you want in less time than you thought possible

But before we get into the details—and there are a *lot* of details—I want to take a moment to explain why they matter, and why it's worth your time to focus on them.

Going Beyond Newbie Gains

Everyone who picks up a barbell or dumbbell quickly learns the importance of two variables: volume and intensity. Do more sets and reps (volume) with heavier weights (intensity or load), and more often than not, you'll see better results than if you do less work with lighter weights.

If you work hard enough and consistently enough, you'll make impressive gains. You'll get bigger and stronger, and at first you may also get leaner at the same time. That's the magic of newbie gains. The less trained your body is, the greater your potential for fast, dramatic results.

But then two things happen: Your strength gains slow down significantly as your body gets closer to its peak potential, and muscle growth often seems nonexistent. You also max out your time, energy, and ability to recover. You can't keep adding volume to your workouts, or workouts to your schedule. And if you focus on intensity, trying to lift heavier and push yourself harder in the time you have, you'll eventually learn a simple fact of physiology: The harder you work, the more recovery you need.

I set out, many years ago, to find new or forgotten ways to trigger muscle growth without adding volume or impeding the body's ability to recover. My first breakthrough came when I tried manipulating sets and reps. What would happen if, instead of doing the classic 3 sets of 10 reps, you did 10 sets of 3? You would

- spend more time doing the primary movement patterns—presses, pulls, squats, deadlifts—and less time doing accessory exercises,
- do more work with heavier weights without increasing your injury risk, and
- improve your strength and skill on key exercises.

Some of this was old-school stuff. Pre-steroid-era bodybuilders spent most of their time doing basic barbell and dumbbell exercises, with the goal of getting stronger rather than chasing the pump. But it wasn't what I saw in gyms or read about in magazines or websites.

My second breakthrough came when I manipulated frequency. Most people, when they're starting out, will train all their muscles two or three times a week. But some muscles recover faster than others, and as I discovered, they respond better when they're trained more often.

My experiments with high-frequency training led to my third breakthrough: figuring out when and how to use more advanced training methods.

Those methods were developed by people who were trying to solve specific problems. But in my experience, most of the people using them didn't have the problem the methods were created to address.

Instead, I saw people who grabbed onto the latest thing they came across because they were bored or frustrated with their current programs. Over time, their workouts became the fitness equivalent of a potluck dinner: lots of stuff to sample, some of which would be excellent on its own, but nothing a professional chef would ever combine and offer to the same person at the same meal. I wanted to find systematic ways to incorporate the right techniques at the right time to get the best possible results for my clients and readers.

That brings me to you.

Building the Right Program for Your Needs

I wrote this book for four types of lifters:

- The ones who never fully achieved their newbie gains. They moved on to advanced programs even though the basics were still working for them. They still have lots of potential to gain strength and size by returning to simple, progressive routines.

- The ones who maxed out their gains on beginner or intermediate programs but continued doing them long after they stopped working.

- The ones who refuse to accept their bodies' unique abilities and limitations. They get hurt, recover, and then return to the exact same exercises and techniques that caused the injury in the first place.

- The ones who took advantage of their newbie gains and learned from their mistakes and injuries. They work out consistently and intelligently. But they're stuck in a cycle of gaining and losing the same 5 to 10 pounds (2.3 to 4.5 kg) of muscle and fat.

The last thing any of these lifters need is a book filled with random exercises to plug into random programs. That's why my book begins with a series of self-assessments, including the functional strength standards, which I developed with John Rusin. It's probably a lot more detailed than any assessment you've seen or used. But once you complete it, you'll understand your strengths and weaknesses and also have an accurate baseline for tracking your progress.

From there you'll learn what to do with that information, choosing the right program for your needs and goals. You'll find guidance for building mass, getting lean, and bringing up specific body parts.

The final two chapters cover nutrition and joint health—what you can do to get leaner and more muscular now, and what you can do to stay that way for the rest of your life. Talk to anyone who's been lifting for two decades or more, and they'll tell you they wished they'd known more about these areas when they started.

No matter how long you've been lifting, whether it's a few weeks or many years, you'll find in these pages a system that will help you get bigger, leaner, and stronger—and stay healthy while you're doing it.

PART I

PLAN FOR MUSCLE

CHAPTER 1

Assess to Impress

The information in this chapter gives you the opportunity to perform an honest assessment of yourself. This will help you establish a starting point to more accurately gauge your progress, beyond looking in a mirror. We go through a series of assessments ranging from posture to strength and endurance. Even if your primary goal is to build muscle and burn fat, these assessments are valuable tools for monitoring your orthopedic health, a key to long-term wellness and performance. The goal is to determine which area(s) of your body might need soft tissue work or less fat, and which muscles might need more strength or endurance.

Before we begin, it is worth mentioning that a joint or muscle we don't test here could be causing a problem in your body or negatively affecting one of your exercises. If you experience pain in any joint during or after exercise, it's imperative to get it checked out by a licensed therapist. There is no honor in working through pain, because it will probably get worse.

Posture

Most of us think of the general term *posture* as standing tall with your shoulders pulled back and eyes straight ahead, like a good soldier. As kids, we were told not to slouch. Even though this might have seemed like unnecessary disciplinary tactics, there is merit to the relationship between posture, health, and well-being (Golec de Zavala, Lantos, and Bowden 2017). There is no doubt that posture is directly related to performance and health.

The way you normally stand can reveal key orthopedic issues. For example, a hunched upper back can indicate stiffness in the thoracic spine or weak abdominals. If one shoulder is higher than the other it could mean the high side has a stiff upper trapezius or the low side has a stiff latissimus dorsi, which can pull that shoulder down. Even though you might not have the education or background to understand what all the various nuances in posture mean, it is helpful to know if your right arch is more flattened than your left or if your right shoulder is anteriorly rotated. These visual cues help determine which muscles could use some soft tissue work by a masseuse or yourself, or it can also tell you what to correct throughout the day while standing and moving.

For example, if your left shoulder is anteriorly rotated, meaning your left palm naturally rests more anteriorly on your thigh than your right, work on keeping your left shoulder pulled back throughout the day. The goal is to see an improvement over the weeks and months in your relaxed standing posture, indicating an improvement in structural alignment. The good news is that once you know how far you stray from ideal posture, which we're about to cover, you can correct the difference simply by practicing good posture throughout the day—no physical therapy or chiropractic visits necessary.

Standing Static Posture Assessment

To assess your standing static posture, have someone take the following photos of you wearing nothing but snug shorts, with your feet bare.

Front and Rear Views

Stand completely relaxed with your arms hanging down at your sides. Get photos from the front and rear views, which is the frontal plane. Ideal posture consists of eyes, shoulders, and pelvis parallel to the ground and an equal arch on each foot; a vertical line can be drawn through the center of the eyes, sternum, and pelvis (see figure 1.1).

There are postural compensations that make the subject fall out of proper alignment in the key areas just mentioned. Common causes of stiffness or weakness that correspond with these compensations from top to bottom are as follows:

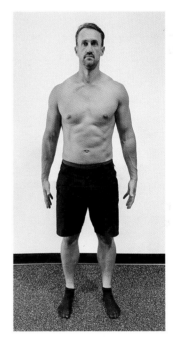

FIGURE 1.1 Frontal plane ideal posture.

- *Tilted or rotated head position:* stiffness in the sternocleidomastoid, levator scapulae, or suboccipitals
- *Elevated or depressed shoulder position:* stiffness in the upper trapezius or levator scapulae (elevated) or latissimus dorsi (depressed)
- *Flattened (i.e., pronated) foot:* weakness of the posterior tibialis or stiffness of the lateral shin muscles

Right and Left Side Views

Stand completely relaxed with your arms hanging down at your sides. Get photos of the right and left side views, which is the sagittal plane. Ideal posture consists of physical alignment that allows a straight vertical line to be drawn from the center of your ear through the center of your shoulder, hip, and knee and through the posterior portion of the lateral malleolus (see figure 1.2).

There are postural compensations that make the subject fall out of proper alignment in the key areas just covered. Common causes of stiffness that correspond with the compensations from top to bottom are as follows:

- *Anterior head position:* stiffness in the suboccipitals
- *Anteriorly rotated shoulder:* stiffness in the pectorals
- *Anterior knee position:* stiffness in the soft tissue of the posterior knee (i.e., posterior joint capsule or popliteus)

Finally, when having the aforementioned photos taken, it is imperative to stand as you normally would without any cues. If you stand more erect than you normally would, with your shoulders pulled back, it can hide your true orthopedic issues.

There's a third possible viewpoint, from overhead. That view of the transverse plane is not necessary since the frontal and sagittal planes reveal what needs to be corrected from our basic assessment.

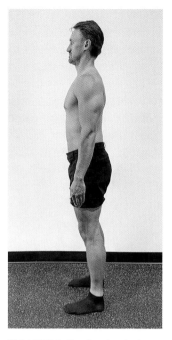

FIGURE 1.2   Sagittal plane ideal posture.

Balance

Balance is an essential aspect of life and performance, controlled by three systems within the body (see figure 1.3). First, the visual system transfers information from your eyes to your brain's cortex to regulate body orientation and self-motion.

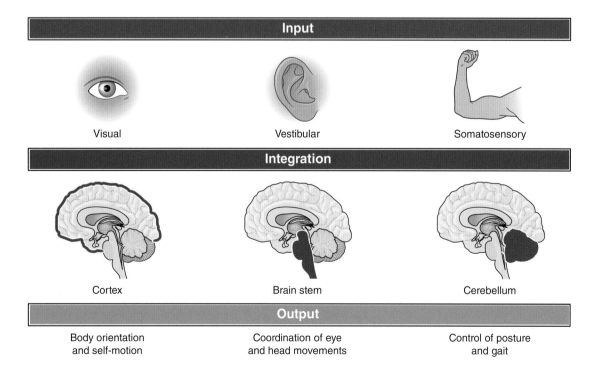

FIGURE 1.3   Three systems that control balance in the body.

Tricking Your Balance

Balance is controlled by three different systems: visual, vestibular, and somatosensory. Put another way, it's your eyes, inner ears, and feet that keep you from falling over, and you never know which could be throwing off your balance. As a physical therapist, I remove sensory input from each system one at a time by using the modified Romberg test to assess how my patient responds (Agrawal et al. 2011). I also use this test to assess the balance of patients who have trouble standing on one leg.

First, you will stand on a firm surface, feet together, with your eyes open. This allows all three systems (i.e., visual, vestibular, and somatosensory) to contribute to the task. If you are able to easily maintain balance in this first step, the second step is to close your eyes while maintaining the same posture. If your body immediately starts swaying, this means your visual system is playing a huge—often excessive—role in your balance. If your balance is still maintained, the third step is to stand on a thick, soft pad with your eyes open, thus requiring input from the visual and vestibular systems. Finally, you'll stand on that soft pad with your eyes closed, which limits sensory information to the vestibular system. This final step is where I want to see my patients able to maintain their balance (i.e., minimal trunk sway) for at least 20 seconds. Any duration less than that and your risk of falling significantly increases by more than threefold (Agrawal et al. 2011).

Research indicates that somatosensory information from your feet is the preferred way for your body to maintain balance (Shumway-Cook and Horak 1986). Here is a list of test conditions as they correlate with each sensory system:

Test condition	Sensory input
Firm surface, eyes open	Visual, vestibular, somatosensory
Firm surface, eyes closed	Vestibular, somatosensory
Soft surface, eyes open	Visual, vestibular
Soft surface, eyes closed	Vestibular

Second, the vestibular system transmits information from your inner ear to the brain stem to coordinate head and eye movement. Third, the somatosensory system feeds information from proprioceptors, joints, and cutaneous nerves in your feet to your cerebellum to control posture and gait, among many other functions.

Sufficient single-leg balance will help you perform better in the gym, and it's also necessary for preventing falls out in the real world. This assessment determines how well you can maintain balance and postural control while standing on one leg (Riemann 2002). If you find this difficult, there's still good news. All forms of exercise, from light to vigorous intensity, have a positive impact on balance (Loprinzi and Brosky 2014).

Single-Leg Balance Assessment

For this assessment, you will need a partner with a stopwatch or a clock or timer that counts seconds. The goal is to stand 16 seconds on each leg with the eyes closed.

To assess single-leg balance, stand tall with your feet together and arms held out to the sides far enough so they're not touching the body. Lift your right knee up in front until it's the same height as your hip, and try to maintain that position for 16 seconds (see figure 1.4). The test stops if you significantly sway your trunk to one side or move the foot of the stance leg.

If you didn't make it to 16 seconds while standing on your left leg, make a note of your time for future reference. Now test your single-leg balance while standing on your right leg with the left knee elevated. If you made it to 16 seconds while standing on each leg, repeat the exercise with your eyes closed.

There are numerous scenarios that could pan out here. Here are a few:

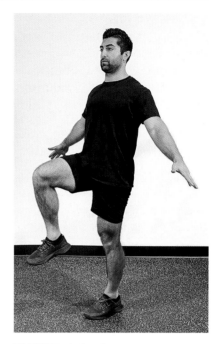

FIGURE 1.4 Single-leg balance test.

- You fell short of 16 seconds on one or both legs with your eyes open. Keep practicing the test until you reach 16 seconds with your eyes open, and then work to achieve the same duration with your eyes closed.

- You passed on one side with your eyes closed but fell short of 16 seconds on the other. If you practice the test for that leg a few times each day, combined with the training programs in this book, you might pass the test in four weeks. Keep at it until you do.

- You were able to maintain single-leg balance on each leg for 16 seconds with your eyes closed. Retest every six weeks to make sure you're maintaining it.

You might be wondering why 16 seconds was the chosen goal for this assessment. That duration is based on data collected from approximately 20,000 amateur golfers by Greg Rose and his team at the Titleist Performance Institute (2019).

Mobility

The goal of this book is to teach you how to build an impressive physique that also performs well during any sport. Indeed, most guys and gals want to build a body that looks *and* performs better than it does now. A key aspect of performing well in the gym is mobility, the ability of your joints to work through a normal range of motion. For example, if your ankles are stiff it will be difficult, if not impossible, to perform a full squat with good form (Kim et al. 2015). Or if your latissimus dorsi muscles are stiff, it will negatively affect your ability to reach your arms overhead, thus setting you up for a shoulder or low back injury in the gym during an overhead press. Sometimes doctors or physical therapists use mobility jargon that can lead to more confusion than solutions. When it comes to mobility, it's often best to look at the big picture. For example, can you touch your toes and fully extend both arms overhead? If you can, you're probably fine to perform most activities you need in life.

For the purposes of this book, we focus on key areas that are typically stiff in an active population of gym-goers: spine, hips, ankles, and shoulders. We look at big, multisegmental movements instead of isolating each joint individually, which should be done by a physical therapist if you see a problem. Let's start with the spine and hips.

Normal Might Not Be Optimal

Elite athletes often have physical demands different from what a typical weekend warrior might need. Consider the dorsiflexion range of motion test we cover in this chapter. For an Olympic weightlifter who needs to drop into a deep squat with a heavy barbell overhead, the recommended value for dorsiflexion might be too low. On the other hand, a normal level of dorsiflexion for an elite sprinter might be too high.

According to world-renowned sprint coach Stuart McMillan, "If we increase dorsiflexion range of motion past what is appropriate to generate a stiff, reflex response on the ground, it will ultimately decrease sprint performance." In other words, elite sprinters benefit from having stiff ankles, usually on the order of 0 degrees of dorsiflexion, compared with the 20 degrees recommended in physical therapy for the general public.

Indeed, there are exceptions to many guidelines for strength and mobility. Elite basketball players benefit from stiffer than normal hamstrings because it gives them more explosiveness when jumping or driving around an opponent. According to McMillan, "More mobility is not necessarily a good thing. It is about what is appropriate mobility for the given task."

Hip Hinge

The hip hinge is an essential movement pattern, necessary for everything from picking up something from the floor to ideal alignment during a deadlift to a proper setup in your golf stance. The inability to touch your toes can identify problems in the hip hinge pattern. The problem could be due to stiffness in the hamstrings, pelvis, hips, or spine.

Multisegmental Flexion Assessment

To assess multisegmental flexion, you will perform a standing toe touch. This assesses the mobility of the posterior chain—a band of muscles that runs from your calves up through the center of your posterior trunk to the base of your skull—and of the pelvis, hips, and spine. The goal is to touch the toes without pain.

To perform this assessment, stand with your feet together and toes pointed straight ahead. Bend forward and try to touch your toes while keeping your legs locked straight (see figure 1.5). If you can touch your toes without pain, move on to the multisegmental extension assessment.

If you can't touch your toes, the next step is to determine if it's a unilateral or bilateral problem. To determine this, stand with all your weight on your left leg, with your right knee slightly flexed and heel elevated, to test the mobility of your left hip (see figure 1.6). Then repeat on the right side by standing with all your weight on your right leg, with your left knee slightly flexed and heel elevated, to test the mobility of your right hip. If you can touch your right foot while standing on your right leg, it's a unilateral problem in the left hip. If you can touch your left foot while standing on your left leg, it's a unilateral problem in the right hip. If you still can't touch your toes on either side, it's a bilateral problem. Soft tissue work for the posterior chain by a qualified therapist is recommended.

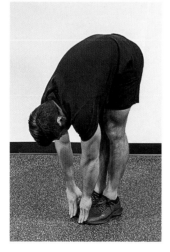

FIGURE 1.5 Multisegmental flexion correct form.

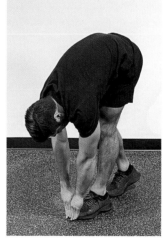

FIGURE 1.6 Multisegmental flexion on the left leg.

Spine and Hip Extension

Most people have more problems extending the hips and spine than they do flexing them. This problem is likely due to long periods of sitting and performing activities that promote poor posture, such as texting on a smartphone or working on a computer (Yang, Cao, et al. 2019). Therefore, the next assessment is to determine how well your hips and spine extend as an integrated unit.

Multisegmental Extension Assessment

This test assesses mobility of the anterior chain—a band of muscles that runs from your quadriceps up through the abdominals to the pectorals—and of the pelvis, hips, and spine.

Ask someone to take a photo of the side view while you are performing this assessment. Stand with your feet together and toes pointed straight ahead. Lift your arms overhead and then lean and reach as far backward as possible. The photo is taken at the end range of movement (see figure 1.7).

There are two things to look for here. First, does the top of your pelvis move past your toes? If not, muscles in your anterior chain might be stiff. Second, do the tops of your shoulder blades move past your heels? If not, your thoracic spine extension might be stiff. If you achieved both, and it didn't cause pain, you passed this test. Check with a physical therapist if you had any problems passing the test.

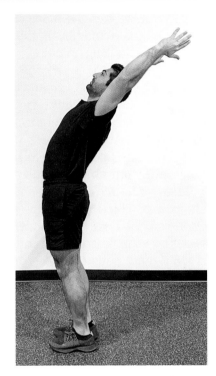

FIGURE 1.7 Multisegmental extension correct form.

Spine and Hip Rotation

At this point we've looked at how the spine and hips flex or extend. Now it's time to look at how those joints rotate. Being able to rotate your body is important for everything from throwing a baseball or punch to reaching for your seatbelt. Sufficient mobility of trunk and hip rotators is important to prevent low back pain (Masharawi, Haj, and Weisman 2020; Roach et al. 2015).

Multisegmental Rotation Assessment

This test assesses the mobility of the muscles that rotate the trunk and hips and the rotational mobility of the spine, pelvis, and hips.

Ask someone to take a photo of you from the back (at the end range of movement) while you perform this test. Stand with your feet together and toes pointed straight ahead. Rotate your trunk to the right as far as possible, as if you're trying to look over your right shoulder (see figure 1.8). Repeat by rotating your trunk to the left as far as possible.

The goal is to rotate far enough so your opposite shoulder can be seen from the rear view. So if you're rotating to the right, your partner standing behind you should be able to see the front of your left shoulder. If you did not pass on one or both sides, get some soft tissue work on the trunk and hip rotators until you pass.

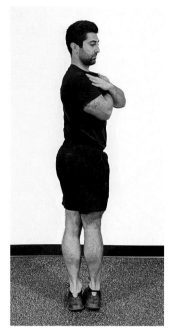

FIGURE 1.8 Multisegmental rotation correct form.

Dorsiflexion

Ankle mobility is often overlooked when assessing a person's ability to squat with proper form. However, your ankle health and squat depth are closely linked (Kim et al. 2015). Here we cover a basic assessment to determine if your mobility is up to par.

Dorsiflexion Assessment

This test assesses mobility of the calf muscles and ankle joint. The goal is for the knee to travel at least four inches (10 cm) past the toes on each side.

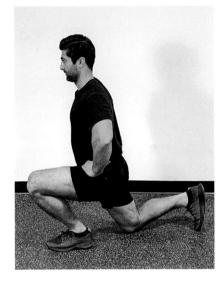

FIGURE 1.9 Dorsiflexion correct form.

To perform this assessment, have a partner nearby with a straight stick and tape measure. Drop into a half-kneeling position with your right knee on the ground and push your left knee as far as possible past the front of your left toes (see figure 1.9). The partner places the stick against the front of the left knee and perpendicular to the ground, and then measures the distance of the knee past the toes. Repeat by performing the same test for your right ankle, with your left knee resting on the floor.

It is easy to cheat during this assessment by collapsing the arch or pushing the knee inward, instead of forward, while testing the ankle. Make sure your knee pushes directly forward over the center of the foot and you maintain an arch. It is important to get an accurate gauge of your ankle mobility because the ability to dorsiflex each ankle through a normal range of motion is essential for performing a squat, deadlift, or lunge with proper form.

Overhead Mobility

The ability to reach both arms fully overhead is necessary for a wide variety of tasks, from lifting your suitcase into overhead storage to performing a shoulder press at the gym. A lack of overhead mobility, sometimes caused by stiffness in the shoulder extensors and internal rotators, can indicate an underlying injury or increase your risk of a future one (Cools et al. 2015; Page 2011). Although the possible culprits for poor overhead mobility can go beyond muscle stiffness, such as stiffness in the joint capsule or a bony impingement, it is important to determine if you're at risk of a shoulder injury, even if you currently don't feel any pain. A simple way to assess your overhead mobility is with the overhead reach test with your back against a wall.

Overhead Mobility Assessment

To assess overhead mobility, you will perform an overhead reach. This assesses the mobility of the shoulder extensors and internal rotators and the upward rotation of the scapulae. The goal is to touch both thumbs to the wall without pain.

To perform this assessment, assume a quarter squat with your low back pressed against a wall. Hold your arms straight in front with elbows locked and thumbs pointing up. Lift your arms overhead as high as possible, and attempt to touch your thumbs to the wall without arching your low back or bending your elbows (see figure 1.10). If you are able to touch both thumbs to the wall, you passed the test. If one or both sides fell short, see a licensed therapist to correct the problem.

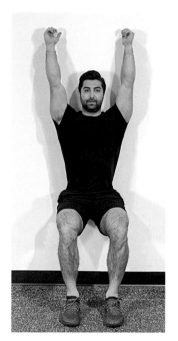

FIGURE 1.10 Overhead mobility correct form.

Cardiorespiratory Fitness

How much cardio do you need? The Center for Disease Control recommends that adults perform at least 150 minutes of moderate-intensity activity, or at least 75 minutes of vigorous-intensity activity, each week (U.S. Department of Health and Human Services 2018). Preferably, this duration of aerobic activity is spread throughout the week. Later in this book we cover workouts, consisting of both resistance training and cardiorespiratory conditioning, that meet those guidelines. For now, the goal is to find a simple way to measure how well your cardiorespiratory system is working to drive your endurance, as well as a way to test your progress.

You can test your cardiorespiratory fitness one of three ways, depending on your current level of fitness. The least taxing option is the 1-mile (1.6 km) walk test (Rockport walk test); the most challenging is the 1.5-mile (2.4 km) run, part of the Navy Physical Readiness Test (Whitehead et al. 2012). Both of these distance-based tests accurately correlate with an increase in $\dot{V}O_2$max, a measure of how well your body uses oxygen during exercise (Weiglein et al. 2011). The third option is the 12-minute walk/run test popularized by Kenneth Cooper, founder of the Cooper Institute (1968). All three tests are valid measures of cardiorespiratory fitness (Mayora-Vega et al. 2016; Weiglein et al. 2011).

A key with any form of testing is to keep the variables as consistent as possible. When you retest in the future, wear the same shoes and run on the same surface. Indeed, there are significant metabolic differences between running on a treadmill versus over ground (Miller et al. 2019). Neither is necessarily better, so use whichever is most convenient for you, and stick with it for future testing. For any of the following three tests it is important to first get clearance from your physician.

1-Mile Walk, 1.5-Mile Run, or 12-Minute Walk/Run

These tests assess the health of the heart, lungs, and blood vessels as well as the endurance of the lower extremities and respiratory muscles. Regardless of the test you choose, perform it with as much effort as possible, as follows:

- For the 1-mile (1.6 km) or 1.5-mile (2.4 km) run, make a note of the time it takes from start to finish.
- For the 12-minute walk/run, begin running and walk only when you don't have the energy to run during the test; make a note of the distance you traveled.

There are a few key points to mention here. First, if you choose to run on a treadmill, set the incline to 1 percent, which better mimics the demand of running over ground. Second, there is little consensus for recommended times or distances for the aforementioned tests. Therefore, the best option is to compete against yourself. Third, there are other ways to test your cardiorespiratory fitness that might be more conducive to the activities you enjoy. For example, you could test your distance using a stationary bike or rower over the course of 12 minutes, thus mimicking the 12-minute walk/run test. Whatever test you choose, work to increase your distance or time every four to six weeks.

Endurance Strength

There are typically two ways to describe endurance. One on hand, it's the ability to complete an hour-long hike at a pretty good clip with your buddy. That task requires your cardiorespiratory fitness to be up to par, which we just covered. On the other hand, the ability to do, say, 20 squats with 50 percent of your body weight also requires endurance. Since that type of challenge requires more strength and doesn't rely as heavily on cardiorespiratory fitness, it is referred to as endurance strength or muscular endurance. For example, a guy might be able to run three miles (4.8 km) at a 6-minute-mile pace, which would be a sign of terrific cardiorespiratory fitness, but he might not be strong enough to carry a 100-pound (45 kg) dumbbell in each hand for 30 seconds, indicating poor full-body endurance strength.

Also, it is likely you've had a buddy challenge you to a push-up contest at one time or another. If he was willing enough to challenge you to this test of endurance strength, it's also likely he could do more than 12 of them with perfect form. Indeed, the National Strength and Conditioning Association (NSCA) recommends performing more than 12 repetitions per set to build endurance strength. In other words, if you're working against resistance—in the form of either body weight or weights—it is necessary to complete at least 12 repetitions of that load before you stop.

Here, we cover four ways to test your endurance strength, ranging from upper body to lower body to full-body challenges.

Push-Up to Exhaustion

For this endurance strength assessment, you will perform push-ups through a full range of motion to exhaustion. This assesses endurance strength of the pectorals, triceps, deltoids, rotator cuff, and abdominals. The goal is to complete 40 push-ups before failure. According to research by Harvard University, being able to perform at least 40 push-ups is associated with a significant reduction in cardiovascular disease over the subsequent 10 years (Yang, Christophi, et al. 2019).

To perform this assessment, begin in the top position of a push-up, with your hands slightly wider than shoulder-width apart and directly below your chest (see figure 1.11a). Lower until your chest touches the ground while keeping your body perfectly straight from neck to ankles (see figure 1.11b). Push your body up to the starting position until your arms are completely straight. Repeat for a maximum number of repetitions.

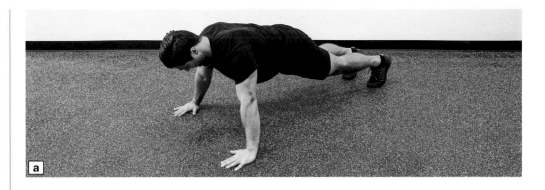

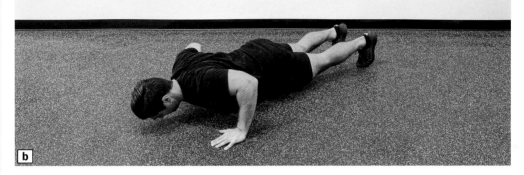

FIGURE 1.11   Endurance strength assessment: push-up to exhaustion.

Goblet Squat

The goblet squat assesses endurance strength of the lower extremity, trunk, biceps, and upper back. The goal is to complete 20 repetitions of the goblet squat with a dumbbell that weighs 50 percent of your body weight.

Compared with a barbell back squat, the goblet version is easier and safer to perform. Because you hold a dumbbell against your chest with both arms, it's easier to unload the movement instead of having a barbell across your upper back that needs to be re-racked. Furthermore, this front-loaded movement allows you to sit back more than a barbell back squat without losing your balance, which is excellent for learning how to correctly execute a hip hinge.

To perform this assessment, stand with your feet slightly wider than shoulder width and angled out slightly while holding a dumbbell in the goblet position (see figure 1.12a). Hold your elbows against your sides, brace your midsection, and then push your hips back and bend your knees until your elbows touch the top of your thighs (see figure 1.12b). Reverse the motion, keeping your midsection braced, until you reach the starting position. Repeat for a maximum number of repetitions.

For some of you, it might be impossible to perform even one repetition holding a dumbbell that is 50 percent of body weight. If that is the case, make a note of the heaviest dumbbell you can use to complete 20 perfect repetitions. After months of completing the resistance training programs in this book, your body will get stronger, allowing you to use a heavier dumbbell. The goal is to boost your strength to the point where you can perform 20 perfect repetitions of the goblet squat with a dumbbell that is 50 percent of body weight (e.g., 100-pound [45 kg] dumbbell for a 200-pound [90 kg] guy). A kettlebell works great for this exercise if a dumbbell isn't available.

(continued)

Goblet Squat   *(continued)*

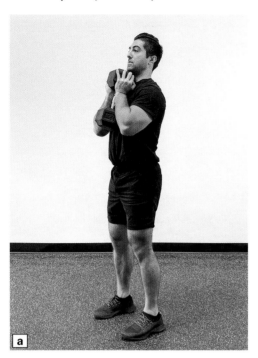
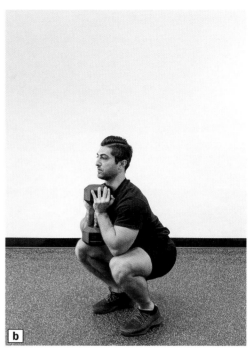

FIGURE 1.12   Endurance strength assessment: goblet squat.

Two-Arm Loaded Carry

For this endurance strength assessment, you will perform a two-arm loaded carry, also known as the farmer's walk. Let's say you decide one evening to google just how strong a guy should be. Or maybe you would like to find some scientific research that indicates how strong a college running back should be. In either case, you'd be out of luck. Currently, no reputable research demonstrates how much a running back should be able to squat, or how much weight a swimmer should be able to row, or any other strength recommendation for athletes, let alone active gym-goers. There is one exception: a peer-reviewed paper on the two-arm loaded carry (i.e., farmer's walk) by Scotty Butcher and John Rusin (2016), which we're about to cover.

This exercise requires high levels of stability strength throughout the trunk, pelvis, hips, and ankles as well as a strong grip. Indeed, this functional full-body exercise provides numerous benefits to athletes, including strengthening the *pillar complex*, a term used to describe

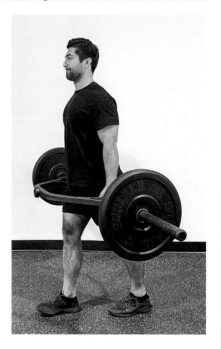

FIGURE 1.13   Endurance strength assessment: two-arm loaded carry with trap bar.

the synergistic activation of the shoulders, hips, and core. It is also an effective test of full-body strength and an exercise to enhance it. According to physical therapist and performance expert Dr. John Rusin, "For testing, developing, and displaying functional core strength, nothing beats the loaded carry and many of its derivatives. The loaded carry has the ability to identify and strengthen weak links simultaneously, as the test and training many times is the corrective fix."

In most cases, it is simplest to use a trap bar to perform the loaded carry There are two reasons. First, many gyms don't have dumbbells or kettlebells that are heavy enough to challenge the strongest gym-goers. Second, it's relatively easy to load and unload a trap bar during testing. However, it's perfectly fine to use heavy dumbbells, kettlebells, or anything else if a trap bar isn't available. For the general population (i.e., nonathletes), the goal is to carry 100 percent of body weight for 30 seconds. The goal for elite athletes is to carry 200 percent of body weight for 30 seconds (Butcher and Rusin 2016). If you're not strong enough to pull the load from the ground, it can be elevated in order to start the carry.

To perform this assessment, stand tall while holding a loaded trap bar with palms facing each other. Walk for 10 steps with a load you would rate as a 5 on a scale of 1 to 10, with 10 being the highest intensity (see figure 1.13). Rest 2 minutes, then walk for 10 steps with a load you would rate as a 7. Rest 3 minutes, then based on the load in your second attempt, guesstimate how much load you could carry for 30 seconds.

One-Leg Standing Calf Raise to Exhaustion

Research in physical therapy demonstrates that athletes and nonathletes alike should be able to perform 25 repetitions of a one-leg standing calf raise (Lunsford and Perry 1995). Sufficient endurance strength of the calves is necessary for a range of activities from descending stairs to running, cutting, and decelerating. Plus the principles for increasing the strength of your calves carry over into new muscle growth, which we cover later. One quick preview: The solution to new calf growth can be as simple as performing one set to failure from the floor through a full range of motion, twice each day (morning and evening), until you can perform 25 consecutive reps.

This test assesses endurance strength of the gastrocnemius and soleus muscles. The goal is to complete 25 one-leg calf raises, through a full range of motion, from the floor.

To perform this assessment, stand on your left leg, with your right knee bent so the right foot is off the floor (see figure 1.14*a*). Push through the base of your left big toe to elevate that heel as high as possible while keeping your left leg perfectly straight (see figure 1.14*b*). Perform as many repetitions as possible with a tempo of 1 second up and 1 second down. Repeat the test while standing on your right leg.

During this test it is very easy to reduce your range of motion as you fatigue. Each repetition should elevate your body as high as the first repetition: Any height short of that and the test stops. Some of my athletes who are seriously motivated to increase their calf girth place a marker above the head, such as the plastic wall slider used to measure your height, to use as a tactile reference for each repetition. In other words, the top of the head must touch the plastic slider for the repetition to count.

(continued)

One-Leg Standing Calf Raise to Exhaustion   *(continued)*

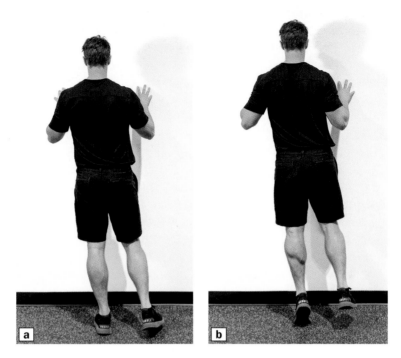

FIGURE 1.14   Endurance strength assessment: one-leg calf raise.

Maximal Strength

Maximal strength is a measure of a person's peak voluntary muscular force. This specific type of strength requires maximal activation of the largest motor units, which can typically sustain their activity for only 5 to 10 consecutive seconds. Maximal strength is important for an athlete who requires full-body power such as a running back, MMA fighter, or hockey player, just to name a few. Training with maximal loads requires high levels of synaptic input to the motor neuron pool, which recruits the high-threshold motor units that produce the most force (Kandel et al. 2013).

Generally speaking, maximal strength forms the foundation for all other types of strength. Lifting heavy loads strengthens the muscles, tendons, and bones, which are then capable of transferring more power to any sport or activity. Indeed, you can't develop high levels of power in the gym unless you have sufficient maximal strength.

Developing maximal strength can also help you increase your endurance for high-intensity activities. For example, improving your one-repetition maximum (1RM) in the bench press from 270 to 315 pounds (122 to 143 kg) will allow you to perform more reps with 225 pounds (102 kg), a common test in the NFL combine. Or consider an athlete who maxes out at three reps for the pull-up. If a few months later he's able to do those three reps with 50 pounds (23 kg) attached to a belt, he'll be able to perform significantly more reps of a body weight pull-up. One reason is because maximal strength development increases an athlete's work capacity, which then allows submaximal exercises to be performed at a lower relative intensity.

More Maximal Strength Is Not Always Better

Maximal strength is a major component of an athlete's overall fitness, but not every athlete needs more of it. The journey toward greater and greater maximal strength can come at a very high cost for athletes because it can wear down their joints, cause neural fatigue, and possibly expose them to unnecessary risks. Keep in mind that there's a limit to how much strength an athlete needs. More is not always better.

There's little doubt that superstar quarterback Tom Brady would fail to beat the vast majority of NFL players in a maximal-load bench press or squat test. Yet he possesses the physical attributes he needs to excel at his sport, all in proper balance. If Brady tried to add 100 pounds (45 kg) to his squat, it might throw off that balance. Or consider an NFL running back who can squat 450 pounds (204 kg), an impressive number for any athlete who's not a heavyweight powerlifter. It's highly unlikely that increasing his squat to 550 pounds (249 kg) would make him run faster or jump higher. In fact, it might have the opposite effect by causing joint pain or strain that, in turn, decreases his speed. Consult with a coach or physical therapist to determine whether or not you would benefit from more maximal strength.

Overview of Testing Your Maximal Strength

When determining your initial level of maximal strength, take great care not to push yourself beyond your physical capabilities. The number one factor in avoiding injury is to maintain ideal form while performing the test, so if you're new to lifting weights, or haven't lifted in months, have a reputable trainer analyze your form. You'll use the Borg CR10 scale, which measures your rating of perceived exertion (RPE). This 10-point scale is a valuable tool for determining how you're working. A rating of 1 should equate to complete rest and relaxation, as if you were lying on the couch, while a rating of 10 is all-out maximal effort. Values within that range are important to know, as we're about to cover.

It is important to not psyche yourself up before or during these tests. That mandates willpower, which is not what you're testing. A maximal strength test, and any other test in this chapter, should measure what you're capable of lifting without extra stimulation to get an accurate value. Now let's move on to the ways you can determine your one-repetition maximum (1RM) in the least stressful way possible.

How to Determine Your One-Repetition Maximum (1RM)

It has never been easy to accurately determine the maximum amount of weight you can lift for one rep. You expend a ton of time and energy as you lift, rest, increase the load, lift, rest, add or reduce the load—judging, missing, and guessing your way throughout the haphazard journey. This cycle continues until you find a true 1RM. This process usually takes 15 to 20 minutes per exercise, at best, and it can be exhausting, not to mention it puts you at risk of injury (Mazur, Yetman, and Risser 1993).

But knowing your 1RM for various lifts is beneficial for two reasons, even if you're not a competitive powerlifter, Olympic lifter, or strongman competitor.

First, some of the programs in this book use percentages of your 1RM to determine how much load you should put on the bar in each workout. Therefore, you'll need to know your 1RM to get those training loads dialed in correctly. Second, it's helpful to calculate 1RM because it's not easy to determine whether your maximal strength is increasing when you're using submaximal loads, which you'll be using for virtually every workout. Last month you were using 60-pound (27 kg) dumbbells for 8 reps; this month you're lifting 50-pound (22 kg) dumbbells for 13 reps. Did you get stronger? You won't know unless you have a good formula.

The most precise way to determine maximal strength is with a 1RM test, which you would rate as 10 on the Borg CR10 scale for a single repetition. A 1RM test, however, can be risky, time consuming, and exhausting. There are simpler, faster, and easier ways to determine your 1RM without overly taxing your mettle and joint integrity, as we cover shortly. For now, just know that a 1RM test is usually unnecessary. But if you decide to use it, stick with exercises that require little skill, such as a pin press, one-arm row, or lat pull-down. Avoid 1RM testing for complex lifts such as Olympic lifts, or exercises that put a lot of strain on the spine, such as a squat, deadlift, and standing overhead press, unless you're an advanced athlete who has been attempting maximal lifts for many years.

Table 1.1 represents the minimum number of steps before performing a maximal strength test. Perform at least three warm-up sets of two reps (3 × 2) with progressively heavier loads that correspond with the proper RPE. If you feel you need additional warm-up sets, perform as many as necessary. Your RPEs can vary slightly from what was just covered. What is important is that your RPE progressively increases and ends around 8 with your last warm-up set. If additional maximal-load attempts are necessary, rest at least 5 minutes in between. Never compromise your form in order to lift a heavier load, and avoid psychological stimulation. The recommended steps are as follows:

- *Set 1:* The first set should be with a load you rate as moderate, or an RPE of 4 or 5 on the Borg CR10 scale, followed by 1 minute of rest.
- *Set 2:* The second set should be rated 6 or 7, followed by 3 minutes of rest.
- *Set 3:* The third set should be approximately an 8, followed by 5 minutes of rest.
- *Set 4:* This is the maximal-load attempt.

Now let's cover three different ways to determine your 1RM without the risk of performing an actual 1RM attempt.

TABLE 1.1   Steps for Testing Maximal Strength

Set	Reps	RPE	Rest
Set 1: warm-up	2	4 or 5	1 min
Set 2: warm-up	2	6 or 7	3 min
Set 3: warm-up	2	8	5 min
Set 4: maximal attempt	X	10	5 min (if necessary)

2 or 3 Repetition Maximum or 5 Repetition Maximum (2RM or 3RM or 5RM) Test

The 2RM or 3RM test is my preferred method of estimating an athlete's 1RM because it relies on a range of reps, which increases your chances of finding the right load in minimal time. Start by following the warm-up protocol shown in table 1.1. Here you'll need to guesstimate what your 2RM or 3RM is, based on the warm-up. If you're unsure, choose the lightest load that seems close. Often a load that's approximately 15 percent heavier than the last warm-up set, if it was rated as an 8 RPE, is a good place to start. Ideally, you will achieve a 10 RPE at rep two or three, which would end the test.

If you failed to hit a 10 RPE on the second or third repetition, rest 5 minutes, and then repeat the 2RM or 3RM test until you get it right. Now you can do some simple math to determine your 1RM, as shown here:

2 reps = 90%-92.5% of 1RM

3 reps = 87.5%-90% of 1RM

You'll simply divide the load by the percentage to find the estimated 1RM. For example, if you maxed out at three reps with 150 pounds (68 kg), your 1RM for that lift is 167 to 171 pounds (76-78 kg). The math looks like this:

150 pounds/0.875 = 171 pounds

150 pounds/0.90 = 167 pounds

Now you have a range that estimates your 1RM. So which value should you use: 87.5 percent or 90 percent? It doesn't matter as long as you stay consistent with future tests. I recommend always using the lower value: 87.5 percent, in this case. I've found it's usually better to err on the lower end of the spectrum, since it helps manage fatigue. Furthermore, the difference between 167 and 171 pounds is relatively small in terms of the effect it will have on your strength and neural development. Put another way, 167 and 171 will both get the job done equally well, so use the lower value to help manage fatigue as much as possible. But also understand that your true 1RM might be closer to 171 pounds. If you're more comfortable attempting a 5RM, or if you end up doing a set that ends with an RPE of 10 on the fifth rep, you can consider that load to be 85 to 87.5 percent of your 1RM for that exercise. The values that correspond to a 2RM, 3RM, or 5RM are shown in table 1.2. These values are estimations that have been shown to be relatively reliable. The only way to get a completely accurate 1RM value is to test it. However, a competitive powerlifter or Olympic lifter is probably the only athlete who benefits from performing a true 1RM test every few months.

Table 1.2   Relationship Between RM and the Corresponding Percentage of 1RM

Repetition maximum (RM)	Percentage (%) of 1RM
2RM	90%-92.5%
3RM	87.5%-90%
5RM	85%-87.5%

Data from J.M. Reynolds, T.J. Gordon, and R.A. Robergs, "Prediction of One Repetition Maximum Strength From Multiple Repetition Maximum Testing and Anthropometry," *Journal of Strength and Conditioning Research* 20, no. 3 (2006): 584-592, and B. Richens and D.J. Cleather, "The Relationship Between the Number of Repetitions Performed at Given Intensities Is Different in Endurance and Strength Trained Athletes," *Biology of Sport* 31, no. 2 (2014): 157-161.

8 to 12 Repetition Maximum (8RM-12RM) Test

The submaximal 8RM-12RM test is a clinically sound way to estimate your 1RM, but it has shortcomings. For one, the further you get from a true 1RM, the less accurate the estimation will be (Macht et al. 2016). As soon as you perform six repetitions, other qualities beyond maximal strength are required to complete the set. I prefer a 2RM or 3RM test since it's the most accurate estimation without all the challenges associated with a true 1RM test. Nevertheless, if you're trying to avoid very heavy loads, the 8RM to 12RM test will sufficiently estimate if your maximal strength is increasing. Let math spare your joints.

Once again, you'll start with the same three warm-up sets in table 1.1. The good news is that it's usually much easier to guess what load you can lift no more than 8 to 12 times. I've found that by aiming for your 10RM you'll have a good chance of falling within the 8- to 12-repetition range on the first attempt. If you miss it, however, adjust the load accordingly, rest 5 minutes, and repeat the test. Once you find the right load, plug it into the following equation:

$$(\text{Load} \times \text{Reps} \times 0.03) + \text{Load} = 1\text{RM}$$

Let's say you tested the dumbbell press using 70-pound (32 kg) dumbbells. You performed 9 repetitions but failed to complete the 10th repetition. Or you rated the 9th repetition as a 10 on the RPE scale and stopped before attempting the 10th rep. In either case, 9 repetitions was your maximum, so the calculation will look like this:

$$(70 \times 9 \times 0.03) + 70 = 1\text{RM}$$

$$19 + 70 = 89 \text{ pounds}$$

The calculation estimates that you can do one repetition of the overhead press with 89-pound (40 kg) dumbbells. Keep in mind that calculations from an 8RM to 12RM test can underestimate your true 1RM. But that's fine, as long as you use this same test to assess progress in the future.

In summary, the way you determine your 1RM is up to you. Now, let's move on to recommended exercises to test your maximal strength.

Functional Strength Standards

The purpose of the functional strength standards is to determine how closely your maximal strength is to recommended values. As mentioned earlier, there is no evidence-based way to determine how strong a person should be for basic lifts in the gym such as a squat or deadlift. Therefore, the following strength recommendations, devised by Dr. John Rusin and me, are based on anecdotal evidence, as well as consultations with elite strength coaches from around the world. Importantly, none of these functional strength standards should be viewed as "pass" or "fail"; instead, they are general guidelines that might improve your performance in your favorite sport. Importantly, the following guidelines apply specifically to males.

So how much maximal strength is enough? There's no answer that fits all athletes or all populations. For example, a competitive powerlifter should be able to squat much heavier loads than a long-distance swimmer. And a soccer player doesn't need to be able to do as many pull-ups as a professional rock climber.

Romanian Deadlift

A strong hip hinge is a fundamental movement pattern that can benefit virtually every athlete, regardless of the sport. That's because the ability to generate speed or power in any movement comes from the core. Fitness magazines like to promote core training programs, which usually consist of abdominal exercises. But if we take into account the true definition of core, the "central or most important part of something," it tells us two things. First, the human body's core is actually the pelvis since it's the *central* part, the place where the trunk and lower limbs connect. Second, that definition also tells us the pelvis is arguably the most important part of the skeleton. Any single exercise, therefore, that challenges muscles that attach to, or help support, the pelvis can potentially be beneficial to you.

There are 45 different muscles that attach to the pelvis, not to mention other muscles that provide indirect support, such as the lats. Of particular importance to full-body power and athletic prowess is the posterior chain, a collection of muscles that runs from the traps down to the hamstrings, with the erector spinae, glutes, and many other muscles in between. If the pelvis is the core of the skeletal system, the posterior chain is the core of the muscular system. To paraphrase an old-school strength proverb, "A strong man is strong in the back of his body."

Of course, there are many exercises that develop the posterior chain, from a good morning to a bent-over row to a power clean. Not all of those exercises, including many others I didn't mention, are essential to a solid resistance training program. A basic hip hinge, however, is essential to sport and life. That's why the Romanian deadlift, one of the purest forms of a hip hinge, is the recommended exercise to test. The other reason is that it's extremely rare for a person to lack the mobility to do it correctly, unlike pulling a deadlift from the floor. Testing the Romanian deadlift is not recommended for some athletes, however, such as a pitcher who has excessive downward rotation of the scapulae; an alternative test is a quarter squat using a barbell.

To perform this exercise, use a barbell or trap bar, or hold a dumbbell in each hand. The strength goal is a 1RM of approximately 180 percent of body weight, calculated by the 2RM, 3RM, or 5RM test. For example, let's say you weigh 200 pounds (91 kg) and have determined your 3RM for the Romanian deadlift. In this case, if the goal is to achieve a 1RM of 180 percent of body weight, you should be able to perform three reps with approximately 315 pounds (143 kg), as outlined in table 1.2.

Lunge

The lunge is a functional movement pattern that requires a combination of single-leg and split-stance strength. It requires sufficient stability strength in the trunk, pelvis, hips, and ankles.

The reverse lunge is the ideal movement pattern to test, rather than a forward lunge. A reverse lunge allows the hips to perform more work, and it's a more stable movement. Alternatively, a forward lunge is essentially a forward "fall" that requires deceleration of the front leg. The question is how to load the reverse lunge during testing. Holding a dumbbell or kettlebell in one or both hands with the arms hanging down at the sides is a smart choice for safety reasons. Contra-

(continued)

Lunge *(continued)*

lateral loading, meaning the weight is held on the side of the leg that's stepping back, has been shown to increase activation of the trunk stabilizers in the frontal plane, as well at the gluteus medius and vastus lateralis of the primary leg (Stastny et al. 2015). Since strengthening those muscles is beneficial for virtually any athlete, the reverse lunge with a contralateral load held down at the side is the recommended exercise to test. The strength goal is approximately 40 percent of body weight 1RM, calculated by the 2RM, 3RM, or 5RM test. For example, for a 5RM test, a 180-pound (82 kg) athlete should be able to perform five reverse lunges while holding a 60-pound (27 kg) weight on one side. Remember, a 5RM is 85 to 87.5 percent of the 1RM.

Horizontal Push

A horizontal push, such as a bench press or push-up, primarily challenges muscles that protract the scapulae, horizontally adduct the shoulder, and extend the elbows. Having adequate strength in those muscles increases upper body pushing and punching power, as well as stability of the shoulder complex.

One of the best exercises to strengthen the horizontal push pattern is the push-up with a band stretched across the upper back. The problem, however, with testing that exercise is that it's difficult to translate the resistance of the band into pounds, and the resistance changes throughout the movement. A seated cable chest press is an excellent exercise to test since it requires shoulder stability and allows the scapulae to move freely. However, that machine isn't available in many gyms and weight rooms. Therefore, a good alternative is the close-grip barbell bench press since it's typically less stressful on the shoulders than a standard barbell bench press. Use a grip width that's three to four inches (8 to 10 cm) wider than the width of your hips, when measured between index fingers. The strength goal is a 1RM of approximately 125 percent of body weight, calculated by the 2RM, 3RM, or 5RM test.

Horizontal Pull

A horizontal pull, such as a chest-supported row or one-arm dumbbell row, primarily challenges muscles that retract the scapulae, horizontally abduct the shoulder, and flex the elbows. Note that those movements are the mirror opposite of what a horizontal push strengthens. Since the shoulder complex typically functions best when there's more strength in the horizontal pull pattern, it's important to determine if there's a significant discrepancy between it and a horizontal push. Having adequate strength in the upper back increases upper body pulling power, as well as stability of the shoulder complex.

A seated or chest-supported row is the recommended exercise to test. However, the problems with an exercise such as the incline dumbbell row are that the bench can get in the way when large dumbbells are being used. Therefore, a seated row is a good option, but keep in mind that it requires plenty of strength in the spinal erectors, unlike a chest-supported row. The ideal exercise to test is a chest-supported row on a machine with a pad that can be adjusted to rest against the abdomen. In any case, perform the row with your elbows close to the trunk during the movement to ensure the lats get sufficient activation. The strength goal is a 1RM of approximately 140 percent of body weight, calculated by the 2RM, 3RM, or 5RM test. If testing a one-arm row variation, use half the recommended percentage.

Vertical Push

A vertical push, such as a military press or dumbbell shoulder press, primarily challenges muscles that upwardly rotate the scapulae, abduct the shoulders, and extend the elbows. When the exercise is performed standing, it requires sufficient stability strength of the trunk and hips. Having adequate strength in these muscles increases overhead strength and stability, as well as upper body pushing and punching power.

First, choose a standing vertical push exercise since it's a better indicator of the full-body stability necessary to press a load overhead. The barbell standing overhead press is a common exercise to test. However, many athletes find the dumbbell overhead press easier on the shoulders since it allows the wrists to move freely. Furthermore, a split stance provides more stability, which can be useful when determining the actual strength of the muscles that perform a vertical push. It's also less stressful on the shoulder because of the position of the rib cage. Therefore, one ideal exercise to test is the split-stance one-arm overhead press using a dumbbell since it will have a greater range of loads to choose from.

In terms of strength goals, for the standing barbell overhead press, aim for a 1RM of approximately 80 percent of body weight, calculated by the 2RM, 3RM, or 5RM test. For the split-stance one-arm overhead press, aim for half that since just one dumbbell is being used. So it's a 1RM of 40 percent of body weight. For example, a 200-pound (91 kg) male should have a calculated 1RM of approximately 80 pounds (36 kg) for the split-stance one-arm overhead press for each side, which equates to a 5RM of around 70 pounds (32 kg).

Vertical Pull

A vertical pull, such as a pull-up or lat pull-down, primarily challenges muscles that downwardly rotate the scapulae, adduct the shoulders, and flex the elbows. Having adequate strength in the upper back increases upper body pulling power as well as stability of the shoulder complex.

Earlier it was mentioned that it's a good idea to aim for a balance of strength between a horizontal push and pull. But that balance doesn't carry over between a vertical push and pull. The reason is that a vertical pull engages significantly more muscle mass, making it a naturally stronger movement than a vertical push.

If you have sufficient strength to do a pull-up, the hammer-grip version works well for most people since it's typically easier on the shoulders and wrists. If you don't have the strength to do a pull-up, a hammer-grip lat pull-down with the hands shoulder-width apart is recommended. The strength goal is a 1RM of approximately 140 percent of body weight for males calculated by the 2RM, 3RM, or 5RM test.

Remember, the aforementioned strength guidelines aren't appropriate for all athletes or the general population. For example, it's not necessary for a pitcher or marathon runner to be able to bench-press 125 percent of his body weight, and it might even be detrimental. But a powerlifter would typically need a lot more than that to win a meet. And a rock climber would likely require significantly more upper back strength than a soccer player. Consult a coach or physical therapist to determine what's best for you.

With all those caveats out of the way, if you choose to test any, or all, of the six aforementioned exercises you'll not only get a good understanding of your general strength but also potentially expose any significant imbalances. For example, if you can bench-press 250 pounds (113 kg) but can row only 150 pounds (68 kg), that strength imbalance could decrease your overall performance and increase your risk of a shoulder injury. Or maybe you performed well on all tests except the reverse lunge. Adding that exercise into your program until you can perform it with 40 percent of body weight could significantly increase your strength where you need it most, which will likely increase your overall sport performance.

Explosive Strength

Explosive strength is the ability to express maximal force in minimal time. Force is measured in newtons, which, not surprisingly, are named after Sir Isaac Newton. One newton (N) is the force required to accelerate one kilogram of mass at one meter per second squared in the direction the force is applied:

$$1N = 1 \text{ kg} \times m/s^2$$

Another way to write that equation is F = ma, where *F* stands for force, *m* stands for mass, and *a* is acceleration. (If we're splitting hairs, *mass* is not the same as *weight*, but you can think of them as being the same for resistance training purposes.)

Consider twin guys who are performing the concentric phase of a deadlift as fast as possible with 315 pounds (143 kg). Athlete A takes 2 seconds to complete the lift; athlete B lifts it in 1 second. In this case, athlete B has more explosive strength than athlete A does. The rate at which an athlete can reach peak levels of force is his rate of force development (RFD). An athlete builds his explosive strength by increasing his RFD. It takes in excess of 0.3 to 0.4 seconds to reach peak levels of force, but many explosive movements such as a jump, shot put, or javelin throw occur in less time than that (Komi 2003). An athlete, therefore, doesn't have enough available time to reach his highest level of muscular force. This is why it's essential to improve your RFD: You will reach higher levels of force in less time. When you hear a basketball announcer mention that the older athlete with the ball has "lost his first step," what he's technically saying is "His RFD has decreased." For any sport that requires lightning-fast movements, from baseball to karate to football, RFD is one of the most important qualities to develop and sustain, as shown in figure 1.15. Increasing the RFD of your calves will also reduce the likelihood of an unexpected fall (Hester et al. 2020).

There are two simple ways to test your explosive strength. You could perform a vertical jump or a standing long jump test. This section covers the particulars of both tests.

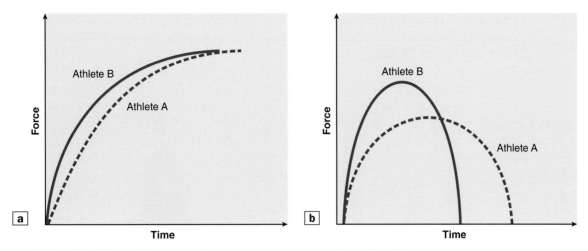

FIGURE 1.15   Rate of force development and explosive strength: *(a)* Both athletes achieve the same level of force, but athlete B produces more force at any given time before the peak. *(b)* Athlete B produces a higher level of force and then turns it off faster than athlete A. In either case, athlete B has a higher RFD and more explosive strength than athlete A.

Vertical Jump Test

The vertical jump test, or countermovement jump as it's known in research, is a reliable, practical, and valid way to measure lower body explosive strength (Markovic et al. 2004). For this test, you'll need chalk and a smooth, flat wall that's at least 11 feet (3.4 m) high, more or less based on your height, or a Vertec device that consists of horizontal vanes.

Perform two warm-up vertical jump tests, with 60 seconds of rest between each trial. These are submaximal trials to prepare the nervous system and joints for the test (maximal effort should not be attempted until the actual test). Then, place the fingertips of your dominant hand in chalk. Standing with your dominant hand as close as possible to the wall, reach up and touch the highest point of the wall (see figure 1.16). This is the reference point for the vertical jump.

In science, all possible variables must be kept consistent through subsequent trials or the data will be skewed. This need for accuracy, of course, is just as important when testing yourself. The biomechanics of the jump must be as consistent as possible. In subsequent trials, if you use a wider or narrower foot placement, or wear different shoes, or jump from a different surface, you won't get an accurate measure of your change in performance. Here are the key variables:

- *Foot placement:* When you're ready to perform the jump, have a partner measure the distance between the inside of your heels and place two marks on the floor with tape so your heels are the exact same width with each subsequent attempt. Whichever foot placement feels most natural to you is what you want to test. That stance width will be slightly different for everyone.

- *Attempts, measuring, and calculations:* Perform a maximal vertical jump test, using as much arm swing as feels natural. Perform three attempts, with 90 seconds of rest between each. Record the highest point, meaning the largest difference between the standing chalk mark and the maximal vertical jump mark (see figure 1.17).

- *Testing frequency:* It's recommended to test the vertical jump every four to six weeks. Ideally, you'll test it on the same day at the same time with the same warm-up, if you choose to use a warm-up. Just 10 jumping jacks performed a minute before the first jump is usually sufficient. The key is to keep whatever warm-up you're doing consistent over time.

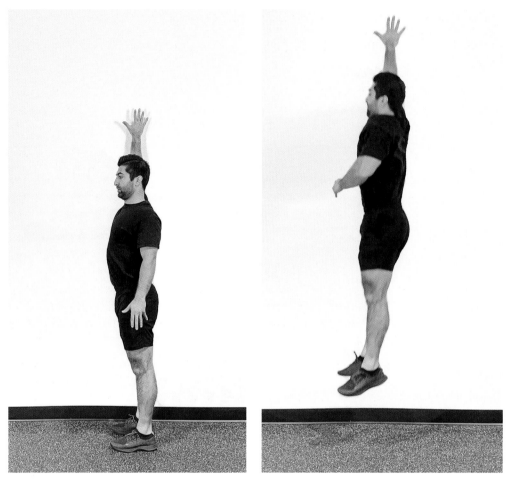

FIGURE 1.16   First, mark the wall with chalk.

FIGURE 1.17   Vertical jump.

Standing Long Jump

The standing long jump, also known as the broad jump, is a versatile tool in athletic settings to measure explosive strength (Peterson, Alvar, and Rhea 2006). It is not only an accurate way to test your potential increase in RFD but also a good measure of which young athlete might be genetically predisposed to being a great power athlete. The kid with the best standing long jump is often the one chosen by an Olympic coach who's looking to build his resume (Castro-Piñero et al. 2010). The primary difference between a vertical jump and a standing long jump test is that the latter challenges balance, which is necessary for sticking the landing. This also means the standing long jump is probably a better test of explosive strength for athletes, compared with the vertical jump. For this test, you'll need a flat surface at least 15 feet (4.6 m) long.

Perform three warm-up standing long jump tests, with 60 seconds of rest between each trial. These are submaximal trials to prepare the nervous system and joints for the test (maximal effort should not be attempted until the actual test).

Again, the biomechanics of the jump must be as consistent as possible. Here are the key variables:

- *Testing surface:* Ideally, you'll jump from a hard surface and land on a slightly softer one. Think of a basketball court floor for the takeoff and a hard rubber surface like you see in gyms for the landing. It's not imperative that you land on a softer surface, but it's a good idea if one is available. A surface that's too soft, however, isn't recommended because it's difficult to make a solid landing.

- *Footwear:* Test the standing long jump with shoes that have minimal cushioning, if possible. Avoid wearing shoes with thick, cushioned soles because they will absorb some of the force you're trying to produce.

- *Foot placement:* When you're ready to perform a broad jump, have a partner measure the distance between the inside of your heels and place two marks on the floor with tape so your heels are the exact same width with each subsequent attempt. Like the vertical jump, whichever foot placement feels most natural to you is what you want to test.

- *Attempts, measuring, and calculations:* Perform three standing long jumps, with 90 seconds of rest between each attempt. If you lose your balance on the landing, it doesn't count. Wait 90 seconds and perform another attempt. Measure from the line (front of your toes) at takeoff to the back of your heel(s) at landing. Measure to the heel that's closest to the takeoff line if your feet aren't perfectly even. The longest jump is the one that counts in your data (see figure 1.18).

- *Testing frequency:* It's recommended to test the standing long jump every four to six weeks. Ideally, you'll test it on the same day at the same time with the same warm-up, if you choose to use a warm-up. Just 10 jumping jacks performed a minute before the first jump is usually sufficient. The key is to keep whatever warm-up you're doing consistent over time.

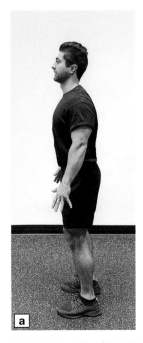 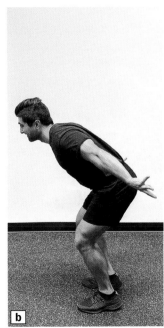 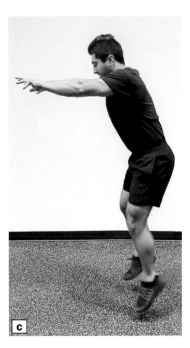 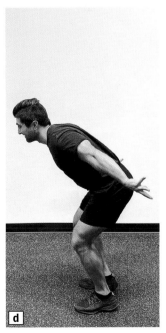

FIGURE 1.18   Standing long jump.

For either test, refrain from any heavy weight training for two days prior. If you perform the assessment two days after a heavy deadlift the first week and then do a retest one day after a heavy deadlift the fourth week, you're going to skew your data because of fatigue. Be smart with your timing of the test, and try to keep all variables as consistent as possible. It would be easy to get into a scholarly discussion over what constitutes an ideal vertical jump or standing long jump distance, but what matters most is that your performance is consistently increasing over time.

Body Composition

At this point we've covered all the tests to analyze your posture, mobility, and performance. Now it's time to outline the details that might matter most to you: how you look in the mirror. The gold standard for measuring your body fat percentage has one unfortunate obstacle: You need to be dead. Cadaver analysis works only on cadavers (Wells and Fewtrell 2006). Assuming that isn't appealing to you, you have a few more options (Duren et al. 2008), although each has its drawbacks.

Take DEXA, for example. Dual-energy X-ray absorptiometry is the most accurate way to measure a living person's body fat and lean muscle mass. This full-body scan takes about 10 to 20 minutes to complete and is highly sensitive to changes in your body composition. But unless you participate in a fitness or nutrition study at a local university that includes before-and-after DEXA scans, you aren't likely to have access to the technology. And if you do have access, it would be prohibitively expensive for most people, since it wouldn't be covered by insurance.

Skinfold measurements are somewhat more accessible. But they require expensive calipers, and it takes a highly skilled practitioner to get accurate data. Someone who's not as experienced or well trained can measure at the same sites (usually your triceps, navel, upper back, outer chest, and front thigh) and come up with very different results.

A doctor will often use body mass index (BMI), a simple calculation based on height and weight (BMI = kg/m^2), to determine if a person needs to drop a few pounds. If you score 25.0 or higher, you're considered overweight. At 30.0 or more, you're considered obese (Rothman 2008). You don't need a medical degree to see the flaw in that logic. A relatively lean athlete or bodybuilder with a lot of muscle mass can easily have a BMI in the overweight range, and some will even cross over to obese.

Since virtually every method to measure your body fat has shortcomings (and I haven't even mentioned several others that are either impractical or inaccurate), the best and easiest solution is to take simple measurements at home and track them over time. You can't use them to calculate your body fat percentage, but you'll have the next best thing: an accurate, inexpensive system to track your progress. To do this, you'll need three tools:

- A cloth tape measure, which you'll use to measure your abdomen every four weeks.
- A high-quality digital bathroom scale, which you'll use once a week. Regardless of all the "Throw away your scale!" chants you hear in late-night informercials, weighing yourself at the right time, under the right conditions, can be a valuable tool, especially if your goal is to lose a lot of weight.

- A camera, which you already have in your phone, to chronicle your progress every four to six weeks. The one complication is that you'll need a friend or partner to take those photos for you, as I'll explain in a moment.

Abdominal Circumference

One thing we can all agree on is this: If your midsection is getting larger, and you aren't pregnant, you're gaining fat. And if your waistline is shrinking, and you haven't recently delivered a baby, you're losing fat. Logically, measuring the circumference of your abdomen is one of the most meaningful ways to determine if you're gaining or losing fat.

To measure your abdominal circumference, plan to measure once per week first thing in the morning, after emptying your bladder. Remove all your clothes except your underwear. Take a cloth measuring tape, wrap it around your low back, and place it across your navel. Using the mirror as your guide, make sure the tape is perfectly parallel to the floor and even on both sides of your abdomen. The tape should be snug enough to

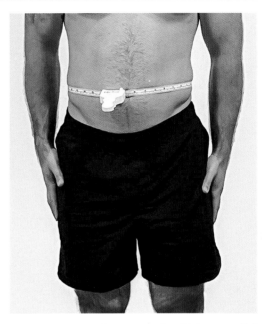

FIGURE 1.19 The tape should be parallel to the floor and snug, but not so snug that it sinks into your skin.

eliminate any gaps, but not so tight it digs into your skin (see figure 1.19). Make a note of the circumference, and then weigh yourself, as we cover next.

Body Weight

The scale is valuable for monitoring your progress, but it can also be maddening. How can you wake up in the morning four pounds (1.8 kg) lighter than you were the night before? How can your weight fluctuate so much from day to day?

The reason isn't all that mysterious. It mainly comes down to your hydration, or lack thereof. Let's assume the human body is about 70 percent water. (The actual percentage can vary from person to person and study to study.) That means a 200-pound (91 kg) male carries an average of 140 pounds (64 kg) of water, which can change quite a bit throughout the day. An hour-long hike on a hot day can easily reduce your body weight by 3 or 4 pounds (1.4-1.8 kg)—all from water, none of it fat.

Despite these daily fluctuations, we know *consistent* self-monitoring of scale weight helps people lose fat (Butryn et al. 2007). The recommended frequency is once per week (Madigan et al. 2016). Monday morning is typically the worst time to step on a scale. Most of us eat and drink more on weekends, causing water retention, which is bad for our confidence even if it's ultimately meaningless. Your body weight typically returns to normal by Wednesday, which is why it's the best day to weigh yourself. We know this from a study that weighed 40 people a total of 2,838 times over the course of a year (Helander et al. 2014).

To get an accurate body weight, plan to weigh yourself once per week first thing in the morning, after emptying your bladder. Remove all your clothes except your underwear. Measure your weight using the same high-quality scale each week when you measure your abdomen.

Comparative Photographs

You can look at yourself in the mirror every day and never see the small changes taking place over weeks and months, even if you have data showing your steady progress. But as they say, a picture can be worth a thousand data points. When you take photos every four to six weeks, you can see visual proof of your progress—proof you can't always detect in the mirror.

Ask someone to take photos of you in good lighting, first thing in the morning, wearing nothing but snug shorts. Take one set of photos from the front, side, and back with your arms hanging relaxed at your sides. Take another set from the same angles while doing a double-biceps pose, contracting all the muscles in your upper body and torso.

Take photos every four to six weeks, ideally at the same time you measure your abdomen and weigh yourself. If your partner isn't available then, at least try to get pictures before you've had the biggest meal of the day. You want your measurements and your photos to combine to form an accurate statistical and visual record of your progress.

Final Thoughts

In this chapter, we talk about how to assess where you are now and how to track your progress over time. You can certainly do all the tests and track all the measurements. There's no better or cheaper way to get an honest, objective understanding of your overall fitness and abilities. But most of you probably won't go to that much trouble. Instead, you'll focus on what matters most to you. And that's fine; effective time management is important for someone whose living doesn't depend on their strength or appearance. Only you can decide what's worth tracking, based on your goals. That said, I recommend *most* readers test and track their body composition and at least one of the three measures of strength.

Here's why I say that: Muscle mass is hard to measure. If you're gaining strength, you're probably also gaining lean mass. Tracking your weight and waist size tells you if the new muscle mass is improving your body composition. If you gain a couple of pounds without increasing your waist size, you've almost certainly improved your body composition. And if you have any doubt, taking new photos every few weeks will show if the increased strength and new muscle mass are giving you the bottom-line result you wanted when you bought this book: a better physique.

CHAPTER 2

Man With a Plan

In this chapter we cover strategies for setting realistic goals and expectations while staying motivated. Four steps are outlined to help you achieve those goals. You will learn the importance of knowing why you want to achieve a goal and of determining how much time you can realistically devote to exercise each week. Then we cover ways to gauge your progress, so you'll know you're on the right track. Finally, we discuss how to make the most of visualization strategies to stay motivated. By the end of this chapter, you will have the tools to be a man with a plan for success.

Setting Realistic Goals and Expectations

You must be realistic about the goals you set and about what you expect from the programs in this book. Many guys want to *simultaneously* lose enough fat to have six-pack abs, gain enough muscle to look like Dwayne Johnson's body double, and build the strength to squat three times their body weight, not to mention achieve a 40-inch (102 cm) vertical jump. But in reality, those goals can interfere with each other. Indeed, it is difficult to build muscle and strength unless you eat a surplus of calories, which counteracts the fat loss you need for that six-pack. Any elite powerlifter will tell you that a thick, fat midsection helps him squat heavier weight. And a heavily muscled physique is much more difficult to elevate 40 inches from the ground than the wiry, lean physique you see on virtually every NBA player who competes in the slam dunk contest. The point here is that many of you probably want the programs in this book to achieve more than one goal at the same time. The likelihood of that happening depends on which goals you seek.

As mentioned earlier, building muscle and strength is best achieved by consuming more calories than your body needs to maintain your current weight; and losing fat requires consuming less calories than your body needs, which slows muscle and strength gains (Aragon et al. 2017). There is no doubt that if your primary goal is to lose fat, any increases in your strength and muscle mass will suffer. That is the "glass is half empty" angle. Someone who sees the glass as half full can say research demonstrates that performing resistance training while losing fat will help preserve your muscle and strength (Cava, Yeat, and Mittendorfer 2017).

For explosive athletes there's more good news: Losing fat can increase your jumping and sprinting performance because you have less weight to move through space (Huovinen et al. 2015). Since gaining muscle or losing fat each requires its own type of diet, you'll need to prioritize which one you seek every six to eight weeks of the program.

How much muscle and strength you gain, or fat you lose, depends on a myriad of factors (Institute of Medicine 2004; Pedersen and Febbraio 2012; Pion et al. 2017). Some of those factors are in your control, such as how many times per week you train, as well as your adherence to the nutrition principles we cover in chapter 11. Other aspects are beyond your control, such as genetics and age (Pion et al. 2017). It is clear that some people can more easily gain muscle or lose fat because they were blessed with the right parents. The same is true with gaining strength and speed. And a middle-aged person will most certainly have a more difficult time transforming his physique than he did when he was 21. A typical guy in his 30s has less muscle mass and testosterone than he did in his 20s, which negatively affects his overall metabolism as well as what he sees in the mirror (Tsametis and Isidori 2018). With each decade past his 30s, the problem only worsens, unless he makes healthy training and lifestyle interventions.

The good news is that you can gain muscle and strength at any age with a proper resistance training regimen. A lower level of testosterone, on the other hand, is not as easy to correct. Stress is certainly a key factor for plummeting levels of testosterone, even if that stress comes from exercise or nutrition. Indeed, training and dieting hard for months leading up to a competition can result in a natural bodybuilder's testosterone level dropping to one-third of what it was before dieting (Schoenfeld et al. 2020). Fortunately, testosterone will return to its higher precompetition level within a month after a normal diet is resumed. The point here is that extreme stress on the body, even if it's ostensibly healthy, can

Are You Setting the Right Kind of Goals?

You need to know what your goals are and why you want to achieve them in order to stay motivated. For some people, however, that might not be enough. Underlying psychological factors you're not even aware of could be sabotaging your results. If you're someone who has a tough time achieving goals, it doesn't necessarily mean you need to see a psychiatrist. Most people struggle with the discipline required to stop eating before they're full, or to skip dessert, or to make it to the gym four times per week for months at a time. If we didn't struggle, we'd all have six-pack abs and bulging biceps.

This is where the advice of John Berardi, author of *Change Maker*, becomes especially valuable. One of his steps for achieving success, whether in the gym, home, or office, is to turn outcome goals into behavior goals. An *outcome goal* is what you want, such as losing 15 pounds (7 kg) of fat. A *behavior goal*, Dr. Berardi states, "is an action that you'd do or practice to move toward that outcome, such as putting down your fork between bites, or practicing your running technique three to four times a week." So as you embark on this journey toward your best physique and performance, Dr. Berardi recommends focusing on behavior goals, since "they're the things we can control."

have a negative effect on your sex hormones (i.e., testosterone). So you can imagine how challenging it will be to gain muscle and lose fat if you have to combat work, family, or financial stressors. You must consider these factors when setting goals for yourself. Expect your best results to occur only during the times you can adhere to the program, manage emotional stress, and get at least eight hours of sleep each night, which we cover in greater detail in chapter 12.

Prioritizing Your Goals

So now it's time to prioritize. If you see plenty of fat around your midsection, losing it should be your priority because a host of benefits will follow. When you lose fat, you will look more muscular in the mirror even if you didn't add any muscle tissue. And losing belly fat will improve your insulin sensitivity, which makes it less likely that you'll gain fat in the future (Clamp et al. 2017). If you're lean enough to see all but your lower abdominals, and if you haven't been doing much resistance or aerobic training, the guidelines in this book to gain muscle and conditioning might be sufficient to remove that last bit of fat around your lower abdomen without drastically changing your diet (assuming it's a relatively healthy one). In any case, you need to be realistic. Decide whether you want your primary goal to be more muscle or less fat. And if you're unsure, the following steps will help you start on the right path.

Step 1: Determine why you want to achieve the goal.

Many of you reading this book will want to achieve six-pack abs so you can look great with your shirt off. But in my 25 years of experience transforming physiques, I've learned that *knowing* your goal isn't enough. You must understand *why* you want that six-pack. This is the time to think deeply and have a clear answer, regardless of how inane it might seem to someone who's not in your shoes.

In my early years as a personal trainer I assumed everyone wanted a ripped midsection just to look better to a potential mate. I was definitely wrong. There are countless examples I could give here, but one worth mentioning is a guy I trained who, as usual, wanted a six-pack midsection. When I asked why, he replied, "I've spent $20,000 on a wardrobe I currently can't wear, so I need my midsection slim enough to once again fit into all those clothes."

Step 2: Determine how much time you can realistically devote to exercise each week.

One of the first questions I ask my patients is, how many days per week can you guarantee you will be able to train, barring any catastrophe? That training frequency is what I use to create the program, even if I know more sessions per week would provide quicker results. Indeed, there is no use in having a program that requires four workouts per week if you can guarantee that you'll do only two.

But many people have unrealistic expectations of their own capabilities when excited about embarking on a new program. They'll say things such as, "Well, I can find a babysitter for an extra evening each week to get to the gym" or "My boss will probably let me leave work early on Fridays so I can fit in my workout." These are the times I see the potential for problems. Words such as *if* and *probably* are red flags.

In chapters 8 through 10 we cover programs with a range of frequencies, from two to six days per week. Choose the program you know you will be able to

Training at Home Versus at a Commercial Gym

Given the COVID-19 pandemic, many people have expanded their home gyms to include a variety of training equipment. Commercial gyms, on the other hand, allow access to a vast array of equipment, from power racks to sleds to pull-up machines that provide assistance. The one challenge with a commercial gym is that other people can occupy a piece of equipment you need. This can be especially problematic with the circuit style of training recommended in this book, which requires you to constantly transition between different exercises. If someone is using a piece of equipment you need, with no plans of leaving anytime soon, you can break up the circuit. For example, if a guy is hogging the pull-up bar, complete your sets of the deadlift and dip, and then return to the pull-up bar when it's free. At that point, pair the pull-up with another exercise that works other muscle groups (e.g., dumbbell bench press). In any case, just be sure to rest at least 3 minutes before repeating an exercise. If you're short on time, perform your pull-up as a drop set, which will be covered in chapter 8. For example, if four sets of the pull-up are programmed that day, perform all sets at the end of your workout, with 30 seconds of rest between each set.

consistently follow from week to week, because consistency is one of the most important components of success in the gym.

Another important factor in choosing the right program is the amount of time you can devote to each workout. Many of the recommended workouts in chapters 8 and 9 take around 30 to 45 minutes to finish, which might be more time than you have available on a hectic day. If your day gets jammed up and you have only enough time to do three rounds of a circuit instead of five, you will still get a positive result. Conversely, when you have more free time than normal to train and sleep, you might want to train twice each day or add high frequency training (HFT) to build a lagging body part or two. In chapter 8 we cover strategies to get the most out of your workouts when training time is limited or when it's plentiful. For now, just determine how much time you can realistically devote to each workout throughout the week.

Step 3: Determine how you will gauge progress.

In chapter 1 we cover ways to assess your current level of mobility, performance, and body composition. You will use those same tests and measurements to gauge your progress. For example, if your primary goal is weight loss, use your scale weight, abdominal circumference, and photographs as your guide. Remember, photographs are valuable because they don't lie. Neither do your clothes. If it's difficult to see a slimmer version of yourself in a photo, but your pants are fitting more loosely around the waist, you know progress is being made. The same can be said about muscle growth. Maybe your arms appear the same in the mirror after four weeks of training, but the sleeves of your dress shirt fit more snugly. That's progress.

We all would like to achieve results much quicker than we know is probably possible. When a guy asks me how much muscle he can gain in three months, my typical response is "What's the most muscle you've ever gained in three months?" If you gain any more than that, you're making excellent progress. From a research standpoint, significant muscular growth has been demonstrated over the course of 12 weeks (Hubal et al. 2005). Significant strength gains have been demonstrated in as little as 8 weeks (Schoenfeld et al. 2019).

How quickly your abdominal circumference will decrease depends on how much you have to lose. A guy with significant abdominal fat will lose inches faster than a guy who's trying to bring out his lower abdominal definition for the beach, as any competitive bodybuilder preparing for a contest can attest to. Or a guy who is new to resistance training will boost his Romanian deadlift much faster than if he had been intensely devoted to that exercise for many years. In any case, here are two realistic goals for anyone:

- See visual improvement in the mirror every four weeks.
- Significantly improve your performance in the gym every six weeks.

Step 4: Use visualization to help achieve your goal.

Your likelihood of success is positively correlated with your motivation. Once you determine *why* you want a ripped midsection or bigger arms or twice the strength you have now, stay focused on it until that goal is achieved. Two helpful strategies to stay motivated are *outcome* visualization and *process* visualization (see figure 2.1).

Outcome visualization is imagining yourself the moment you achieve your goal. This process has been used by many of my clients, including the guy who wanted to fit back into his expensive wardrobe. For him, outcome visualization consisted of imagining himself and his wife dining out at their favorite Italian restaurant while wearing the Armani suit that hangs in his closet. He would imagine this scenario numerous times throughout the day; and when he was feeling less than motivated, it would provide a psychological boost. Or maybe your goal is to jump six inches (15 cm) higher or squat 100 more pounds (45 kg) than your current personal record (PR). In any case, imagine what it will feel like when you achieve the goal, and hold that image as long as possible.

Process visualization is imagining yourself performing the necessary steps to achieve your goal. With regard to the squat, here are some examples to make process visualization as realistic as you can:

- Imagine the smell of your gym or garage when you're in the squat rack.
- Imagine loading the plates onto the barbell that correspond to your target PR.
- Imagine how your feet, legs, and core feel when the heavy load is across your upper back.
- Finally, imagine yourself straining a bit to achieve that new PR instead of lifting it with pure ease.

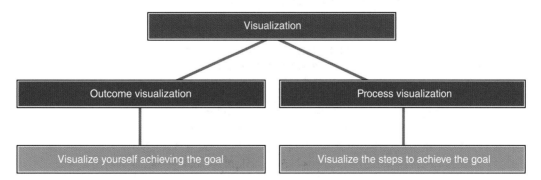

FIGURE 2.1 Outcome versus process visualization.

The more realistic you can make the visualization, the more likely it will help. Visualization can be used for more than just your sets and goals. Use it to also imagine yourself getting up early, and preparing your preworkout meal when everyone else is still asleep, so you can fit in your workout on a busy day, if that is a challenge you'll face moving forward. Many of my athletes have successfully used visualization, as have countless other star athletes such as Michael Jordan and Tiger Woods.

The ABCs of Motivation

As a physical therapist, I know how difficult it can be to keep my patients motivated. It doesn't matter if it's a professional athlete, celebrity, or CEO: They all have bad days. Sometimes they have bad weeks or even months. One of my duties is to help get them out of that rut, or at the very least, get them through a successful session with me. During these times I focus on the ABCs of motivation (see figure 2.2):

- *Autonomy:* This is the sense of control and independence. For example, I would let my client choose which exercise he prefers that day to warm up, or where he'd like to go to lunch after the session.
- *Belonging:* This is the need to feel included, accepted, and connected with others. For example, I would ask my client to tell me about her tennis game or what's going on in the storyline of her favorite TV show.
- *Competence:* This is the need to feel capable of doing something successfully. For example, I would choose exercises that I know my client is capable of performing well that day. There are times to push a client to achieve a new PR in the squat, or perform a balance exercise longer than normal, but this day isn't one of them.

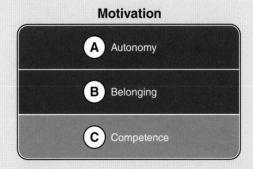

FIGURE 2.2   ABCs of motivation.

My goal is to help my patients experience the ABCs during each session, especially when they are struggling with life. You can use this same approach the next time your significant other, child, or friend needs a boost.

Final Thoughts

In this chapter, we talk about ways to get an intelligent plan in place. Oftentimes, people start on a journey without a clear destination, which in this case is a leaner, stronger physique that performs as well as it looks. Achieving that goal requires dedication and focus, so the steps in this chapter are as important as how you train and eat. As the saying goes: If you fail to plan, you plan to fail.

CHAPTER 3

Muscle Rules

Over the last 25 years I've had the pleasure of working with numerous professional athletes, from all-stars in the NBA to world champions in the UFC. The primary reason I was hired by the team or agent was to improve the athlete's performance or help in recovery from an injury. But all these male and female athletes had one thing in common: They all wanted to build a more impressive physique in the process of working with me, even if that wasn't the goal of their coach.

Your primary goal might be to build a more impressive physique, regardless of how well it performs. In most cases, however, you'll want your newly sculpted physique to also perform better during a game of flag football or softball with your buddies. That is why this chapter covers the principles of building bigger muscles while also making your body stronger and faster in the process. These principles can apply to any training program, whether you follow what's in this book or create your own plan. The chapter starts with an overview of muscle and motor units and then explains the importance of a proper movement progression. Then it covers guidelines for warming up before training, as well as ways to choose the right equipment and workout structure. You will learn the optimal training frequency to stimulate muscle growth and the importance of adequate sleep. We discuss your protein needs, and then finish with a section on progressive overload. By the end of this chapter, you will have learned nine rules to build a body that performs as well as it looks.

Muscle Fiber Types and Motor Units

The human muscular system includes some 650 muscles. The stapedius, located in the middle ear, is the smallest muscle in the body, which makes sense because it's attached to the stapes, the smallest bone in the body. The gluteus maximus is the largest muscle. Not surprisingly, it's also connected to the largest bone: the femur.

Muscles are categorized as three primary types: cardiac, smooth, and skeletal. Cardiac muscle makes up the walls of the heart; its contractions allow blood to circulate. Smooth muscle, found throughout the body, does the thankless work of keeping your organs and blood vessels running on autopilot. Skeletal muscle is the contractile tissue that produces voluntary action and reflex action. Since this book is about building a better physique and performance, our focus is on the actions of skeletal muscle (see figure 3.1). So for the rest of this book, the word *muscle* will relate specifically to skeletal muscle.

Your speed, power, and endurance rely heavily on the type of fibers that make up your muscles. Humans have three primary types of muscle fibers: type I, type IIa, and type IIx. Type I slow-twitch fibers are the main fiber type for an activity that can be sustained for long durations at a low intensity, such as walking or jogging for 30 minutes. Type IIa fast-twitch fibers work with type I fibers during a moderate-intensity activity such as climbing 10 flights of stairs or walking up a long hill. Type IIx fast-twitch fibers come into play mainly during short, quick bursts of high-intensity activity such as a maximum vertical jump or heavy squat.

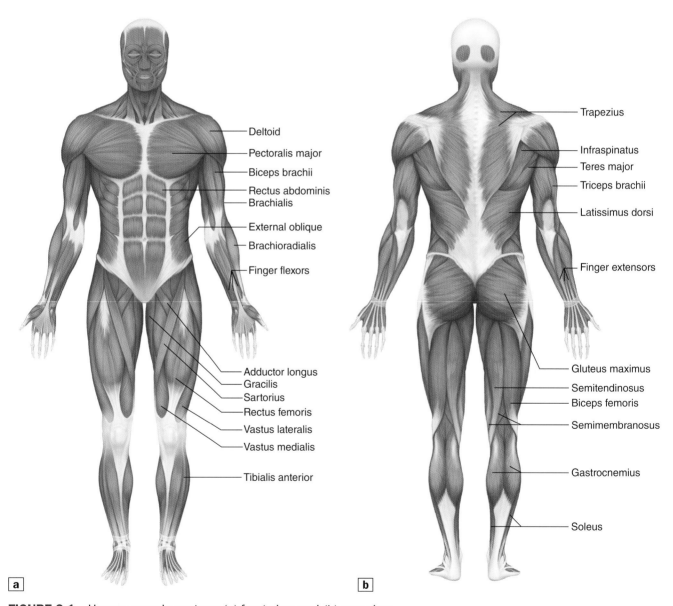

FIGURE 3.1   Human muscle system: *(a)* front view and *(b)* rear view.

Muscle fibers are arranged in bundles, ranging from around 10 fibers in muscles around your eyes to thousands of fibers in large muscle groups (e.g., hamstrings). Each bundle of fibers is connected to one motor neuron, which sends a signal to contract all those fibers. The combination of the single motor neuron and all the muscle fibers it activates is a motor unit. Since there are three primary types of muscle fibers there are three types of motor units (see figure 3.2):

- Slow (S) motor units that contain type I fibers
- Fast fatigue-resistant (FFR) motor units that contain type IIa fibers
- Fast fatigable (FF) motor units that contain type IIx fibers

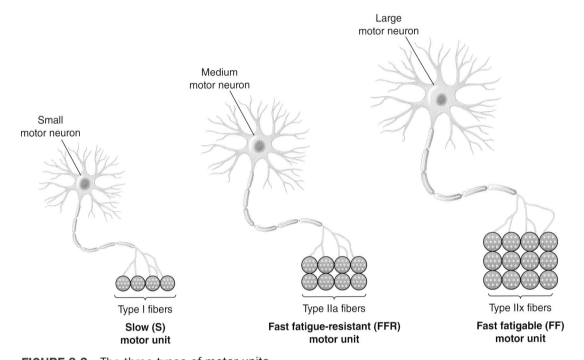

FIGURE 3.2   The three types of motor units.

Your nervous system recruits motor units in an orderly fashion, from smallest (S motor units) to largest (FF motor units). When a muscle contracts, the S motor units fire first, producing small increments of force. As more force is needed, larger motor units are recruited, each contributing progressively more force, with that force increasing in progressively larger increments:

- Low force activity = S motor units
- Medium force activity = S + FFR motor units
- High force activity = S + FFR + FF motor units

This orderly recruitment of motor units is known as the size principle (see figure 3.3) and was first proposed by neurophysiologist Elwood Henneman (1957).

When the nervous system determines that a muscle requires relatively little force, it activates relatively few motor units, and the ones it activates deploy the muscle's smallest fibers. When higher levels of force are required, the nervous system brings in larger motor neurons, which activate more and bigger fibers. Once all motor units are recruited, the brain sends a stronger signal to the motor

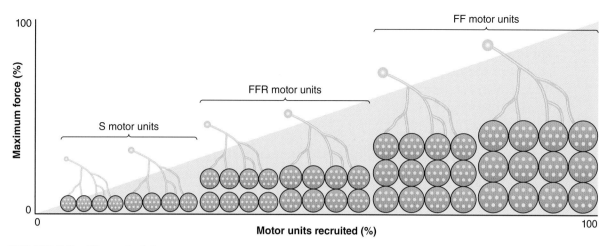

FIGURE 3.3   Size principle.

unit to increase its firing rate (i.e., rate coding), resulting in even greater levels of force (Kandel et al. 2013).

The goal of resistance training is to recruit the most motor units possible during each set. Put another way, it's necessary to produce high levels of force during each set of an exercise to recruit all the motor units, which in turn builds the most muscle mass and strength. There are three primary ways to accomplish that goal:

- Lift a heavy load, meaning a load you can't lift for more than five repetitions.
- Lift a submaximal load, which is a load you can lift for more than five repetitions, and take that set close to, or to, momentary muscular failure (i.e., muscle exhaustion).
- Lift a submaximal load as fast as possible, which produces higher levels of force compared with lifting it more slowly.

Fundamentals of a Movement Progression

The purpose of resistance exercise is to create metabolic and structural disruptions that, when recovered from, improve your strength, power, and muscle mass. This is best achieved when you follow the fundamental aspects of a movement progression: movement competency, strength, and power (Liebenson 2014). Movement competency is the ability to move well, requiring a combination of mobility and stability throughout the body. You learn proper mechanics of basic movement patterns with minimal load, such as a squat or overhead press with an empty barbell. In this stage it's recommended to consult with a reputable trainer to ensure proper lifting technique. Once this is achieved, load is added to basic movement patterns such as the squat, hip hinge, and overhead press. Load is increased over the course of months until a respectable level of strength is developed, which, depending on the person, may or may not be close to the functional strength standards covered in chapter 1. From that point, you can add high-velocity exercises such as a jump squat or medicine ball throw to develop power.

There will often be carryover between movement competency, strength, and power. For example, when you develop strength it can also improve your movement competency and power. But the first goal is to perform an exercise properly before load is added, and then movement velocity is increased after a foundation of strength is achieved (see figure 3.4).

It is imperative to always maintain perfect technique when performing an exercise. Adding load or lifting faster requires skill that must first be developed with lighter loads.

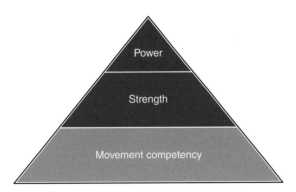

FIGURE 3.4   Fundamentals of training progression.

Exercise Preparation

Before a workout, game, or match it's important to prepare your body for training. As a general rule, a warm-up will cause mild sweating without accumulating fatigue. There are two primary goals of a warm-up:

- To enhance your muscles' dynamics so they can perform better
- To prepare you for the demands of exercise

Research demonstrates virtually no relationship between a warm-up and injury prevention. However, there's strong evidence that certain types of preparation can improve your performance in the gym or on the field (McCrary, Ackermann, and Halaki 2015), thanks to the following four physiological benefits:

- An increase in the speed and force of muscle contractions
- Greater oxygen delivery to working muscles
- Faster nerve transmissions, which can improve muscle speed and reaction times
- Increased blood flow through active tissues

A dynamic warm-up starts with general activity followed by more specific movements that mimic what the workout or sport requires. Here are two examples—one for a baseball player and another for a powerlifter—to help you better understand a dynamic warm-up.

A baseball player jogs for 3 minutes, then perform arm circles and high kicks for 3 minutes, and ends with 5 minutes of throwing a baseball, starting with a relatively low intensity and then increasing it over time. A powerlifter who needs to perform a barbell squat for the first exercise in his workout might prepare by doing the following: 3 minutes of pedaling on an exercise bike, followed by 3 minutes of body weight lunges and push-ups, and then three or four sets of progressively heavier barbell squats with a submaximal load before his first work set.

These examples demonstrate a graduation from general activity to more specific movements the athlete needs. Some athletes might need considerably more time and activity to get the physiological benefits of a warm-up, while others might need less. The bottom line is that warming up is highly individualized to the athlete and sport. With those points in mind, we now cover the three components of a dynamic warm-up that can benefit you before training: general activity, dynamic stretches, and sport-specific activity.

General Activity

As just mentioned, a dynamic warm-up often starts with general activity. Some examples are walking, jogging, skipping rope, doing jumping jacks, pedaling on a bike or arm ergometer, or using an elliptical machine. Many athletes, ranging from baseball players to jiu-jitsu practitioners to soccer players, start with some form of jogging. One way a jog might be improved is by alternating between jogging forward, jogging backward, and side shuffling in each direction. This can be performed either on or off a treadmill. Another ideal general activity for many athletes is skipping rope, since it requires coordination and balance while working the upper and lower body simultaneously. In most cases, approximately 3 to 5 minutes of general activity is sufficient to increase heart rate, blood flow, and neural transmission, but a longer duration might be required.

Dynamic Stretches

After the general activity is finished, the next common step is to perform dynamic stretches. The goal is to rapidly move your joints through their full range of motion to the point where a light stretch or slight tension is felt at the muscle's end range. Examples include arm circles through a large range of motion, high front kicks, and side kicks. The goal of dynamic stretching is to increase tissue extensibility and enhance neural transmissions, which can then carry over to greater performance in the gym or sport. Approximately 3 to 5 minutes is generally sufficient, but go longer if you think it's necessary.

Sport-Specific Activity

The third component of a dynamic warm-up is sport-specific activity. At this stage you'll perform movements that mimic, or closely mimic, what your training requires. For example, if your first exercise is a dumbbell row, start with a few light sets of that exercise. Or a soccer athlete could perform a series of short sprints and cuts in each direction, mimicking what the sport requires. The sport-specific activity should start at a relatively low intensity, around 50 percent of maximal effort, and then steadily increase over the course of 5 to 10 minutes.

> **MUSCLE RULE 3:**
> Perform a dynamic warm-up before training.

You might prefer to shorten the duration of the dynamic warm-up if it's a day you're doing a short workout in the gym or lengthen it if you're preparing for a softball game in your summer league. In any case, make a point to spend at least a few minutes performing each category of exercise, and avoid accumulating any fatigue. Now that we've covered the key components of a dynamic warm-up, let's move on and discuss ways to structure your workouts.

Training Equipment and Workout Structure

Everyone benefits from training efficiently, from a guy who might have only 30 minutes of available workout time to an athlete who needs to devote many hours throughout the week to practicing his sport. Therefore, it is often wise to choose exercises and workouts that stimulate the largest number of muscles with the fewest exercises possible. In this section we cover those options.

Free Weights Versus Machines

If you walk into any major gym you'll likely see a combination of free weights and exercise machines. Generally speaking, resistance that's free of any restrictions is recommended for two reasons. First, an unrestricted load allows the joints to move freely, reducing stress to those vulnerable tissues. Second, a dumbbell or kettlebell requires greater muscle activation since it requires control in all three movement planes. Indeed, it takes more skill to perform a barbell squat than a squat on a Smith machine, which fixes the barbell in one plane. Movement in life and sport requires stability and coordination in all three planes, which is why many coaches favor free weights over machines. Because free weights require greater activation of stabilizer muscles, such as the rotator cuff when pressing a dumbbell overhead, they theoretically have a better transfer to life and sport. Here are some of the most popular forms of external loading that allow unrestricted joint motion:

- Dumbbell
- Kettlebell
- Barbell
- Cable or band
- Sled

- Medicine ball
- Sandbag
- Weighted vest
- Large tire

In some cases, however, a body weight load is sufficient to provide resistance. This is especially true for exercises such as the pull-up, dip, handstand push-up, and one-leg squat. With a little ingenuity, virtually any movement or muscle group can be strengthened using nothing but body weight for resistance. And using gymnastics rings is another way to make any upper body exercise more challenging. For example, performing a push-up from rings requires more muscle and neural activation than performing it with your hands on the ground. One caveat here: Avoid making an exercise so unstable that your training load must be drastically reduced, thus limiting your strength gains.

Exercise machines can be useful to an athlete or the general population, and many companies these days are building versions that are much more joint-friendly than in decades past. Just keep in mind the goal of the exercise is to determine if a machine or free weight is a better option. When training efficiency is the goal, a free weight is often the better choice since it stimulates more motor units.

Full-Body Versus Split Workouts

There are two primary ways to design a workout. On one hand, you can perform a full-body workout, which usually consists of at least three exercises:

- Upper body pull (e.g., row or pull-up)
- Upper body push (e.g., bench press or overhead press)
- Lower body–dominant exercise (e.g., squat, deadlift, lunge or swing variation)

Examples include a workout consisting of a circuit of the pull-up/dip/deadlift or row/overhead press/lunge or lat pull-down/bench press/squat. On the other hand, a split workout consists of exercises that target a specific region of the body, such as arms and back in one workout and chest and shoulders in another, which we cover later.

Basically speaking, a full-body workout activates and strengthens the majority of muscle groups in the body. This can also be accomplished with two exercises. For example, a workout consisting of only the deadlift and bench press challenges enough muscles to be considered "full body." Even though this combination lacks a pure upper body pull, such as a row or pull-up, the deadlift requires significant activation of the upper back muscles. Variations of the clean and the squat also develop upper back strength, especially the Zercher squat. Since a horizontal push works more muscles than a vertical push (i.e., greater activation of the pectorals), some variation of a bench press, push-up, or dip is often recommended when choosing only two exercises. However, a vertical push can also work if you lack strength in that movement.

There are numerous other combinations as well. Basically, any squat or deadlift variation combined with an upper body push will target the majority of muscles in the body. If you have the mobility and coordination to correctly perform a clean and jerk, it alone can train most of the muscle groups since it consists of an upper body pull, squat, and vertical push. Any variation of a clean (e.g., power clean, hang clean) could be combined with an upper body push. If you want more chest development, use a horizontal push. The Turkish get-up (TGU) activates all the major muscle groups except the upper back. Therefore, you could perform a TGU with a pull-up or row. Another popular combination is the TGU paired with a kettlebell swing since it strengthens the upper back as well as the posterior chain. The key point is that sometimes it's optimal for a full-body workout to have the fewest exercises possible. This is especially true when you're short on time or energy. Here are a few examples of exercise combinations that can form a full-body workout:

- Upper body pull + upper body push + squat or deadlift or lunge or swing
- Upper body push + squat or deadlift or swing or clean
- Horizontal upper body push + snatch
- Upper body pull or kettlebell swing + Turkish get-up

Other exercises, whether another multijoint movement or an isolation exercise, can be added, depending on what you're trying to build or strengthen.

A split workout, as mentioned earlier, focuses on training specific regions of the body. For example, one workout trains the upper body, and another workout trains the lower body. This upper–lower split is also known as a two-day split because it takes two workouts, or two days, to work the entire body. A three-day split trains each major muscle group over the course of three workouts. There are numerous variations, but here is one popular version:

- *Workout 1:* legs and abs
- *Workout 2:* chest, triceps, and deltoids
- *Workout 3:* back, biceps, and forearms

It is possible to break up those muscle groups even further and follow a four-day, five-day, or six-day split, where each workout is devoted to fewer muscle groups (Schoenfeld, Grgic, and Krieger 2019). In most cases, however, any training split beyond a two-day upper–lower routine is used by professional bodybuilders who want to train each muscle group with a very high volume. Most of you will not have the luxury to spend hours each day in the gym to isolate every major muscle group. Furthermore, a three-day training split is inefficient.

With full-body training you can stimulate all the major muscle groups in a single workout, which is advantageous for almost anyone. Indeed, a systematic review on training frequency demonstrates that two sessions per week per major muscle group is the minimum recommendation for achieving optimal muscle growth (Schoenfeld, Ogborn, and Krieger 2016). Why split your training up so you have to do six workouts when you can do it in only two?

Training Frequency

Most people train a muscle group anywhere from one to three times per week, depending on their program. As we just covered, training each muscle group twice per week appears to be the *minimum* frequency for muscle growth. For building strength, up to four sessions per week per muscle group has been shown to be superior to one or two (Grgic et al. 2018). With those points in mind, that is why the recommended structure for training is three full-body workouts per week, as covered in chapter 8. In my experience, that structure hits the sweet spot for most people. The frequency is high enough to optimally build muscle and strength with only three trips to the gym each week.

What research hasn't yet demonstrated is the upper limit of training frequency per muscle group per week when hypertrophy is the goal (Dankel et al. 2017). Since there is no scientifically backed research to say that training a lagging muscle group six times per week is better than three, I turn to real-world observations. It is clear that most athletes who train a given muscle group almost daily—let's call it six days per week since even professional athletes take a day off—have built that muscle to a proportionally large degree. For example,

- professional cyclists have proportionally large thighs,
- gymnasts who perform the rings have proportionally large biceps, and
- swimmers have proportionally large upper back muscles.

You can probably think of numerous other examples. Importantly, the afore-mentioned athletes are training those muscles with a relatively high intensity. A marathon runner doesn't build big thighs, even though those muscles are being trained daily, because the intensity is too low to stimulate growth (i.e., a low level of motor unit recruitment).

Early in my career I started experimenting with high frequency training (HFT), which I define as training a muscle group four or more times per week. I did this to accelerate growth in my clients' lagging muscle groups. After much experimentation, I found that for small muscle groups (e.g., calves, biceps, deltoids), 12 sessions per week was optimal. This meant my clients performed one set to failure in the morning and evening of, say, a standing one-leg calf raise six days per week. They continued with that frequency until the intended growth was achieved and then maintained it with three sessions per week, at the beginning of their three full-body workouts when they were fresh and could stimulate that muscle with a high intensity.

I attribute their success with my HFT protocols to the fact they were able to expose those lagging muscles to a significantly higher volume of work each week, which research has shown to be important for hypertrophy (Schoenfeld, Ogborn, and Krieger 2017). Indeed, they would not have been able to perform all 12 sets in one workout with the same repetitions and intensity as they were able to do one set at a time, many hours apart spread throughout the week. This brings up an important point: When volume is equated, more sessions per week isn't advantageous for hypertrophy (Schoenfeld et al. 2019). For example, let's say you were going to do six sets of eight repetitions (6 × 8) of the bench press with 225 pounds (102 kg). Whether you did three sets on Monday and Thursday or one set per day for six days straight, the hypertrophy effect would be the same.

Sleep Hygiene

There is an old adage that states, "Muscle is built outside the gym." Sure, you need to train hard and intelligently program your workouts, but you will not achieve optimal results if you lack sufficient sleep. The recommended sleep duration for adults is seven to nine hours per night (Mukherjee et al. 2015). However, people who consistently perform challenging resistance training will likely need even more than seven hours. So if we split the difference, your mother was right when she told you to sleep eight hours each night. There are numerous deleterious effects of sleep deprivation. Here is a list of some that pertain to athletes:

- Increased cortisol (a stress hormone) and decreased growth hormone (Mougin et al. 2001)
- Decreased maximal and submaximal strength for the deadlift, bench press, and leg press (Reilly and Piercy 1994)
- Poorer cognitive function and decision-making ability during athletic performances (Killgore 2010; Reilly and Deykin 1983)
- Increased susceptibility to obesity and diabetes (Patel et al. 2006)
- Decreased muscular power output (Souissi et al. 2013)

Many of these negative effects are demonstrated with as little as two hours of sleep deprivation, and caffeine the following day didn't help (Reyner and Horne 2013). The good news is that restoring sleep to eight hours per night can solve all these problems, including your anabolic hormones (Chennaoui et al. 2016). If you can't manage to get sufficient sleep during the night, a short (e.g., 30 minute) nap

How to Improve Your Sleep Quality

Some people have the available time to sleep eight or nine hours, but they toss and turn most of the night. If you fall in that category, here are 10 strategies from the University of California San Diego Center for Pulmonary and Sleep Medicine to improve your sleep hygiene:

- Don't go to bed until you are sleepy. If you aren't sleepy, get out of bed and do something else until you become sleepy.
- Regular bedtime routines/rituals help you relax and prepare your body for bed (reading, warm bath, etc.).
- Try to get up at the same time every morning (including weekends and holidays).
- Try to get a full night's sleep every night, and avoid naps during day if possible (if you must nap, limit to 1 h and avoid nap after 3 p.m.).
- Use the bed for sleep and intimacy only; not for any other activities such as TV, computer or phone use, etc.
- Avoid caffeine if possible (if must use caffeine, avoid after lunch).
- Avoid alcohol if possible (if must use alcohol, avoid right before bed).
- Do not smoke cigarettes or use nicotine, ever.
- Consider avoiding high-intensity exercise right before bed (extremely intense exercise may raise cortisol, which impairs sleep).
- Make sure bedroom is quiet, as dark as possible, and a little on the cool side rather than warm (similar to a cave).

University of California San Diego Center for Pulmonary and Sleep Medicine

will significantly help (Hayashi, Motoyoshi, and Hori 2005; Waterhouse et al. 2007). The goal is to get those eight hours of sleep each day, even if it requires a short nap after lunch.

Protein Intake

A list of rules for building muscle would not be complete without a discussion about protein intake, as any bodybuilder can attest to. We delve deeper into the fundamentals of nutrition in chapter 11, but for now, it's important to cover one rule that relates to protein. Because if you're not getting enough of it, improvements in body composition and performance will suffer (Campbell et al. 2018).

Let's say you want to build a brick house. You will need plenty of bricks in a variety of shapes and sizes to complete the task. This analogy works for building muscle too. But instead of bricks, your muscles are constructed of 20 different amino acids. One of those amino acids, categorized as a branched-chain amino acid (BCAA), is leucine. It is particularly important for triggering protein synthesis, the necessary step for building muscle (Moro et al. 2016).

At this point you might be tempted to run to your supplement store and buy the biggest bottle of leucine pills they have. However, it would be a lesson in futility. You also need two of the other branched-chain amino acids, valine and isoleucine, to elicit a better response (Osmond et al. 2019). In fact, you need all 20 amino acids to provide your metabolism with the necessary building blocks it needs for hypertrophy. Since you never know which amino acid(s) your body will need at any given time, it's a wise choice to eat foods that contain all 20: animal proteins (i.e., meat and fish), eggs, and dairy. There are vegetarian options as well, such as soy, quinoa, rice, and beans; however, they all lack the level of BCAAs contained in meat, eggs, and dairy.

The million-dollar question that everyone wants to know is, How much protein do I need? In 2014, a systematic review of resistance trained lean athletes on a caloric deficit recommended 2.3 to 3.1 grams of protein per kilogram (kg) of fat free mass (Helms et al. 2014). For this equation you would first need an accurate determination of your body fat percentage, preferably by a DEXA scan. Let's say a guy weighs 200 pounds (91 kg) and the DEXA indicated he has 20 percent body fat. That means he has 160 pounds (i.e., 72 kg) of fat free mass, which equates to 166 to 223 grams of protein each day. That's a lot of food to eat considering it takes four whole eggs or four ounces (120 g) of steak to get 28 grams of protein.

A more recent recommendation is a minimum of 1.6 grams per kg of body weight (not fat free mass), spread evenly across a minimum of four meals per day (Schoenfeld and Aragon 2018). So this same 200-pound guy would need to eat at least 146 grams each day, or 36 grams in each of his four meals, which is a more realistic and viable goal for anyone not married to a chef. This same research suggests an upper limit of 2.2 grams of protein per kilogram of body weight per day (i.e., 200 grams for a 200-pound person). In my experience, it's best to start at the low end of any protein recommendation to analyze how you look, feel, and perform. From there, increase your protein intake if you believe you could benefit from more.

MUSCLE RULE 7: Eat at least 1.6 grams of protein per kilogram of body weight.

Finally, getting that protein from food is always recommended; however, you can make up any difference by consuming a high-quality protein powder such as cold-processed whey protein concentrate.

Deload

If you've been lifting for a while, you know there are times when your body seems to give up on you. Your bench press and deadlift haven't improved in months. You cut your workouts short because you just don't have the energy. Your motivation sinks, and you start looking for excuses to skip workouts.

Some of this is inevitable. The stressors of work and life compete for your energy and compromise your recovery. But sometimes the problem is your program. You've been pushing too hard for too long, and your body simply needs a break.

That's why most strength and conditioning coaches include a deload in their athletes' training programs. The concept is simple enough: You train with less volume and intensity for a week. How often you deload depends on your training experience. If you're an advanced lifter, you might need a deload every third week. Complete novices might not need to back off until they've trained consistently for two or three months. Everyone between those two extremes will probably do well with a planned deload every four to six weeks. The key word is *planned*. A deload week should be scheduled in advance.

But you never really know when you're going to hit a wall, which means it's hard to predict exactly where in your program you'll need a deload. Even experienced lifters can underestimate how hard they're working, and how much time they need to recover between workouts, and find they need to back off before their scheduled deload.

MUSCLE RULE 8:
Deload when
necessary.

Conversely, a scheduled deload might be a waste of time for someone whose training is less consistent and who ends up with more recovery time between workouts than the program anticipated.

In either case, your body's needs should overrule your program's timetable. If you don't need the deload when it comes up in your schedule, postpone it until you do. And if you feel burned out before your scheduled deload, just follow the two-thirds rule. You have three ways to do it:

- *Put in two-thirds of the effort:* Do the workouts as programmed, but instead of finishing each set with maybe one repetition in reserve, stop with two or three reps in the tank.

- *Use two-thirds of your training load:* Again, you'll do the programmed workouts, but you'll use a third less weight on each set of each exercise.

- *Perform two-thirds of your sets:* If the workout calls for three sets of an exercise, do two sets instead. If the math doesn't work out that neatly—the routine gives you four or five sets of key exercises, for example—add up the total sets in the workout and cut a third of them. Just don't cut entire exercises. Do at least one set of every exercise, and cut at least one set from each one.

Regardless of which option you choose, that temporary one-third reduction in volume or intensity should allow your body to recover from its residual fatigue, which means you can return stronger the following week. And if that doesn't work, it's time to change your program.

What Causes Muscle Soreness and Is It Necessary for Growth?

The discomfort you feel 24 to 72 hours after a hard workout is delayed-onset muscle soreness (DOMS), an umbrella term used to describe the muscular pain, stiffness, and tenderness that can follow exercise. It's most often caused by three circumstances. First, when you perform an exercise for the first time or haven't performed that exercise in weeks or months. Second, when you significantly increase your training intensity, such as adding 10 percent more load or pushing a set to failure. Third, when the volume of exercise significantly increases, such as doing six sets instead of three.

Decades ago, some scientists thought lactate, a by-product of muscle metabolism indirectly associated with the burn you feel after 50 push-ups, might be the cause of DOMS. However, lactate levels return to normal within one to two hours after training ends, which refutes that theory (Goodwin et al. 2007). Soreness is actually caused by microtears within the muscle, which are a normal part of the training process. Your body will repair the damage and make the muscle stronger within a few days.

Another common myth is that a workout must make you sore in order to trigger muscle growth. Although muscle damage is one mechanism of hypertrophy, it's not the only one (Schoenfeld 2010). Many high-level athletes rarely experience soreness but are nonetheless able to keep building new muscle. Soreness shouldn't be viewed as a training goal but as an inevitable side effect of adding a new exercise or changing the training parameters. So if you like to get sore after a workout, keep mixing things up.

Progressive Overload

One of the most important components for programming your training is progressive overload, which is a gradual increase in stress that's placed on the body in order to elicit a positive adaptation. The act of purposefully lifting ever-heavier loads dates back to the sixth century B.C. when Milo of Croton trained for wrestling. The legend states that each day Milo would carry a calf to build his strength. As the calf grew, so did Milo's strength. These days, the progressive overload principle is credited to Thomas DeLorme, an Army physician who helped rehabilitate soldiers during World War II (Todd, Shurley, and Todd 2012). His system was simple:

- Perform 3 × 10 for basic resistance exercises (i.e., 1 × 10 with 50 percent of 1RM, 1 × 10 with 75 percent of 1RM, 1 × 10 with the heaviest load possible).
- Try to increase the load of the third set each workout.

How to Use Postactivation Potentiation to Become More Explosive

The way exercises are arranged in a workout can have a positive influence on performance in subsequent sets or similar movement patterns. For example, research demonstrates that some athletes can jump higher or sprint faster after a few heavy sets of a squat or deadlift, thanks to postactivation potentiation (PAP) (McBride, Nimphius, and Erickson 2005). There are two practical applications here.

First, a PAP conditioning set can be used to increase performance (i.e., rate of force development) of an explosive activity such as a vertical jump or 40-meter sprint. A study in the *Journal of Human Kinetics* compared two potential PAP protocols on national- and regional-level soccer players (Sanchez-Sanchez et al. 2018). One protocol consisted of performing a squat with 60 percent of 1RM, while the other protocol was 90 percent of 1RM. In either case, the soccer athletes rested 5 minutes and then performed 20-meter sprints. Athletes who performed the squat with 90 percent of 1RM experienced greater improvements in sprint velocity. The trick is to manage the balance between PAP and fatigue. For example, one or two sets of a heavy deadlift at the beginning of a workout followed immediately by a maximal vertical jump or sprint attempt could work well. Or a few sets of a heavy bench press before a javelin or medicine ball throw. When a heavy load with low volume (e.g., 2 × 2 with 90 percent of 1RM) is used, the PAP effect is almost immediate. Second, a squat or deadlift can be placed before a power exercise in a circuit to potentially induce PAP (e.g., a heavy set of the deadlift before a set of box jumps). In any case, the act of programming heavy maximal strength exercises with lighter, explosive strength exercises in the same workout is known as contrast training.

Although it's still not clear what induces PAP, it seems to be a temporary enhancement of muscular factors and, maybe more importantly, neural factors (Wallace et al. 2019). The potential benefits of PAP to improve explosive performance appear to be mainly limited to experienced power athletes. In other words, PAP is less likely to work for a young or relatively weak athlete (Rixon, Lamont, and Bemben 2007).

Research indicates that the effect of PAP is very individualized, some athletes got a positive response and others experienced a decrease in performance (Lim and Kong 2013; Seitz and Haff 2016). Nevertheless, there appears to be enough positive research on PAP to give it a try. Perform a heavy set of a squat or deadlift, then wait 15 to 30 seconds and see if you can jump higher. If you can, keep this contrast training in your program to increase your explosive power.

Since that time there have been numerous improvements in the way you can program progressive overload. We start by covering the components of volume and intensity, as well as the relationship between the two. Note that this section on progressive overload contains the most technical information in this book, and it may not be of interest to you. If you want to better understand the relationship between volume and intensity, read on. However, if you're just an avid lifter who wants to build a better physique, you can skip to the next chapter. With that caveat out of the way, let's cover the components of progressive overload.

Volume

Volume is the amount of load that can be calculated in pounds or kilograms for each workout, week, or training cycle. Volume affects neural, hypertrophic, hormonal, and metabolic responses to exercise (Schoenfeld, Ogborn, and Krieger 2017). The simplest definition of volume, as it applies to resistance training, is the total number of reps multiplied by load as shown in this equation:

$$\text{volume} = \text{total reps} \times \text{load} \tag{3.1}$$

If an athlete squats 5×6 (i.e., 30 total repetitions) with 250 pounds (113 kg), the volume is 7,500 pounds (3,400 kg) ($30 \times 250 = 7,500$). One way to program progressive overload is by steadily increasing exercise volume. This helps improve your work capacity while preparing your muscles, tendons, and ligaments for the strain of high-impact activities that are common in sport. Equation 3.1 allows you to determine a change in volume when different parameters are performed. For example, an athlete performs 30 total reps of the squat with 250 pounds (113 kg) in one workout, and 40 total reps with 200 pounds (91 kg) in the next session. Even though the load decreased, his actual exercise volume increased from 7,500 pounds (3,400 kg) to 8,000 pounds (3,630 kg). This volume calculation can be paired with the intensity calculation we're about to cover so you can determine how they're related in a training cycle.

Intensity

Intensity is a measure of effort as it relates to time or load. There are four ways to increase intensity:

- Use a higher percentage of 1RM.
- Increase speed of movement.
- Decrease rest periods between exercises.
- Work closer to momentary muscular failure.

To calculate intensity, divide exercise volume by total number of reps. Keeping with the earlier example, the squat volume is 7,500 pounds (3,400 kg), consisting of 30 total repetitions. In this case, exercise intensity is 250 (7,500/30 = 250), as shown in this equation:

$$\text{exercise intensity} = \text{exercise volume/total reps} \tag{3.2}$$

The Secret Formula of the Soviet Union's Success

From the late 1960s to 1990, athletes from the Soviet Union dominated weightlifting competitions. Although many theories can be put forth as to why, the most logical explanation pertains to the way they organized their strength training sessions. One striking difference, compared with the way Olympic weightlifters trained in the United States, was the large amount of time Soviet athletes spent training with submaximal loads. Indeed, training with loads greater than 90 percent of 1RM made up only 5 to 6 percent of their total reps over the course of years (Zatsiorsky 1992). This is surprising considering the goal of Olympic weightlifting events (i.e., the snatch and the clean and jerk) is to lift the heaviest load possible for a single repetition.

Thanks to intense research by a few of the top Russian sport scientists who analyzed the training schedules of the most successful Soviet weightlifters over the course of four Olympic training cycles (i.e., 16 years), we now know how much time those athletes spent training in each loading zone:

Percentage of 1RM (intensity zone)	50%-60%	61%-70%	71%-80%	81%-90%	91%-100%
Percentage of reps in intensity zone	10%	25%	35%	25%	5%

So if you're looking for a novel year-long program to build your squat, deadlift, or snatch, just follow the guidelines in this table. First, figure out how many total reps you'll perform over the course of a year for, say, the squat. Second, plug in the loads for the squat, making sure you'll perform the correct percentage of total repetitions by the end of the year. For example, if over the course of 12 months you plan to perform 1,000 total repetitions, 350 of them should fall within 71 to 80 percent of your 1RM. Third, vary the volume around 20 percent between training sessions, which means it will fluctuate higher and lower over time to create a wavelike pattern. This is a project I make all my graduate students at the University of Southern California complete by the end of their semester with me. But don't worry, I won't be grading you.

Volume–Intensity Relationship

At this point, calculations for volume and intensity might seem arbitrary. However, it's important for some people, such as strength coaches, to know how to calculate the volume–intensity relationship for lifts that can induce high levels of fatigue, such as work sets for the squat, deadlift, or snatch. Importantly, the calculations are not for warm-up sets, single-joint exercises, or other low-intensity exercises that have a minimal effect on fatigue. For loaded carries, volume equals load multiplied by steps. If an athlete carries 250 pounds (113 kg) for 20 steps, volume is 5,000 (250 × 20).

In North America, it is generally accepted that athletes focus on increasing either volume or intensity from workout to workout—aiming for both can be too taxing, except for short periods. For example, if you performed 4 × 6 for the row on Monday, you could perform 4 × 7 with the same load the following Monday (i.e., volume progression), or you could increase the load 2 or 3 percent and perform 3 × 6 (i.e., intensity progression). Indeed, a good rule of thumb is to perform one less set of an exercise when the load is increased in order to manage fatigue. Research demonstrates that loading increments as small as 0.5 pound (0.2 kg) can be effective for progressive overload (Hostler et al. 2001). However, in Russia and Europe, a 20 percent change in volume between training sessions is often programmed. To be clear, this means the volume can increase or decrease, creating a wavelike pattern. This type of programming requires greater skill and should be reserved for lifters and strength coaches who thoroughly understand the overall strategy. Therefore, a novice lifter or coach is wise to initially focus on increasing either volume or intensity between workouts.

> **MUSCLE RULE 9:**
> Strength coaches and advanced lifters must know how to calculate the volume–intensity relationship.

This information applies specifically to a multijoint exercise an athlete is trying to build. An example is a sprinter who wants to boost his squat so he can run faster. His coach should track the volume–intensity relationship of the squat over the course of his year-long training cycle to determine how changes in that relationship affect his performance.

In summary, progressive overload is achieved by programming any of the following:

- Increase volume (i.e., workout volume or mileage).
- Use a higher percentage of 1RM.
- Work closer to momentary muscular failure (i.e., rep progression).
- Increase velocity of movement (i.e., speed progression).
- Decrease rest periods between sets of the same exercise (i.e., density progression).

Final Thoughts

We cover a lot of ground in this chapter, from preparing for a workout to progressive overload techniques. The purpose of this chapter is to give you a lifetime's worth of tools that can apply to any program. Some of the topics we cover, such as calculating volume and intensity, might not interest you at this point. But someday you might want to learn more in-depth principles that elite strength coaches use for high-performance athletes. Other topics, such as strategies for increasing sleep quality and guidelines for protein intake, are essential for everyone. In any case, you might benefit from reading this chapter a few times to better understand the programs we cover later in this book.

PART II

MUSCLE METHODOLOGY

CHAPTER 4

Building Muscle Versus Burning Fat

Everyone knows you need to train one way to get bigger and another way to get leaner.

When the goal is to increase muscle mass, you need to do a high volume of training, using moderately heavy weights and sets of 8 to 12 repetitions, with some periods of heavier lifting with the goal of increasing strength. And when the goal is to lose fat, you need to use lighter weights with much higher reps. Indeed, those are the recommendations you'll typically hear and read. And it makes sense, especially if you look at the people who have the kind of physiques we aspire to. The most muscular non-steroid-using bodybuilders almost always do high-volume workouts with reps in the traditional hypertrophy range. The leanest people often promote body weight movements and cardiorespiratory exercise while eschewing heavy weights.

But with some thought, you'd see the flaw in using anecdotes as evidence. Generations of young lifters have followed the training routines of elite athletes and contest-winning bodybuilders, but very few have ended up with physiques like theirs. You and I could do the exact same program and get very different results. I might get bigger while you get leaner, even though we're both doing the same exercises with the same system of sets and reps.

That doesn't mean the program is optimal for either goal. It just means the results of a program are determined by factors beyond sets, reps, and exercise selection. Chief among them is your caloric balance, as you'll see in this chapter. You'll also learn the physiological causes of muscle growth. I'll finish with a comparison of my muscle-building and fat-burning programs—why they're similar in some ways but very different in others.

Muscle Growth: What Scientists Know

These days we have handheld phones that are more powerful than computers in the 1960s, which took up entire rooms. That computing power, combined with advances in imaging technology, allows researchers to examine muscle tissue in ways never imagined by the pioneers of exercise science in the 20th century. But for all those advancements, we still don't know much about the physiological and metabolic adaptations that make your muscles grow. Two things scientists are pretty sure of: the roles played by satellite cells and the mTOR pathway.

After a bout of resistance training, your muscle fibers have trauma in the form of microscopic tears through the fibers and surrounding structures. This microtrauma signals the muscle's satellite cells (i.e., muscle stem cells) to activate and move to the site of damage. The satellite cells donate their nuclei, which starts a cascade of events that allow the fibers to increase their size (Egner, Bruusgaard, and Gundersen 2016). The mTOR pathway is thought to be the master regulator of muscle growth (Thomas and Hall 1997). Short for mammalian target of rapamycin, mTOR performs numerous roles involving insulin, growth factors, and amino acids, as well as the muscle's nutrient, oxygen, and energy levels (Hay and Sonenberg 2004; Tokunaga, Yoshino, and Yonezawa 2004).

One question that still baffles scientists is, Can adult muscles split to form new fibers?

To get the idea, think of a stock you bought in a Fortune 500 company. If the stock price increases rapidly, the company may decide to split the stock, so instead of owning one share worth $100, you own two shares, each worth $50. Muscle fibers are like the stock shares in the first half of the analogy. We know they can get larger. But we don't know if a single fiber can split into two smaller fibers (a process called hyperplasia) when it reaches a critical level of growth (Jorgensen, Phillips, and Hornberger 2020).

How Does Muscle Grow or Shrink?

A muscle's physiological cross-sectional area can expand (hypertrophy), shrink (atrophy), or stay the same size. Throughout the day, the body alternates between periods of muscle protein synthesis and muscle protein breakdown. Hypertrophy occurs when synthesis is higher than breakdown over the course of a day or more. The muscle pulls amino acids from the blood, which it then uses to build muscle proteins. Atrophy occurs when protein breakdown is higher than protein synthesis. In this case, muscle proteins break down into amino acids, which are then released into the blood, where they're used for other metabolic processes. These processes are shown in figure 4.1.

After a bout of high-intensity resistance exercise, muscle protein breakdown *and* synthesis increase (Phillips et al. 1997). But during the subsequent 24 to 36 hours, synthesis is greater than breakdown. The result is a net increase in muscle protein (i.e., hypertrophy), assuming the person has eaten enough protein for that to occur (Cermak et al. 2012; West et al. 2016).

As most of us know, increasing a muscle's size through hypertrophy not only makes you look better on the beach but increases your performance as well, assuming you don't also gain a lot of fat. Larger muscles can produce more force, which can then improve your speed, strength, and power. Similarly, smaller muscles are less impressive visually, and more often than not reduce your performance. We usually think of those changes in muscle size taking place in the myofibrils. These are the contractile elements, the ones that generate force. But the volume of noncontractile elements—glycogen and semifluid plasma—can also change. That means two forms of hypertrophy are theoretically possible (see figure 4.2):

- *Myofibrillar hypertrophy:* growth of the myofibrils, which increases a muscle's force potential
- *Sarcoplasmic hypertrophy:* increased volume of glycogen and semifluid plasma, which doesn't necessarily increase force potential

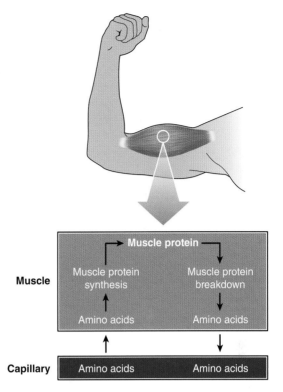

FIGURE 4.1 Muscle protein synthesis and breakdown.

So what triggers muscle growth in the gym? Scientists have several theories to explain how resistance training drives hypertrophy. Research by Brad Schoenfeld (2010) suggests three possible mechanisms:

- *Mechanical tension:* the stress within a muscle and its supporting tissues when it works against resistance
- *Metabolic stress:* the buildup of lactate, protons (H+), and inorganic phosphates during exercise
- *Muscle damage:* disruption of the muscle fibers in response to intense or high-volume exercise

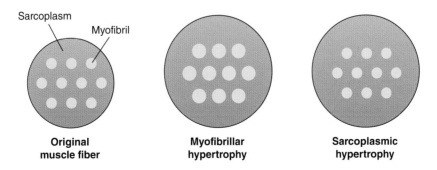

FIGURE 4.2 Myofibrillar versus sarcoplasmic hypertrophy.

The Sarcoplasmic Hypertrophy Controversy

In this chapter we cover two forms of hypertrophy: myofibrillar and sarcoplasmic. Scientists know myofibrillar hypertrophy exists because they have the technology to measure it. Sarcoplasmic hypertrophy, on the other hand, is a little trickier to determine. There is uncertainty whether sarcoplasmic hypertrophy occurs, and if it does, what role it plays (Haun et al. 2019; Roberts et al. 2020).

Old-school lifters assumed that training with heavy loads stimulates myofibrillar hypertrophy, while training with light loads to failure (e.g., 35 repetitions of a push-up) leads to sarcoplasmic hypertrophy. If you were a bodybuilder, the type of hypertrophy didn't really matter, since any growth was good. However, we now know that you can get muscle fibers to grow without heavy or moderate loads (Burd et al. 2010).

The good news is that training with virtually any range of repetitions, from 3 to 30 or more per set, can increase muscle cross-sectional area (Burd et al. 2010; Mitchell et al. 2012). Which range of repetitions you choose for any given workout depends on what goals you're trying to achieve in addition to muscle growth. If you want more strength, sets of fewer than 6 repetitions work best (Jenkins et al. 2016). If you want to increase muscular endurance, you'd choose higher repetitions. Another benefit of low- or high-repetition sets is adding variety to your training, rather than the typical 10 to 12 repetitions for every exercise.

The type and intensity of exercise determine which of the three factors come into play. Evidence suggests that mechanical tension is most likely the primary factor, since hypertrophy often occurs without significant metabolic stress or damage to the muscle (Eftestøl et al. 2016).

Regardless of the trigger, activation of the muscle's satellite cells is important for hypertrophy. When a muscle is at rest, or isn't being challenged to any significant degree, satellite cells sit quietly around the fibers. But once mechanical tension, metabolic stress, or muscle damage occur, satellite cells become active and donate their nuclei to the muscle fibers, causing them to grow (Vierck et al. 2000). Satellite cells also aid other regulatory processes that facilitate repair, regeneration, and growth (Toigo and Boutellier 2006).

Training Principles to Build Muscle or Burn Fat

Most people have one of two goals in mind when they train—to build muscle or burn fat—and in reality, almost any resistance training program can do both. Consider three intelligently designed resistance training programs, based on the muscle rules discussed in the previous chapter. Let's say each of these three programs has a different emphasis:

- Training plan 1 emphasizes heavy loads (3-5 sets of 3-5 reps).
- Training plan 2 emphasizes moderate loads (3-4 sets of 6-12 reps).
- Training plan 3 emphasizes lighter loads (3-4 sets of 18-20 reps).

If you simply look at the sets and reps, and don't know anything else about the programs, you could say with some confidence what each program is designed to achieve. The goal of training plan 1 is obviously to build maximal strength. Plan 2, using the most common hypertrophy parameters, is for someone trying to increase muscle size. And plan 3, with its high volume (up to 80 reps per exercise), would be best for fat loss.

But what if you learned that every set in plan 3 is to be taken to momentary muscular failure to create metabolic stress, a potent stimulus for hypertrophy (Schoenfeld 2010)? Or that plan 1 includes lots of single-joint exercises for muscles that wouldn't typically be emphasized when the goal is pure strength? Or that plan 2 has relatively short rest periods and thus limited recovery between sets, which wouldn't be optimal for hypertrophy? Wouldn't that change your sense of what each program was designed to achieve?

The truth is, any of the three can be a muscle-building or fat-burning program. Training with heavy loads induces greater growth of type II muscle fibers, or equal growth of type II and type I fibers, mainly by myofibrillar hypertrophy. Training with lighter loads for a high volume or to momentary muscular failure causes more growth in type I fibers and might stimulate sarcoplasmic hypertrophy (Haun et al. 2019). What matters most is this:

- All muscle fiber types can grow with the right type of training. In chapters 8 and 9 you'll see programming with repetitions that range from 3 to 30 per set to get maximal stimulation of all muscle fiber types.

- Your daily nutrition is the difference maker. If you consistently consume 500 calories a day above your maintenance level, you'll gain muscle with any of the three programs I just described. If you eat 500 calories below your maintenance level, you'll lose fat with the same programs.

Regardless of your goal—to build muscle or to burn fat—the core component of your elite-physique training programs will be three full-body circuits each week. And you'll prioritize multijoint exercises, since they stimulate more muscle groups with each set than isolation exercises do. But this is where the similarities end. A fat-loss program needs a few modifications because training and eating to burn fat requires a caloric deficit, which imposes stress on your immune system. With too much overall stress, you won't be able to maintain optimal levels of testosterone and other anabolic hormones (Fry and Kraemer 1997; Schoenfeld et al. 2020). The modifications are as follows:

- *Less volume:* You'll do four rounds of a circuit instead of five or more.

- *Less intensity:* You'll stop each set one or two repetitions short of failure to avoid excessive muscle damage (another form of stress).

- *Fewer exercises:* Fat-loss workouts often have three or four multijoint exercises instead of five or more.

- *Shorter rest periods:* With 30 to 45 seconds of rest between each exercise in a circuit, instead of 2 to 3 minutes, you'll elicit a larger cardiorespiratory response (Alcaraz, Sanchez-Lorente, and Blazevich 2008).

- *More metabolic work:* Each workout will end with a metabolic exercise (e.g., sprints or sled work) to stimulate fat loss. You'll also do lower-intensity cardiorespiratory exercise on nonlifting days to promote fat burning and manage fatigue.

The first three changes—lower volume and intensity and fewer exercises—help you limit training-induced physical stress at a time when your body is already coping with the stress of a reduced-calorie diet. If you're relatively new to strength training, or coming back from a long layoff, you may increase strength and muscle mass during a caloric deficit while also losing fat. But if you're an intermediate to advanced lifter who's been training consistently for the past few years, you may be lucky to maintain your muscle mass while losing fat. The more likely outcome is that you'll lose some muscle along with the fat. That said, if you have a lot of fat covering strong and well-developed muscles, you will probably appear more muscular as you get leaner, even though you actually have less total muscle. It's a trade-off most of us will gladly make when the goal is to improve your physique.

The fourth change—shorter rest periods—increases the density of your workout. In other words, you perform more work in less time. Your heart rate will increase, and you'll breathe harder from the greater cardiorespiratory demand (Alcaraz, Sanchez-Lorente, and Blazevich 2008). You'll also have higher levels of EPOC (excess postexercise oxygen consumption), which means you continue to burn calories at a higher rate in the hours following your workout (Greer et al. 2015). Some research suggests EPOC aids in fat loss, although probably not to the extent you often see promoted in fitness marketing (Williams et al. 2013).

Calorie burning is also the reason for the fifth change. Metabolic work is similar to strength training with limited rest periods, in that it raises your heart rate and contributes to EPOC. The low-intensity cardiorespiratory exercise on the days in between strength workouts will also burn calories and train your body to better utilize fat for fuel. So why not do only high-intensity metabolic exercise, like interval training, on nonlifting days? The goal is to limit fatigue and facilitate recovery. High-intensity exercise creates an acid load on the body that must be buffered by your kidneys, which can be stressful if you do too much of it. Simply walking at a brisk pace on those days, instead of remaining sedentary, will increase circulation, which helps your body clear the waste products left over from your strength workouts.

Final Thoughts

In this chapter, we talk about the differences between training for fat loss or muscle gain. To recap what we covered earlier: Almost any well-designed resistance training program has the potential to build muscle or burn fat, to some degree. But you won't gain much muscle when consuming a caloric deficit each day or lose fat when eating a caloric surplus, no matter how hard you try. That's why specific nutrition and training adjustments are often necessary to optimize your results. And if you're unsure which goal to focus on first, take a look in the mirror. If there's any excess fat around your midsection, focus on fat loss first.

CHAPTER 5

Lower Body Training

When it comes to physical development, few things are as visually impressive as a muscular lower body. When you see big glutes, thighs, and calves on a guy it just screams "power!" In this chapter we cover a vast array of exercises and progressions that focus primarily on the lower body muscles. In many cases, the exercises will also work the core and upper back, making the exercises more full-body in nature, which translates to the physical demands of life and sport. You will learn the principles for choosing appropriate lower body exercises. We cover variations that work for novice to advanced lifters, as well as joint-friendly training options for readers whose bodies have a little more mileage on them. By the end of this chapter, you should have a thorough understanding of ways to increase the size and strength of the lower body, as well as a myriad of progressions that can suit all levels of the fitness spectrum.

Development of Lower Body Musculature

Let's start with a fact: Exercises that target the lower body musculature are not easy. It requires a lot of effort and focus to do them correctly because exercises such as the squat and deadlift simultaneously work hundreds of muscle groups, including your largest ones (i.e., glutes, hamstrings, and quadriceps). This is especially true when training with a challenging load. That is why guys often like to skip "leg day" when they're feeling a bit run down. However, the muscles throughout your legs, hips, and pelvis need to be big and strong to build a body that performs as well as it looks.

Your power comes from your hips and pelvis. When you think of an explosive athlete, it's likely you picture a running back sprinting through defenders or a powerlifter pulling a deadlift that's triple his body weight. You might think of an MMA fighter who throws a powerful roundhouse kick. Even the ability to throw a hard knockout punch comes from the hips. Imagine a right-handed puncher standing in a split stance with his left leg forward and right leg behind him. He pushes off his right foot, which generates force that travels up through his hips, trunk, and shoulders and then culminates when his right fist lands on his opponent. Any weakness in that chain, from the right foot to the right fist, will diminish his performance. Put another way, you need a strong lower body to be a powerful athlete.

In a bodybuilding contest, judges look for proportional development between the upper and lower body. From a physique standpoint, there are few things that look as odd as an incredibly muscular upper body paired with skinny legs. Indeed, lower body training is not only necessary to be powerful but also visually impressive.

The glutes get plenty of press these days, and for good reason. Your glutes consist of three muscles: gluteus minimus, gluteus medius, and gluteus maximus (see figure 5.1). Collectively, they perform three actions at the hip: extension, abduction, and external rotation. Weakness in the glutes has been linked to pain in the low back, hip, and knee. Of the three, the gluteus maximus is the largest, strongest muscle in the body. Or it should be, anyway. That's because the maximus is responsible for a myriad of performance and orthopedic benefits, including the overall shape of your butt.

Now let's cover two primary categories of lower body exercises—exercises that emphasize the hip versus the quads and exercises performed on one leg versus two legs.

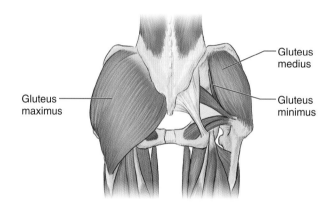

FIGURE 5.1   Gluteal muscles.

Hip Versus Quad Emphasis

The way you perform any given exercise can have a profound effect on which muscles are emphasized. For example, a squat can be performed with a relatively vertical or horizontal trunk angle as shown in figure 5.2.

The trunk angle affects which lower body muscles are emphasized during a squat. When your trunk is more vertical, your knees must travel forward to maintain balance (i.e., quad emphasis). Conversely, when your trunk shifts farther forward, your hips travel backward and very little forward movement of the knees is required to maintain balance (i.e., hip emphasis).

Basically speaking, maintaining a trunk angle of greater than 60 degrees at the bottom of a squat emphasizes the quadriceps more than the hips, while a trunk angle of less than 60 degrees emphasizes the hips. You can use the shin angle as a guide for determining which muscles are emphasized. The shins travel forward to emphasize the quadriceps (see figure 5.2a) but remain mostly vertical to emphasize the hips (see figure 5.2b).

Importantly, this categorization is not limited to the squat: It carries over to all lower body exercises. Two examples are appropriate here. First, a forward lunge emphasizes the quadriceps since the shin travels forward, while a reverse lunge can be performed with a vertical shin angle to emphasize the hips, as shown in figure 5.3. Put another way, a reverse lunge spares the knees, making it a joint-friendly option for those who have knee pain. Second, a deadlift can begin with the shins angled forward to emphasize the quadriceps or remain vertical to put a greater emphasis on the hips, as shown in figure 5.4.

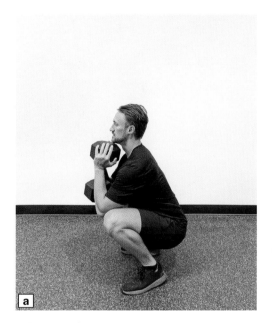
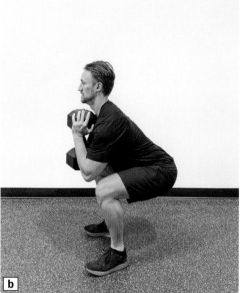

FIGURE 5.2 Squat with *(a)* a relatively vertical trunk angle greater than 60 degrees and forward movement of the shins and *(b)* with a relatively horizontal trunk angle less than 60 degrees and vertical shins.

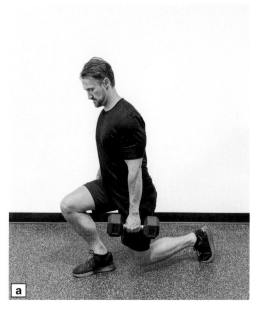
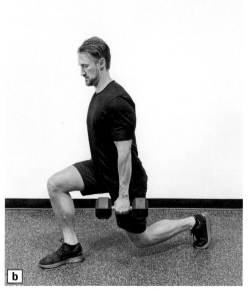

FIGURE 5.3 *(a)* Forward lunge for quad emphasis and *(b)* reverse lunge for hip emphasis.

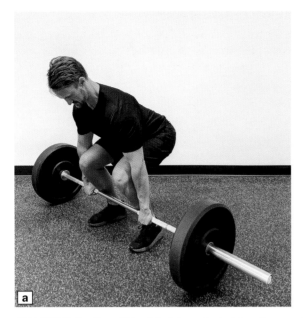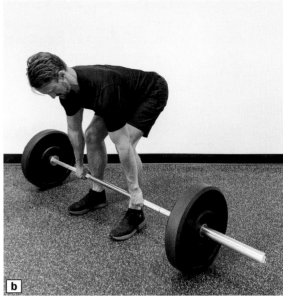

FIGURE 5.4 Deadlift with *(a)* angled shins for quad emphasis and *(b)* vertical shins for hip emphasis.

From a programming standpoint, both quad- and hip-emphasis exercises have their place to ensure complete development of the lower body musculature. That is why you'll often see a hip-emphasis exercise in one workout followed by a quad-emphasis exercise in the next workout in chapters 8 and 9. However, if you have cranky knees, an exercise that emphasizes the hips more than the knees might prove to be a better programming option, as opposed to skipping a lower body exercise altogether, which will impair your results. For example, if a forward lunge is programmed in a workout, you can replace it with a reverse lunge to spare your knees. Conversely, if you want more quadriceps development, you can adjust the technique of any hip-emphasis exercise to have a greater quad emphasis, as covered earlier. Now let's move on to two- and one-leg exercises.

Two-Leg Versus One-Leg Exercises

The logic of one-leg strength exercises is impeccable: Most actions in sports—from running and jumping to throwing and kicking—are produced with force generated by one leg, while the other acts in support. But because the exercises are hard to teach or supervise, especially in a group setting, and because their benefits aren't as easy to quantify as those of bilateral exercises like squats and deadlifts, they're sometimes an afterthought in strength and conditioning programs.

As a general rule, two-leg exercises such as a traditional squat or deadlift are mastered before incorporating one-leg versions of the same movement. Indeed, a one-leg version of a squat or deadlift requires considerably more balance and coordination (i.e., neural activation) to get the technique dialed in. That is one reason it's such a valuable addition to any training program. The other reason is arguably even more important: One-leg exercises reduce compression stress through the spine.

Before we move on it's important to clarify what I mean by a one-leg exercise. Ostensibly, it means that only one leg is on the ground throughout the entire movement, such as a one-leg squat or deadlift. But that's not necessary to reap the benefits we just covered. Any split squat, lunge, or step-up variation will also unload the spine and require greater neural activation than a two-leg exercise. So for the purposes of this chapter, any of the following lower body exercises will be categorized as a one-leg exercise:

- One-leg squat
- One-leg deadlift
- Lunge
- Split squat
- Step-up

In chapters 8 and 9 you'll see that two-leg and one-leg exercises rotate between workouts, meaning if a deadlift is programmed on Monday a lunge, step-up, or similar one-leg variation is programmed on Wednesday. This allows you to keep training your lower body with plenty of load and intensity without straining your intervertebral discs. Performing a two-leg squat or deadlift exercise for each workout can put considerable strain through the spine, which is stressful to your discs and requires a longer recovery.

Lower Body Exercises

In this section we cover a wide range of lower body exercises. Variations that require a machine (e.g., leg press) or any apparatus that limits a movement to one plane are purposely omitted. For optimal muscle stimulation, development, and performance benefits, I've found that free-weight variations carry over to sport while also promoting joint health and integrity better than machines do.

SQUAT VARIATIONS

The squat works hundreds of muscles in ways that have functional and athletic implications. The movement pattern represents a developmental milestone for toddlers; the key to speed and power for athletes; and a vital link to active, independent aging for seniors. But with all those benefits come substantial risks to athletes, especially those who are taller and have less core stability. A lot can go wrong with a barbell back squat if you're not careful. That is why we'll start by covering the goblet squat, arguably the most user-friendly of all squat variations.

MUSCLES WORKED:

quadriceps

glutes

hamstrings

hip adductors

spine extensors

stabilizing muscles of the shoulder girdle
(when using external resistance), core, and hips

calves

Goblet Squat

For the goblet squat the load is held against the chest, which helps novice lifters learn to sit back during the descent without losing their balance. This is a terrific exercise for lifters at any level of experience. The only shortcoming is that a single dumbbell or kettlebell might not be heavy enough for very strong athletes during maximal strength training.

HOW TO DO IT

1. Grab a kettlebell or dumbbell with both hands on one end, and stand holding it against your chest, just below your chin (see figure a). Set your feet about shoulder-width apart, toes forward or pointed out slightly.
2. Push your hips back and lower yourself as far as you can while keeping your lower back in its natural arch (see figure b).
3. Push back to the starting position and repeat.

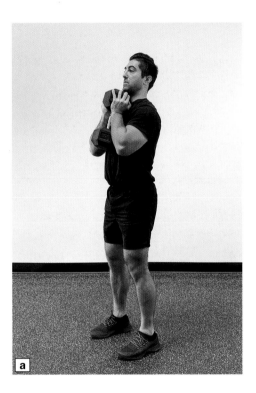
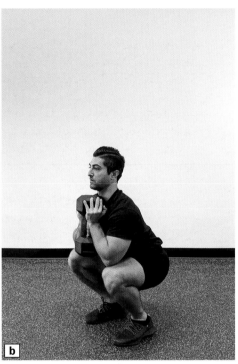

ADVANTAGES

- The load allows a more upright posture, with less risk of lumbar flexion.
- Most lifters achieve a deeper range of motion with goblet versus barbell squats, with more consistent form from rep to rep.

COACHING CUES

- If you are new to this exercise, it's beneficial to have a flat bench or chair behind you. This allows you to sit back without fear of losing your balance.
- Avoid any inward buckling of the knees.

Barbell Back Squat

As mentioned earlier, a lot can go wrong with a barbell back squat if you lack mobility in the ankles, hips, or thoracic spine. This exercise can also be problematic for lifters who are tall or have relatively long legs. Even though a back squat is often considered a beginner or foundational exercise, some people will never be able to perform it through a full range of motion with ideal form. If you happen to be one of them, program another version of the squat that better suits your structure and mobility. That being said, a barbell back squat is a terrific exercise to build strength and muscle mass for those who can perform it correctly.

HOW TO DO IT

1. Load a barbell in the rack and duck under it, positioning the bar on your upper traps (see figure a). Grab the bar with a wide overhand grip.
2. Lift the bar off the rack, take one small step back with each foot, and position your feet about shoulder-width apart, toes pointed out slightly (see figure b).

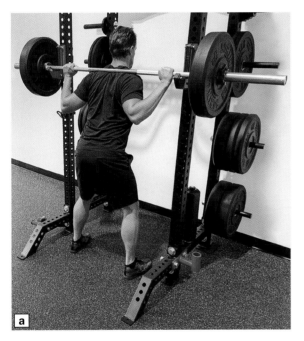

a

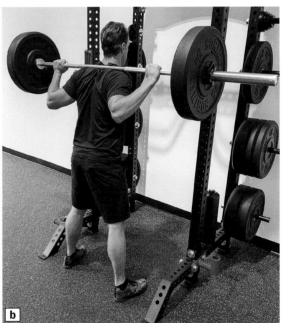

b

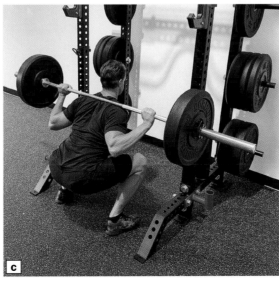

c

(continued)

Barbell Back Squat *(continued)*

3. Push your hips back and lower yourself as far as you can while keeping your lower back in its natural arch (see figure c).
4. Push back to the starting position and repeat.

ADVANTAGE

The barbell back squat has functional carryover to virtually any sport or full-body activity.

COACHING CUES

- The weight *must* stay over the middle of the foot; if it's farther forward, over the toes, this compromises balance and places excess strain on the lower back and knees. Have a partner observe you from the side to make sure the load is properly aligned.
- Athletes with longer femurs will typically achieve better form with a wider stance and toes angled out up to about 45 degrees.
- Pay attention to your neck and chin. If you tend to bend your head back, make a double chin; that will keep your neck aligned and put you in a stronger overall position.
- To make any two-leg squat or deadlift variation even better, wear a resistance band around your lower thighs. The resistance of the band activates additional gluteal fibers, which promotes athleticism while reducing knee pain.

Front Squat

It is common to see high-level athletes perform a front squat with a barbell across the clavicles and elbows held high. However, that version requires more wrist mobility than most lifters have. Holding two kettlebells in the rack position is usually a much better option.

HOW TO DO IT

1. Hold a kettlebell in each hand against your chest, with the elbows bent and held close to the sides (see figure a).
2. Push your hips back and lower yourself as far as you can while keeping your lower back in its natural arch and elbows tucked tightly to the sides of the trunk (see figure b).
3. Push back to the starting position and repeat.

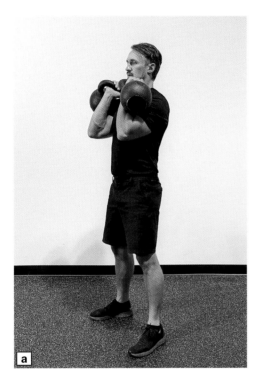
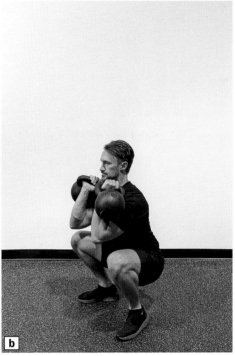

ADVANTAGES

- You can sit back more and therefore maintain a more vertical torso.
- The front squat is often a better option for taller athletes than the back squat.
- Using two kettlebells instead of a barbell reduces strain on the wrists.

COACHING CUE

As in the back squat, the weight *must* stay over the middle of the foot. That means your torso will be more upright.

Zercher Squat

The Zercher squat is named after the late strongman Ed Zercher. Holding a barbell or sandbag in the crooks of your elbows is useful for a wide variety of exercises including the split squat, lunge, and walking.

▶ HOW TO DO IT

1. Place a barbell on the pins in a power rack at a height just below your elbows. Dip underneath the bar and position it in the crooks of your elbows, with your arms bent and palms facing you. Lift it off the rack, step back, and position your feet about shoulder-width apart, toes forward or pointed out slightly (see figure a). Wear long sleeves to minimize skin irritation.
2. Push your hips back and lower yourself as far as you can while keeping your lower back in its natural arch (see figure b).
3. Push back to the starting position and repeat.

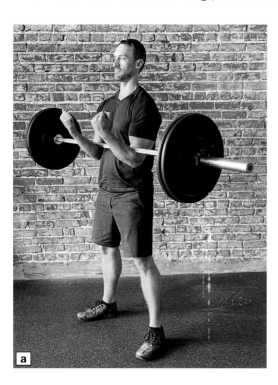
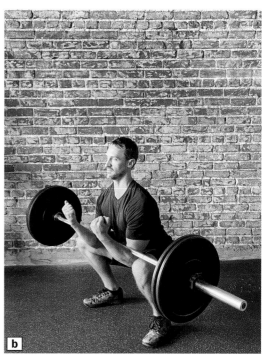

ADVANTAGES

- This variation works more upper back muscles than the back squat, as well as the biceps.
- It works well for people who lack the wrist mobility that's necessary for a front squat.
- The Zercher barbell position can be used for a wide variety of exercises including the split squat and lunge variations.

COACHING CUES

- For most lifters, the goal is to lower until the elbows touch the tops of the thighs.
- Keep your chest held high, knees wide, and shoulder blades pulled together.
- A power rack with the pins set at an appropriate height is necessary to prevent low back strain while removing the barbell after each set.

Jump Squat

The jump squat can be an excellent exercise to build explosive power. The key is to use an external load held down at arm's length or against the chest, which is easier on the shoulders and safer than holding a barbell across the upper back.

❍ HOW TO DO IT

1. Stand with your feet wider than shoulder width while holding a trap bar or a dumbbell in each hand.
2. Perform a quarter squat while keeping the knees over the feet (see figure a).
3. Perform the jump by explosively extending the hip and knee joints as you drive through the center of your feet (see figure b).
4. Land as softly as possible without your knees buckling inward, mimicking the starting position.
5. Repeat the smooth, continuous motion for reps.

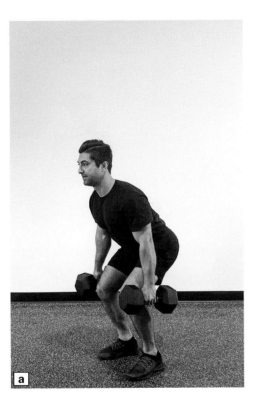
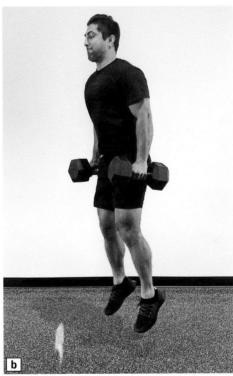

ADVANTAGES

- The jump squat increases explosive power of the lower body.
- It develops deceleration strength during the landing.

COACHING CUES

- The landing should be as soft and quiet as possible.
- Holding a single dumbbell or kettlebell in the goblet position can be a good option for some lifters.
- The transition between the landing and jump should be as fast as possible.
- Wear a weighted vest to increase the load if holding a weight in front isn't an option.

Belt Squat

The belt squat is one of the most underrated squat variations. This terrific exercise allows you to strengthen and build your thighs and glutes while sparing your low back. It is an excellent movement to train with a high frequency or during low back rehabilitation.

HOW TO DO IT

1. Place a kettlebell or plates on a bench in front of you. Loop the chain of a chin/ dip belt through the weight and then attach the clip to your belt. Step back so the weight is hanging freely from the belt (see figure a). Stand with your feet wider than shoulder width and angled out slightly to the most comfortable position.

2. Hold your arms straight out in front of you, push your hips back, and then bend your knees, lowering yourself as far as possible or until the weight touches the floor (see figure b).

3. Push back to the starting position and complete all reps.

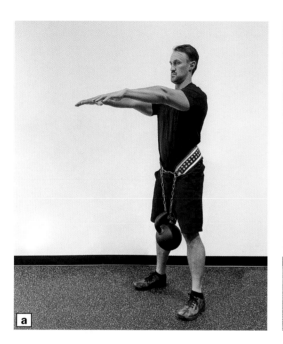

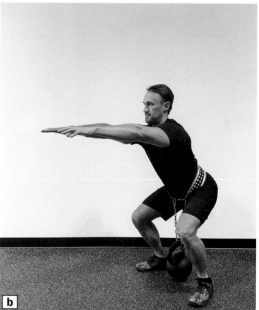

ADVANTAGES

- This squat variation spares the lower back while building the thighs and glutes.
- It can be performed with a high frequency.

COACHING CUES

- Standing with both feet on a short step or box is great for increasing the range of motion.
- Some lifters prefer to perform this exercise as a partial movement from the bottom position to halfway and then back down to keep tension on the quadriceps.
- To progress this exercise, place two short steps or boxes on the floor to stand on to increase your range of motion (see figure c).

One-Leg Squat

You will see many versions of a one-leg squat online that require more mobility and balance than most people will ever have. Those versions might make for good entertainment, but they're impractical from a programming standpoint. The primary problem with a true one-leg squat is the difficulty maintaining a neutral pelvis. Once that neutral position is lost, it can lead to low back, hip, or knee pain. That is why a staggered stance is recommended—it helps maintain a neutral pelvis while providing just enough balance support to keep the exercise from turning into a circus act. Using a bench when performing this exercise allows you to sit back without losing your balance, and the dead spot position is effective for building starting strength. You hold a weight against your chest to provide a counterbalance, making this variation a viable option for many lifters.

○ HOW TO DO IT

1. Start by sitting on a box or bench, knees bent to 90 degrees and feet about four inches (10 cm) apart. Move your right heel forward around 12 inches (30 cm) and rest it lightly on the floor. Hold a weight against your chest, with your elbows tucked to the sides (see figure a).
2. Shift your torso forward and push through the center of your left foot to elevate your body without increasing the pressure through your right heel (see figure b).
3. Slowly lower back to the starting position.
4. Perform all reps on one leg before switching to the other.

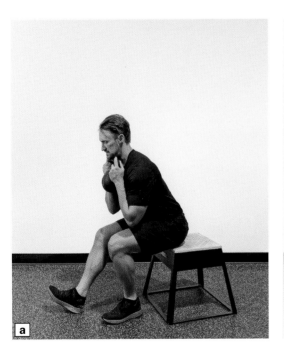
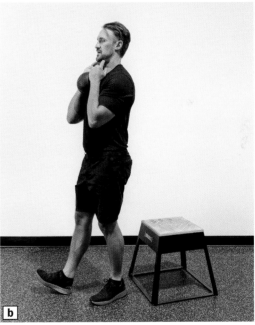

ADVANTAGE

This squat variation increases one-leg strength without requiring extreme mobility of the hips and ankles.

(continued)

One-Leg Squat *(continued)*

COACHING CUES

- Start with a relatively high box or bench if you've never done the exercise before.

- When you can do multiple reps with good form, lowering your body to the box while maintaining a neutral pelvis, you can progress to a lower box or bench.

- The ultimate goal is to increase your strength and stability to the point where you begin the exercise while standing and then lower yourself without resting on the box (see figure c).

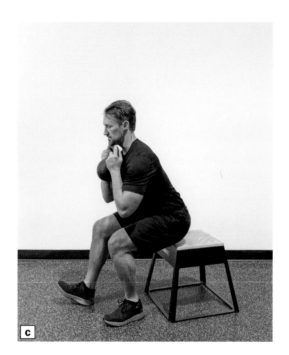

SPLIT SQUAT VARIATIONS

Although the squat puts you in the strongest possible position for lifting, few human movements take place with your feet parallel to each other. Walking, climbing, throwing, and striking all require a split stance. So even though the split squat works the same muscles, it works them in a slightly less stable and predictable posture, one that comes closer to the context in which they'll be used.

MUSCLES WORKED:

quadriceps

glutes

hamstrings

hip adductors

stabilizing muscles of the core and hips

calves

Split Squat

The standard split squat (also known as a stationary lunge) is an excellent squat variation that unloads the spine and emphasizes the quadriceps. It is also useful for developing the vastus medialis, the teardrop muscle on the inner (i.e., medial) side of your knee joint.

HOW TO DO IT

1. Hold a weight in each hand at arm's length. Stand in a split position, with your weight distributed evenly between your front foot and the toes of your trailing leg (see figure a).
2. Bend your knees and lower your body until your rear knee is at or near the floor (see figure b).
3. Push back to the starting position for recommended reps, and then repeat with your opposite leg in front.

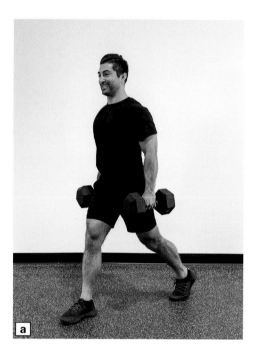 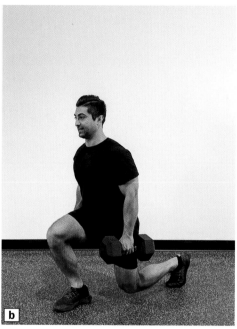

ADVANTAGE

The split squat develops strength and size of the glutes and thighs with minimal stress on the lumbar spine.

COACHING CUE

There's no perfect form for every lifter. The front knee of a person with short femurs may extend a little past the toes, while the knee of someone with long legs may stay well behind, with the shin perpendicular to the floor. Either can be right for that person, as long as the knee and toes remain aligned.

Bulgarian Split Squat

The Bulgarian split squat (also known as a rear-foot-elevated split squat, or RFESS) is a progression from the standard split squat. In this version, your rear foot is elevated, which requires the front leg to work harder during each repetition. An added benefit is that it puts the quadriceps of the elevated leg in a stretch position to increase hip mobility.

HOW TO DO IT

1. Hold a weight in each hand at arm's length, and set the toes or instep of one foot on a bench, box, or step (see figure a).
2. Lower yourself until your front thigh is more or less parallel to the floor (see figure b).
3. Push back up to the starting position for recommended reps, and then repeat with your opposite leg in front.

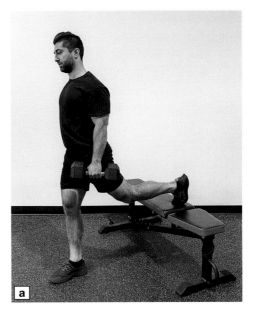

ADVANTAGES

- This variation focuses work on the quadriceps of the forward leg, making it a potent muscle-building exercise.
- It increases flexibility of the hip flexors of the leg that's elevated.

COACHING CUE

The higher the box, the more the lifter will tend to lean forward at the hips, usually in alignment with the thigh of the trailing leg. As with split squats, that leg–torso angle will be more vertical with taller athletes and more diagonal with those who have shorter legs. This means your posture might be different from your training partner's, and that's okay.

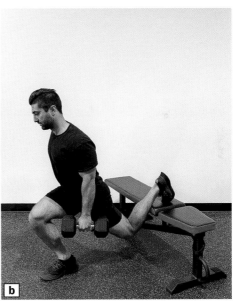

PROGRESSIONS

- Inexperienced lifters: Start with a low step, six to eight inches (15-20 cm), and look to get a full range of motion using body weight only before adding load.
- More advanced lifters: Progress to a higher box or bench. As you do, make sure to rest the instep of the trailing leg on the box rather than the toes.
- To add balance and stability challenges, rest the toes of the trailing leg on a medicine ball, or set the foot of the trailing leg in the loop of a suspension trainer.

Split Jump Squat

This is the most advanced version of the split squat. It requires plenty of strength and power to elevate your body high enough to switch your legs midair and land with the opposite leg forward. The landing phase is especially beneficial to athletes who need to decelerate from a high velocity. For many people, no additional load is required for this exercise.

▶ HOW TO DO IT

1. Stand in a split position, with your weight distributed evenly between your front foot and the toes of your trailing leg. Hold a weight in each hand down at arm's length, or place your hands on your hips.
2. Bend your knees and lower your body until your rear knee is at or near the floor (see figure a). 3. Explosively push through both legs to elevate your feet off the ground, and switch your legs midair (see figure b).
3. Land with your opposite leg in front (see figure c). Each landing counts as one rep (i.e., 10 total reps requires 5 reps with each leg forward).

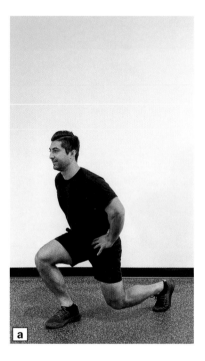
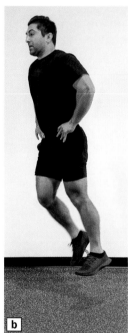
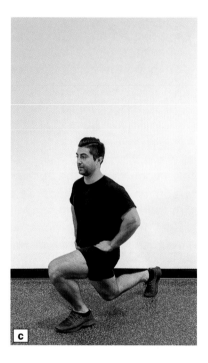

ADVANTAGES

- The split jump squat increases explosive power of the lower body.
- It develops deceleration strength during the landing.

COACHING CUE

If you're strong enough to perform this exercise while holding weights, the key is to use a load that's light enough to get maximum elevation.

LUNGE VARIATIONS

The lunge seems like a simple progression from the split squat, but for some inexperienced lifters, that long step forward or back will be a surprising challenge. You're not only taking a longer step than you normally would but also repeating the movement with identical form. More experienced and better coordinated athletes can use a variety of loading and programming options to challenge strength, balance, stability, and conditioning.

MUSCLES WORKED:

quadriceps

glutes

hamstrings

hip adductors

stabilizing muscles of the core, hips, and ankles

calves

Reverse Lunge

The reverse lunge is a fundamental strength exercise that allows you to use plenty of load. Compared with a forward lunge, a reverse lunge is a much more stable movement because the front leg is always on the ground. There are two primary ways to load the reverse lunge. You can hold a weight on the same side of the leg that's stepping back. This offset load increases activation of the vastus lateralis, gluteus medius, and lateral trunk. The other option is to hold a weight in each hand, which works well for strong lifters who need more load than one weight can provide.

HOW TO DO IT

1. Stand with your feet together while holding a weight in your left hand hanging down at arm's length (see figure a).
2. Take a long step back with your left leg, plant the toes of your trailing leg, and lower your body until your rear knee is at or near the floor (see figure b).
3. Step back to the starting position.
4. Perform all your reps with one leg, and then switch the weight to your right hand and repeat the reps while stepping back with your right leg.

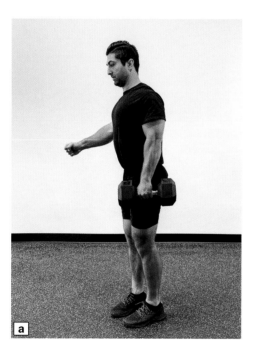
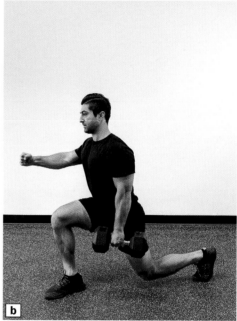

ADVANTAGES

- The reverse lunge is usually a safe option for lifters with a history of knee pain since the shin can remain vertical throughout the movement.
- A large load can be used because it's a more stable movement than a forward lunge.

COACHING CUES

- Avoid any inward buckling of the knee.
- Drive through the heel of the forward leg to increase gluteal activation.

Deficit Reverse Lunge

The deficit reverse lunge is a terrific progression from the standard reverse lunge. Stepping back from a four- to six-inch (10-15 cm) elevation requires a deeper lunge, which increases activation of the glutes, hamstrings, and vastus medialis (i.e., teardrop muscle). The deficit is also an effective progression when a heavier load isn't available.

HOW TO DO IT

1. Stand on a four- to six-inch (10-15 cm) step or short box with your feet together while holding a weight in your left hand hanging down at arm's length (see figure a).
2. Take a long step back with your left leg, plant the toes of your trailing leg, and lower your body until your rear knee is at or near the floor (see figure b).
3. Step back to the starting position.
4. Perform all your reps with one leg, and then switch the weight to your right hand and repeat the set while stepping back with your right leg.

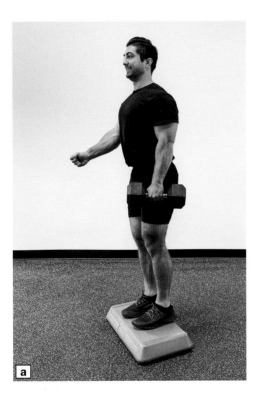
a

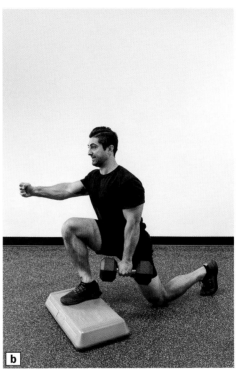
b

ADVANTAGES

- This variation increases activation of the hamstrings, glutes, and vastus medialis.
- It puts a greater stretch on the quadriceps, hip extensors, and adductors.

COACHING CUES

- Avoid any lateral flexion of the trunk.
- Drive through the heel of the forward leg to increase gluteal activation.

Forward Lunge

The forward lunge starts by taking a big step forward with one leg and planting it on the ground before lowering into a deep stretch position. In other words, a forward lunge is essentially a controlled fall, which makes it a more challenging variation. It also places a large emphasis on the quadriceps, making it a great thigh builder for some or potentially aggravating the knee joint for others. As in the reverse lunge, you can perform this exercise with an offset load or with a weight in each hand.

HOW TO DO IT

1. Stand with your feet together while holding a weight in your left hand hanging down at arm's length (see figure a).
2. Take a long step forward with your right leg, and lower your body until your rear knee is at or near the floor (see figure b).
3. Push yourself back to the starting position through the middle of your front foot.
4. Perform all your reps with one leg, and then switch the weight to your right hand and repeat the reps while stepping forward with your left leg.

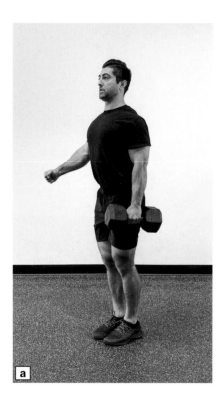
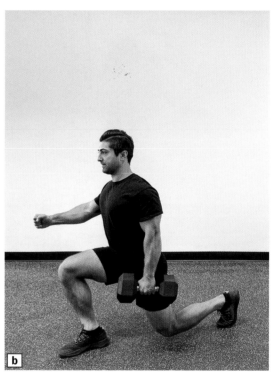

ADVANTAGES

- The forward lunge increases activation of the vastus medialis.
- It increases deceleration strength.

COACHING CUE

You have probably been told that the front knee should never go past the toes. But it's never that simple. You may do well with the knee well past the toes, while someone else will experience knee discomfort with a relatively vertical shin.

Step-Through Lunge

The step-through lunge combines a reverse and forward lunge into one movement. This challenging variation is great for people who want to emphasize the hips and quadriceps at the same time. The large step that's required from the reverse to forward lunge position requires significant balance and stability.

▶ HOW TO DO IT

1. Stand with your feet together while holding a weight in the rack position, arm bent and elbow tucked to your side, in your left hand. Take a long step back with your left leg, and lower your body until your rear knee is at or near the floor (see figure a).
2. Push yourself out of the reverse lunge, moving your left leg forward in the air without touching the floor (see figure b).
3. Continue moving your left leg forward, and plant the foot in front of you in the forward lunge position (see figure c).
4. Push through the middle of your left foot, and return your leg back to the reverse lunge position.
5. Perform all your reps with one leg, and then switch the weight to your right hand and repeat the reps while stepping back and forward with your right leg.

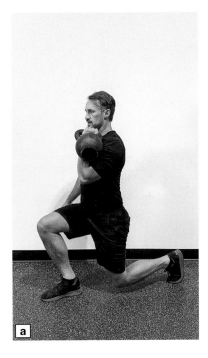
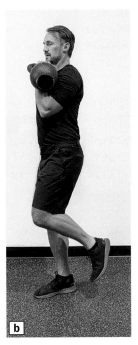
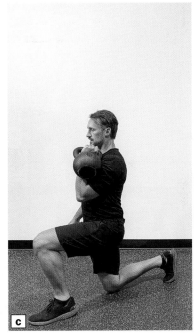

a   b   c

ADVANTAGES

- This variation combines a reverse and forward lunge into one movement.
- It increases deceleration strength.

COACHING CUES

- Start slow with this exercise since it requires a very large step-through. Use the same load you would for a forward lunge.
- For some, it's easier to learn the movement by holding a weight in each hand instead of an offset load as described.

Lateral Lunge

Most lifters train their legs by standing up and down or stepping forward and backward with weight. That misses the lateral movement pattern, which is necessary for all aspects of life and sport. The lateral lunge should be part of any resistance training program because it emphasizes the adductors and increases hip mobility.

▶ HOW TO DO IT

1. Stand with your feet hip-width apart while holding the handle of a kettlebell with both hands in front of you down at arm's length (see figure a).
2. Take a long step to the right with your right leg and plant your foot so it's angled slightly outward, and then lower your body as far as your mobility allows while your trunk shifts forward (see figure b).
3. Push yourself back to the starting position through the middle of your front foot.
4. Perform all your reps by stepping to the right with your right leg, then perform the same number of reps by stepping out to the left with your left leg.

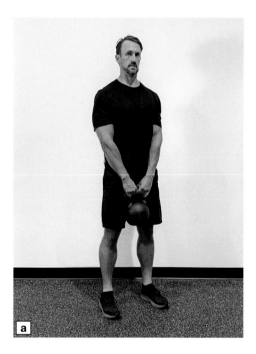
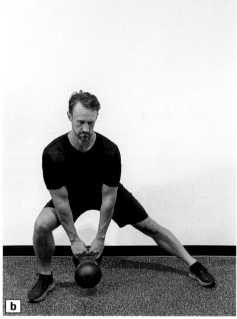

ADVANTAGES

- The lateral lunge emphasizes the hip adductors.
- It increases hip mobility.

COACHING CUES

- How much the foot angles outward for the working leg depends on the genetic structure of the hip. Use the foot position that feels most natural.
- Focus on pushing your hips back, and avoid inward buckling of the working knee during the lowering phase.
- You can also perform this exercise by holding one end of a dumbbell vertically.

STEP-UP VARIATIONS

The step-up is among the most underrated exercises for athletes at all levels. For more advanced athletes working with heavier loads, it produces greater glute activation than squats, and with increasing step height, it can lead to dramatic lower body muscle development. For those recovering from an injury, a low step can help restore balance, strength, and stability.

MUSCLES WORKED:

quadriceps

glutes

hamstrings

hip adductors

stabilizing muscles of the core, hips, and ankles

calves

Step-Up

The step-up allows for a wide range of loading depending on the height of the box. Since the exercise virtually eliminates the eccentric phase, it can be performed with a high frequency because it causes minimal muscle soreness.

HOW TO DO IT

1. Stand with your left foot flat on a box or step and your right foot on the floor behind it while holding a weight down at your side in your right hand (see figure a).
2. Push through the heel of the left foot to lift yourself up until it is straight and the foot of the trailing leg is alongside of it (see figure b).
3. Without putting any weight on the trailing leg, lower it back to the floor.
4. Perform all your reps, then switch sides and repeat the set.

ADVANTAGES

- The step-up strengthens and builds the thighs and glutes with minimal eccentric stress or low back strain.
- It is an excellent option for tall people or those with long legs who can't perform a full squat with proper form.

COACHING CUES

- Do not push off with the toes of the trailing leg. The forward leg should do all the work.
- A lower step—6 to 12 inches (15-30 cm)—is plenty for shorter, heavier, or less experienced people. Younger, taller, and better trained athletes can start with 18 inches (45 cm) and work up to 24 inches (60 cm).
- You can increase step height or increase load, but it rarely makes sense to do both at the same time.
- The loading options are the same as for the reverse lunge, although for strength and muscle development in the most advanced athletes, holding a dumbbell or kettlebell in each hand is often the best choice.

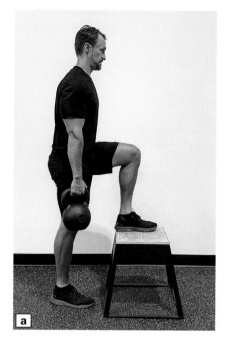

a

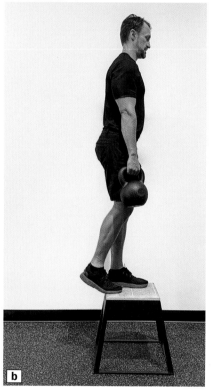

b

Lateral Step-Up

The lateral step-up emphasizes the adductors, which are important muscles to strengthen for a wide array of athletes. That advantage also works in your favor to build the overall size of your thighs.

HOW TO DO IT

1. Stand with one foot flat on a box or step and the other foot on the floor out at an angle (see figure a). Start with no additional weight, or hold a weight in the goblet position.
2. Push through the heel of the top leg to lift yourself up until the leg is straight and the foot of the trailing leg rests on the step (see figure b).
3. Lower the trailing leg back to the floor under control.
4. Perform all your reps, then switch sides and repeat the set.

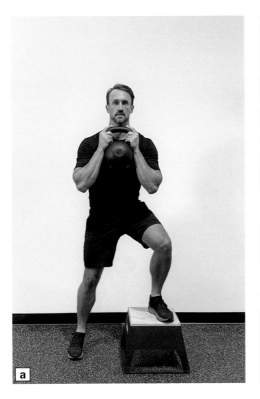 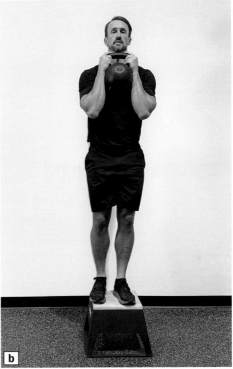

ADVANTAGES

- This exercise is a good choice for developing lateral hip stability in athletes who move laterally in their sport, which is most of them.
- The eccentric portion of the lateral step-up resembles the one-leg squat.

COACHING CUES

- Heavier or less experienced athletes should start with a very low step—four to six inches (10-15 cm).
- Use a higher step if you need it—up to 12 inches (30 cm) if you are tall—but you don't need to go up from there. Progress the movement with load or rep speed.

DEADLIFT VARIATIONS

You won't find a better exercise for building strength and mass in the extensor chain. The deadlift helps young athletes become better athletes and power athletes become more powerful. Moreover, the variations give you many ways to get stronger without increasing the risk of injury.

I recommend the double-overhand grip for deadlifts. Some athletes prefer the mixed grip, usually because it allows them to train with the heaviest possible loads. They're right about the effect of a mixed grip; that's why competitive powerlifters use it. But for strength and conditioning, when the goal is to develop a range of qualities that translate to better performance, the mixed grip has two major drawbacks. First, there's the risk of muscle imbalances. Over time, the shoulder on the overhand side can lose some of its ability to externally rotate, while the forearm on that side can lose range of motion in supination. Second, the biceps on the underhand side absorbs excessive stress due to the near-maximal loads typically lifted with a mixed grip. And of course that stress is uneven, since the biceps on the overhand side isn't challenged in the same way. That's why I recommend using the double-overhand grip 100 percent of the time.

MUSCLES WORKED:

glutes

hamstrings

quadriceps

extensors of the lower and middle back

latissimus dorsi

trapezius

stabilizing muscles of the core and hips

biceps

gripping muscles of the forearms

Deadlift

The barbell deadlift is another fundamental exercise that can work well for virtually anyone. The key is to not limit yourself to pulling from the floor. The exercise is just as effective when the barbell is elevated, say, four or six inches (10-15 cm) higher. This is necessary for taller athletes or people who have low back or mobility deficits. So even though the exercise is shown from the floor, you can elevate the starting position to whatever height is necessary to maintain a neutral spine at the beginning of the pull. Finally, always lower the deadlift relatively quickly, but under control, to avoid unnecessary stress on your discs.

▶ HOW TO DO IT

1. Load the bar and roll it against your shins. Set your feet about shoulder-width apart, toes straight or angled out slightly, and grab the bar overhand, with your arms just outside your legs. Push your hips back, push your chest out, and tighten everything from your hands to your feet (see figure a).

2. Thrust your hips forward and pull the bar straight up the front of your legs until your ankles, knees, and hips are fully extended (see figure b).

3. Pause, lower the bar to the floor along the same path relatively quickly, reset your grip, and repeat.

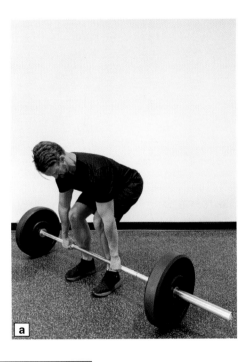
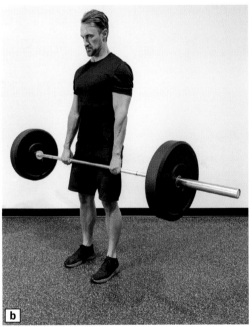

ADVANTAGES

- The deadlift has functional carryover to all aspects of life and sport.
- Most people can perform a deadlift, especially with the load in an elevated position.

(continued)

Deadlift   *(continued)*

COACHING CUES

- You can make the deadlift even more effective by trying to "bend the bar," which activates your lats and helps support your lumbar spine. But if for any reason you need to use a mixed grip, switch hand positions with each set. Pay special attention to which one you use on your heaviest sets, making sure the maximum stress doesn't always fall on the same side.

- As with the squat, the weight should always be over the center of the foot, never out in front of it. There should be a straight line from the shoulders to the barbell to the middle of the foot.

- To get proper alignment of the neck and torso, maintain a neutral head position, meaning your eyes face the same direction as your chest. Do not elevate or lower your chin. At the same time, you want to keep your chest up, with tension in the upper back muscles.

- Form will vary from person to person, with sometimes extreme differences in knee and hip angles. But everyone should keep the lower back in its natural arch.

- Avoid hyperextending the back to complete the movement. It's completely unnecessary and puts the lumbar spine at risk.

- Even with ideal form, not every lifter should pull weights from the floor. If you don't yet have the hip mobility or core stability for a traditional deadlift, pull from an elevated surface, such as short boxes or thick weights (see figure c).

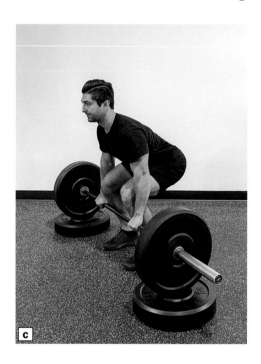

c

Sumo Deadlift

The sumo deadlift uses a much wider stance than a traditional deadlift. This makes it a better option for taller lifters or those who feel more comfortable pulling a deadlift with a more upright torso. The wide stance puts a greater emphasis on the hip adductors, which is beneficial to many athletes.

HOW TO DO IT

1. Load the bar and roll it against your shins. Set your feet beyond shoulder-width apart, toes angled out about 45 degrees, and grab the bar overhand, with your arms just inside your legs. Push your hips back, push your chest out, and tighten everything from your hands to your feet (see figure a).

2. Thrust your hips forward and pull the bar straight up the front of your legs until your ankles, knees, and hips are fully extended (see figure b).

3. Pause, lower the bar to the floor along the same path relatively quickly, reset your grip, and repeat.

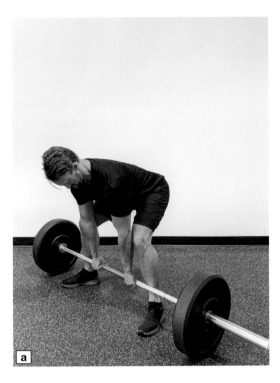
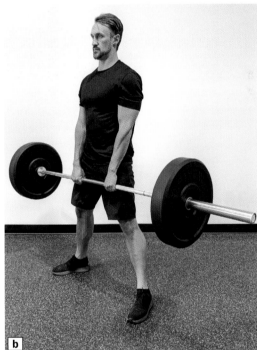

ADVANTAGES

- The wide stance and upright posture are generally more appropriate for lifters with longer legs or shorter arms.
- The wider leg position shifts some of the work to the adductors.

COACHING CUE

Since the legs are wide, it's common for people to let their knees buckle inward (i.e., knee valgus) as they lift the load. To counteract this, pull your knees outward during this exercise.

Trap Bar Deadlift

The trap bar deadlift (also known as the hex bar deadlift) is another excellent option for taller lifters. And the handles allow for a neutral grip, which spares the shoulders for many people. Since the trap bar centers the load more than a barbell, it works well to increase the size and strength of the quadriceps.

HOW TO DO IT

1. Load the bar and stand in the middle. Set your feet somewhere between hip- and shoulder-width apart, toes forward. Grab the handles with your arms just outside your legs. Push your hips back, push your chest out, and tighten everything from your hands to your feet (see figure a).
2. Thrust your hips forward and pull the bar straight up from the floor until your ankles, knees, and hips are fully extended (see figure b).
3. Pause, quickly lower the bar to the floor along the same path, reset your grip, and repeat.

ADVANTAGES

- For many lifters, this is the most back-friendly deadlift option, since the load is always at the center of gravity.
- The high handles are also a boon for athletes who aren't good candidates to pull from the low bar position.
- The trap bar takes some work from the posterior chain (especially the middle and lower back) and moves it to the quadriceps, making this variation a squat–deadlift hybrid.

COACHING CUE

Lifters often stop short of full hip extension during this exercise, so maximally squeeze the glutes when standing tall to avoid that shortcoming.

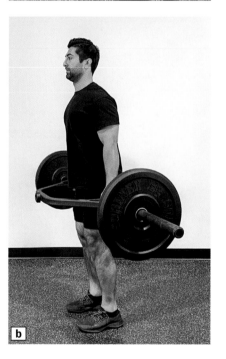

Romanian Deadlift (RDL)

The Romanian deadlift (RDL) is essentially a partial deadlift that starts from the lock-out position. The lifter lowers the weight to around knee level before returning it to the starting position, making it a viable option for virtually anyone, especially tall athletes with mobility deficits. The only potential disadvantage is that you need a power rack to start the exercise. This is one of the deadlift variations where you need to lower the weight relatively slowly to avoid low back strain because a quick drop is very risky to the discs. Dumbbells are just as effective as a barbell, and often preferable to many.

HOW TO DO IT

1. Place two heavy dumbbells on a bench in front of you. Grab them and step back from the bench, with the dumbbells against your thighs, and set your feet between hip- and shoulder-width apart, feet straight ahead (see figure a).
2. Brace your core, and then push your hips back, lowering the dumbbells until they're just below your knees while maintaining a neutral spine (see figure b).
3. Push your hips back to the starting position and repeat.

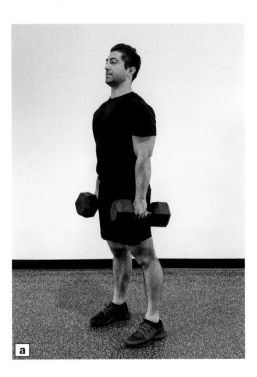
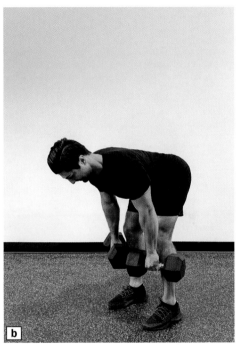

ADVANTAGES

- This eliminates the range of motion in the lower half, which can be the highest risk phase for people with a history of low back pain or poor mobility.
- It is an excellent way to teach the hip hinge.

COACHING CUE

Younger athletes, especially females, will try to lower the weight far below their knees. If you find yourself doing this, slow the movement down and focus on the quality of hip extension rather than range of motion.

Staggered-Stance Romanian Deadlift

The staggered-stance RDL is a terrific exercise for two primary reasons. First, it minimizes stress on the low back. Second, it provides a bridge between a two- and one-leg RDL. This is one of the most underrated deadlift variations, given how many people can perform it without low back strain.

▶ HOW TO DO IT

1. Place two heavy dumbbells on a bench in front of you. Grab them and step back from the bench, with the dumbbells against your thighs, and set your feet hip-width apart, toes straight ahead. Rest the ball of your left foot approximately 12 inches (30 cm) behind you (see figure a).
2. Brace your core, and then push your hips back, lowering the dumbbells until they're just below your knees while maintaining a neutral spine (see figure b).
3. Push your hips back to the starting position, and repeat for all reps with the right leg.
4. Switch your stance so your left leg is performing the work while the ball of the right foot rests on the floor.

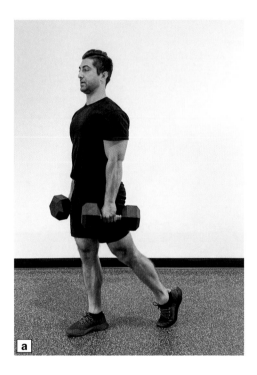
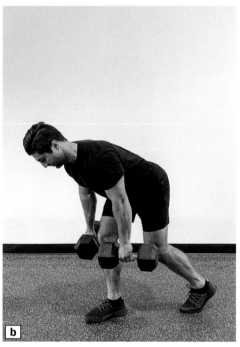

ADVANTAGES

- This variation drastically reduces strain throughout the low back.
- It provides a bridge between the two- and one-leg deadlift.

COACHING CUE

All of the tension should be felt through the front leg and hip. The leg that's slightly bent should have no pressure going through the foot—it's only there to provide minimal balance support.

One-Leg Romanian Deadlift

The one-leg RDL can be performed with a range of loading options. You can hold a weight in each hand, as we're about to cover, or you can use a barbell. Some people like to hold a single weight on the opposite side of the working leg. Choose whichever option works best for your balance and available equipment.

HOW TO DO IT

1. Grab two dumbbells or kettlebells and hold them at your sides as you stand with your knees close together and your left foot slightly off the ground (see figure a).

2. Hinge at the hips as you extend your left leg behind you, lowering the weights toward the floor (see figure b). Pause with your neck, torso, and left leg aligned and your right knee bent slightly. 3. Squeeze your right glutes to pull your body back to the starting position.

3. Do all your reps, switch sides, and repeat the set.

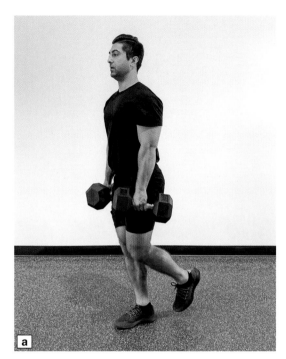
a

ADVANTAGE

This variation builds one-leg strength, which is necessary for a wide range of athletes and nonathletes alike.

COACHING CUES

- Young, inexperienced lifters will absolutely butcher this exercise if they don't move slowly. Work on form first, load later.

- Most lifters will need some practice to reach a full range of motion. No matter your range of motion, maintain one-leg balance with the leg and torso aligned.

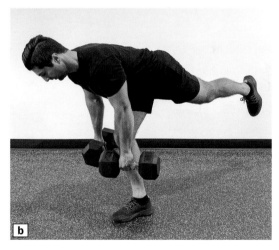
b

POSTERIOR CHAIN VARIATIONS

In this section we cover some effective exercises that don't perfectly fall within a squat or deadlift variation. These exercises emphasize all, or part of, the posterior chain. Some target the entire posterior chain, such as the swing, while others emphasize the glutes or hamstrings.

Kettlebell Swing

The kettlebell swing, popularized by Pavel Tsatsouline, builds explosive power and muscle throughout the entire posterior chain. The key is to start with a relatively light load and maintain perfect form with every repetition throughout this dynamic exercise.

❯ HOW TO DO IT

1. Stand with your feet wider than shoulder width, with a kettlebell resting on the ground about a foot (30 cm) in front of you. Push your hips back, keep your knees directly above your feet, and then reach forward to grab the kettlebell with both hands while maintaining a neutral spine (see figure a). This is only the starting position and is not repeated throughout the subsequent reps.

2. To initiate the swing, explosively pull the kettlebell so it swings back between your legs (see figure b).

3. Explosively thrust your hips forward as you stand, driving through the center of your feet, using minimal assistance from your arms to elevate the kettlebell. Swing the kettlebell up until it's around chest height (see figure c). Your body should be perfectly vertical at the end of the motion.

4. Reverse the motion, and continue for the desired number of reps. To end the set, perform a hip hinge and lower the kettlebell straight down to the floor.

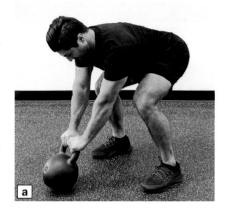

a

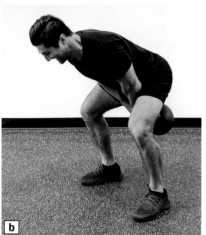

b

ADVANTAGE

The swing encourages high-velocity hip extension, which builds explosive power of the posterior chain.

COACHING CUES

- Maintain a neutral spine throughout the exercise by moving within a range that suits your mobility.
- The arms provide minimal assistance for the swing; the majority of the elevation should come from a powerful hip extension.
- The shoulders should remain down throughout the movement; avoid shrugging.
- The heels should remain on the ground throughout the movement. Drive through your heels to keep them on the ground.
- The most common mistake is leaning the trunk backward as the kettlebell reaches its highest position; your trunk should be perpendicular to the ground at the peak of the swing.

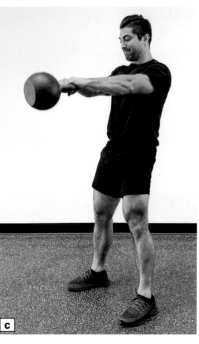

c

Alternating Kettlebell Swing

For this version of the swing, you'll alternate which hand is gripping the kettlebell during each repetition. Switching hands helps develop coordination while activating the core's anti-rotation muscles that protect the lumbar spine.

HOW TO DO IT

1. Stand with your feet wider than shoulder width, with a kettlebell resting on the ground about a foot (30 cm) in front of you. Push your hips back, keep your knees directly above your feet, and then reach forward to grab the kettlebell with the right hand while maintaining a neutral spine.

2. To initiate the swing, push your hips back and let the kettlebell swing in between your legs (see figure a).

3. Explosively thrust your hips forward as you stand, driving through the center of your feet, using minimal assistance from your right arm to elevate the kettlebell. Swing the kettlebell up until it's around chest height, then release it with your right hand as you reach your left hand to catch the handle (see figure b).

4. After catching the kettlebell, your right arm drops to the side of your body and your left arm swings back between your legs (see figure c).

5. During the next ascending phase of the kettlebell, switch from your left hand back to your right. Continue for the desired number of reps.

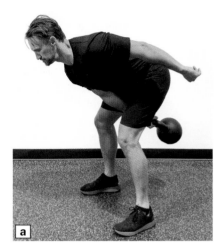

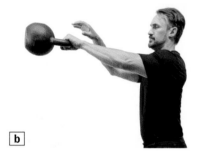

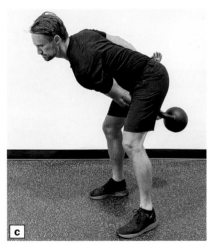

ADVANTAGES

- Alternating the arms develops greater motor and eye–hand coordination than a two-arm swing.
- It requires greater activation of the anti-rotation trunk muscles.

COACHING CUES

- Start with a very light kettlebell, and consider switching hands at a position lower than the chest if you're new to the exercise.
- Limit any rotation of the trunk at the bottom of the swing as much as possible.

Hip Thrust

The hip thrust, popularized by Bret Contreras, is a great way to build size and strength of the glutes and hip extensors with minimal strain to the low back. You can perform the exercise with your upper back resting on a bench if one is available. If not, you can perform it with your upper back resting on the floor.

▶ HOW TO DO IT

1. Place a thick, wide pad around the center of a barbell. Sit on the ground with your legs straight under the barbell, upper back resting against a flat bench. Roll the barbell toward your torso until it's resting above the upper portion of your pelvis, and then bend your knees to 90 degrees with your feet shoulder-width apart. Lift your hips slightly to elevate your glutes off the ground (see figure a).
2. Push through your heels and extend your hips until they reach full lockout while keeping your chin tucked (see figure b).
3. Slowly reverse the motion and repeat.

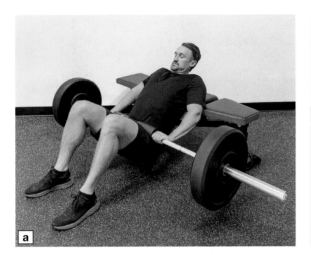
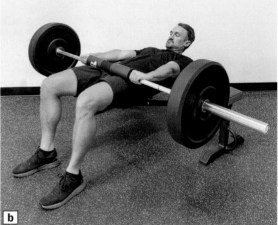

ADVANTAGE

The hip thrust lets you use a heavy load to train the hip extensors without the low back strain of a deadlift or squat.

COACHING CUES

- Use a load that allows full hip extension, where maximum glute activation occurs.
- Keep the chin tucked throughout the movement and the eyes focused on the hips to increase neural drive.

Staggered-Stance Hip Thrust

The staggered-stance hip thrust is a progression that emphasizes one hip at a time. This version provides two benefits. First, since one hip is performing most of the work, you don't have to use as much load as you do with the standard hip thrust. Second, this variation helps build single-leg strength, which is important for any sport.

▶ HOW TO DO IT

1. Place a thick, wide pad around the center of a barbell. Sit on the ground with your legs straight under the barbell, upper back resting against a flat bench. Roll the barbell toward your torso until it's resting above the upper portion of your pelvis, and then bend your knees to 90 degrees with your feet about four inches (10 cm) apart. Lift your hips slightly to elevate your glutes off the ground.
2. Rest the heel of your left foot approximately six inches (15 cm) forward (see figure a).
3. Push through your right heel and extend your hips until they reach full lockout while keeping your chin tucked (see figure b).
4. Slowly reverse the motion and repeat. Perform the recommended reps, then switch your stance so your left hip is doing the work.

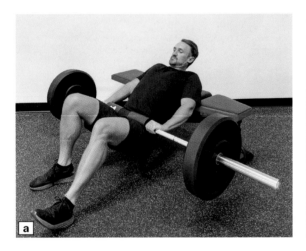
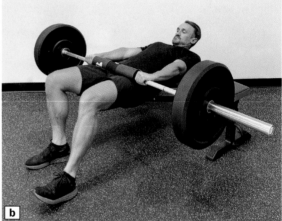

ADVANTAGE

This variation helps increase single-leg strength.

COACHING CUES

- Use a load that allows full hip extension, where maximum glute activation occurs.
- Keep the chin tucked throughout the movement and the eyes focused on the hips to increase neural drive.
- The most common mistake is a hip drop on one side. Your pelvis should remain parallel to the floor throughout the movement.
- The working leg should perform virtually all the work. The resting heel merely provides balance support and should not contribute to hip extension.

Slider Leg Curl

The leg curl is a common exercise in bodybuilding circles that is typically performed while seated on a machine. Here is a version you can perform with sliders, popularized by celebrity trainer Valerie Waters. This exercise helps strengthen and build the hamstrings during knee flexion, instead of their other function, hip extension. Training for both hip extension and knee flexion results in complete development of the muscle group.

◉ HOW TO DO IT

1. For this exercise you'll need a slick ground surface such as a hard floor or slide board. Lie on your back with each heel resting on a slider, heels hip-width apart, arms crossed at your chest or flat on the ground (see figure a).
2. Pull your heels toward your glutes as you simultaneously lift your hips (see figure b).
3. Slowly reverse the motion, focusing on the eccentric phase, and repeat.

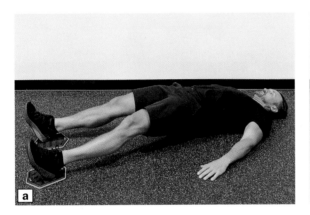
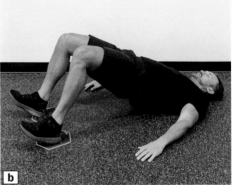

ADVANTAGES

- This version of the leg curl builds hamstring and glute strength while sparing the low back.
- It builds eccentric strength of the hamstrings, which can reduce the risk of a knee injury.

COACHING CUES

- If you get a cramp in your hamstrings, slow the tempo and temporarily shorten the range of motion.
- Go for a full stretch of the hamstrings at end range of motion.

Slider One-Leg Curl

Once the standard leg curl becomes easy, you can progress to the one-leg curl. This variation requires considerably more strength and stabilization throughout the core, hips, and pelvis. The one-leg curl challenges even the strongest athletes.

⦿ HOW TO DO IT

1. Lie on your back with your left heel resting on a slider, right leg held off the ground, and hips slightly elevated (see figure a).
2. Pull your left heel toward your left glutes as you simultaneously lift your hips higher (see figure b).
3. Slowly reverse the motion, focusing on the eccentric phase, and repeat for the desired reps before switching legs.

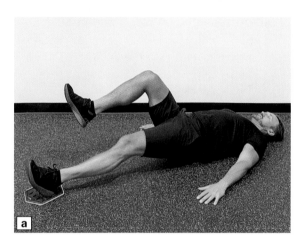
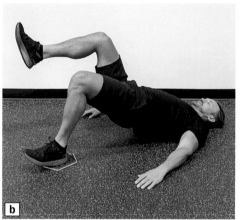

ADVANTAGE

The one-leg curl requires greater activation of stabilizers throughout the trunk and hips compared with the two-leg version.

COACHING CUES

- Maintain a level pelvis during the motion.
- If necessary, perform repetitions through a partial range of motion in the early stages.

Standing Fire Hydrant

The glutes perform three actions at the hip: extension, abduction and external rotation. Hip extension is the action trained by lunges, deadlifts, step-ups, etc. However, hip abduction and external rotation are two actions missed by those traditional lower body exercises. Therefore, the standing fire hydrant is an excellent addition to any program to develop the size and strength of the gluteal fibers that perform abduction and external rotation. Since the glutes are notorious for being difficult to activate, this exercise is performed as an isometric hold, instead of repetitions, to increase your mind muscle connection.

▶ HOW TO DO IT

1. Place a miniband just above your knees and stand with your feet together.
2. Place your hands on your hips, push your hips back, bend your knees slightly, and shift your trunk forward to around 60 degrees. Lift your left foot off the ground and then abduct and externally rotate your left hip as far as your mobility allows.
3. Hold the position for 30 seconds, then switch sides so you're standing on your left leg with your right leg elevated.

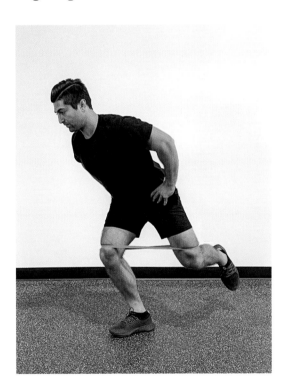

ADVANTAGE

Increases size and strength of the gluteal fibers that perform hip abduction and external rotation.

COACHING CUES

- Maintain a level, unrotated pelvis during the hold.
- Pull the knee of the stance leg outward to increase activation of the glutes (i.e., pull the right knee to the right when standing on the right leg).

CALF TRAINING VARIATIONS

There is an old joke in bodybuilding circles that if you want great calves you need to choose the right parents. The point is that genetically small calves are notoriously difficult to grow. But the truth is, your calves can and will grow with the right type of training. They respond especially well to a very high frequency, up to twice per day for six days per week, as we cover in chapter 10. For now, here are three variations from easiest to most challenging.

One-Leg Calf Raise

Performing a one-leg calf raise from the floor is one of the most user-friendly calf builders you'll find. You can do this exercise literally anywhere, assuming you just want to knock out as many reps as possible and don't need to hold a weight in your hand. This is an ideal high-frequency exercise to build your calves. The goal is to work up to 25 repetitions through a full range of motion with each leg, and then progress to the elevated version covered next. Or you can keep adding reps until you reach 100 or more. There really is no limit.

HOW TO DO IT

1. Stand on your left leg approximately 12 inches (30 cm) in front of a wall, with your right foot elevated about four inches (10 cm) off the ground and behind you. Hold a dumbbell in your right hand, and rest your left fingertips lightly against the wall to maintain balance. If you don't have the strength for extra load, place the fingertips of both hands against the wall (see figure a).

2. Push through the base of your left big toe to elevate your heel as high as possible (see figure b). Focus on getting an intense calf contraction at the top of the movement.

3. Slowly lower back to the starting position.

4. Perform all reps on the left leg, and then switch sides.

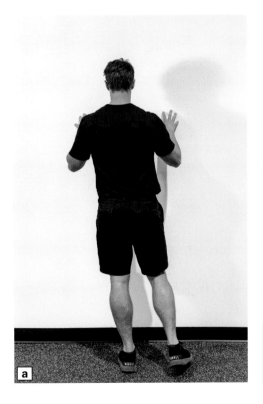
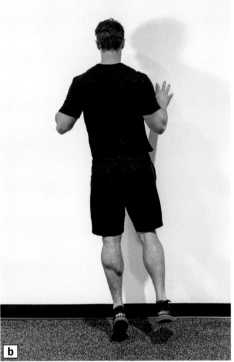

ADVANTAGE

This variation requires twice the muscle activation of the two-leg version.
It increases single-leg strength.

(continued)

One-Leg Calf Raise   *(continued)*

COACHING CUES

- Many people prefer to perform this, or any calf exercise, without shoes because they feel a stronger calf contraction.

- Holding a weight in your hand isn't necessary in the early stages if your strength isn't up to par.

- Perform this exercise with both feet on the ground if you lack the strength to perform the one-leg version.

- To make this exercise more challenging, hold the peak contraction for 1 to 3 seconds for each repetition.

- A weighted vest works well to increase the load when a dumbbell or kettlebell isn't available.

Elevated One-Leg Calf Raise

Once you can perform plenty of one-leg calf raises from the floor, a great progression is to perform them from an elevated surface such as a short box or step in your house. This increases the stretch of the calf muscles, which provides a new stimulus for muscle growth.

HOW TO DO IT

1. Place a short step on the floor against a wall. Stand on the edge of the step, with your left heel hanging off, while holding your right leg off the step. Hold a dumbbell on your right side, and start with your left calf in the deepest stretch position. Rest your left fingertips lightly against the wall to maintain balance. Or place the fingertips of both hands against the wall for the body weight version (see figure a).
2. Push through the base of your left big toe to elevate your heel as high as possible (see figure b). Focus on getting an intense calf contraction at the top of the movement.
3. Slowly lower back to the starting position.
4. Perform all reps on the left leg, and then switch sides.

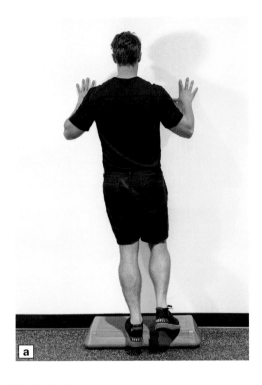 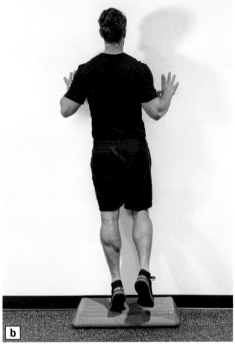

ADVANTAGE

Elevation increases eccentric stress on the plantar flexors during the stretch.

COACHING CUES

- Holding a weight in your hand isn't necessary in the early stages if your strength isn't up to par.
- To make this exercise more challenging, hold the stretch position or peak contraction, or both, for 1 to 3 seconds for each repetition.
- A weighted vest works well to increase the load when a dumbbell or kettlebell isn't available.

One-Leg Hop

Once you have built a good base of strength, which means you can perform 25 elevated one-leg calf raises through a full range of motion, you can start incorporating one-leg hops into your calf-building program. This challenging exercise increases eccentric stress (i.e., muscle damage), which is a potent stimulus for new muscle growth.

▶ HOW TO DO IT

1. Hold a light weight in your right hand, with your arm hanging freely at your side. Stand on your left leg, knee slightly bent, with your right foot elevated from the floor (see figure a).
2. Hop on your left leg, staying on the balls of your foot with each repetition (see figure b). Your left heel should never touch the ground.
3. Perform all reps on the left leg, and then switch sides with the weight in your left hand.

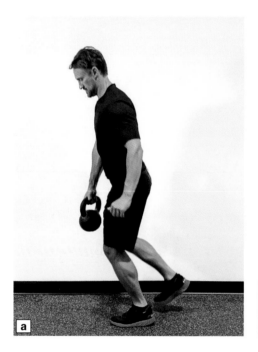
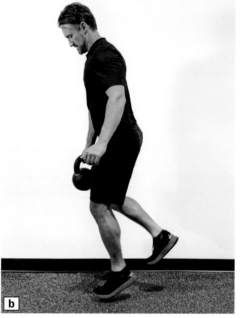

ADVANTAGE

This variation increases eccentric stress on the plantar flexors during the landing.

COACHING CUES

- Holding a weight in your hand isn't necessary in the early stages if your strength isn't up to par.
- Perform the reps with minimal knee bend to keep the tension on the calves without the quadriceps taking over.
- A weighted vest works well to increase the load when a dumbbell or kettlebell isn't available.

CHAPTER 6

Core Training

Bodybuilders, athletes, and warriors have worked to strengthen their midbody muscles for as long as people have trained to improve their physique, performance, or ability to fight. Until recently, most people just assumed the best way to achieve those goals was to focus on the abdominal muscles and work them as directly as possible. They spent countless hours on their backs doing as many sit-ups, leg raises, and twists as they could tolerate.

Sit-ups, like push-ups, became the universal answer to every question a coach, drill instructor, or physical education teacher could ask. Want to turn an also-ran into a champion? Sit-ups. Want to make soldiers tougher? Sit-ups. Want to punish schoolchildren? Sit-ups. Today that seems insane. When University of Waterloo spine specialist professor Stuart McGill tested sit-ups, his research revealed compression forces on the spinal discs at levels documented by the National Institute for Occupational Safety and Health (NIOSH) to elevate back injury rates. (The NIOSH is responsible for setting exposure limits to reduce disease and injury in the American worker.) McGill's research showed there were better ways to enhance abdominal athleticism with less risk (2015). The word quickly spread, and today those exercises are rarely seen in gyms, schools, or military bases.

But it wasn't just the exercises that McGill convinced us to question. He wanted us to change how we viewed the function of the muscles themselves. Instead of looking at the abdominals as muscles we should train in isolation, like the biceps or triceps, he got us to focus on their function within the entire movement chain. The abdominals aren't acting as prime movers when we're running, throwing, or climbing. They act as the link between the upper and lower body. It's their stability and endurance, rather than pure strength, that provide a base for movement while also protecting the spine.

The work of McGill and many others led us to our current understanding of the core: It includes all the muscles that act on the hips and lower back to provide stability to the spine and allow powerful, repeatable movements. Many people equate core training with movements that *create* motion in the spine, like crunches, twists, and side bends. But a core that works to *resist* motion in the spine helps transfer power generated in the hips out to the limbs, which McGill calls "distal athleticism." That approach to core training increases your training capacity, limb speed, and power (McGill 2015). To be clear, many athletes need to not only twist and flex their spines but also do so at a high velocity. And often in one motion. Just picture a pro golfer hitting her tee shot or a baseball slugger knocking one out of the park. A rotational athlete's spine has the resiliency to perform a career's worth of powerful spinal movements, if injury risk outside of sport is minimized. Trainers will sometimes assume that having rotational athletes perform twists, turns, and side bends with a heavy medicine ball will make them stronger. But adding those compression forces usually spells trouble. Your discs are already susceptible to injury during flexion and rotation, and that risk increases exponentially when compression forces are added (Desmoulin, Pradhan, and Milner 2020). There is a time and place to program high-velocity rotational exercises with very light loads, such as a six-pound (2.5 kg) medicine ball. But as a general rule, spend your time in the gym developing your core's ability to resist motion, and let most of your rotational training come from your sport.

This chapter goes deep into the core—to the muscles and the best exercises for appearance, performance, and prevention of low back injuries. I also clear up some mythology about what core training *can't* do: reduce the stubborn fat that keeps your abdominals hidden.

Development of Core Musculature

It is easy to understand the benefits of building strength in your midsection. Stronger midsection muscles support your spine and allow you to squat or deadlift heavier loads. What's less understood is the benefit of building more endurance in the muscles that surround your spine and pelvis (McGill 2015). Those muscles must be able to maintain their activation for extended periods of time, which is why you'll see 30-second holds, and similar durations, programmed later in this book.

But we're getting ahead of ourselves. Let's first talk about your abdominal muscles, and then expand on that to include the entire core (see figure 6.1). Your abdominals include four interconnected muscles:

- The *rectus abdominis* is the "six-pack" muscle that flexes your spine when you bend forward and protects your internal organs.
- The *external obliques* are fingerlike muscles on the sides of your abdomen that assist the rectus abdominis in its functions. But more important, they rotate your spine while also *preventing* rotation.
- The *internal obliques*, as their name suggests, are beneath the external obliques, with fibers running in the opposite direction. Their main role is to provide stability during mundane, low-effort activities like sitting and standing.
- The *transversus abdominis* is the innermost layer of the abdomen. It helps control abdominal pressure to protect your organs and works synergistically with your other midsection muscles.

Those are the four main muscles that make up your midsection—the muscles you think of when you refer to your abs. But those muscles don't work in isolation, no matter how hard you try. Your abdominals are synergistically linked with five other muscles, which are collectively known as the core:

- The *hip flexors* pull your legs up toward your torso.

- The *spinal erectors* extend your spine when you bend backward and also prevent your spine from bending when you need it to remain stable while lifting a heavy load.

- The *gluteus maximus*, your body's strongest muscle, works with your hamstrings to extend your hips when you're bent forward. It also works with the gluteus medius and minimus, among other muscles, to produce a variety of hip movements.

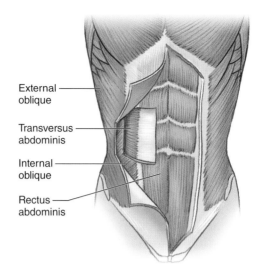

External oblique

Transversus abdominis

Internal oblique

Rectus abdominis

FIGURE 6.1   Abdominal and core muscles.

- The *quadratus lumborum*, which runs diagonally from the tops of your pelvis to the sides of your lumbar spine, both allows and prevents side-bending movements. It also works with the spinal erectors to extend and prevent extension of your lower back.

- The *latissimus dorsi*, your body's largest muscle by square footage, plays a key role in stabilizing your lower back in every pulling exercise, from rows to deadlifts.

Indeed, there's a lot more to your core than you probably imagined. And we've only discussed its muscles. Think about your skeletal structure. Your spine and lower limbs are linked through your pelvis, allowing your body to function as one interconnected unit that can run, jump, or throw a roundhouse kick. In other words, the pelvis is the central part of the skeleton. So if we consider the technical definition of *core*, which according to the Oxford dictionary is "the part of something that is central to its existence," then your pelvis is actually your core. It's all enough to make your stomach hurt.

You Can't Crunch Your Way to a Leaner Midsection

No discussion about the core would be complete without mentioning spot reduction. No reputable research supports the notion that directly training your midsection will make it lean. But you can certainly find research that refutes it. For example, one small study used MRI to compare fat distribution in the arms of young tennis players (Sanchis-Moysi et al. 2019). The researchers found no difference between the fat in their dominant and nondominant arms. Nevertheless, this is where we probably don't need science to support what we already know: Losing fat around your midsection requires a caloric deficit. Exercise, of course, will help. But many people have lost plenty of fat without ever breaking a sweat. In chapter 11 we cover nutrition guidelines to help you combat inflammation and insulin resistance, two of the biggest culprits for keeping fat around your gut.

Core Exercises

The purpose of core training is threefold. First, it increases the strength of muscles that surround the hips, pelvis, and spine. Weakness in any of those muscles impairs athletic performance because the transfer of power throughout your core is lost via energy leaks. Second, it protects your spinal discs from injury. Sufficient strength and endurance of the muscles that attach to the spine and pelvis are necessary to resist abrupt movements that can herniate a disc (McGill 2015). Third, a well-developed midsection will look more visually impressive once you achieve a low body fat percentage.

It might surprise you how much abdominal activation you can get from exercises not categorized as core training. For example, muscle activation during a pull-up is actually highest within the rectus abdominis (Hewit, Jaffe, and Crowder 2018). Other exercises such as a goblet squat and deadlift require high levels of muscle activation within your core to stabilize your spine. If you've ever pulled a heavy deadlift, or performed 20 goblet squats with a challenging load, you already know that's true. No EMG data required.

So why target your core at all? To protect your spine and improve full-body performance. Even though many exercises such as a front squat or back extension will challenge your midsection, muscle activation from those exercises is not as high as it is with direct core training (Bautista et al. 2020). Now let's get to the exercises that will build all the core strength you'll ever need, and spare your spine in the process.

PLANK VARIATIONS

The plank has been a popular pose in yoga and Pilates, but it wasn't until Stuart McGill published research on its benefits that the strength and conditioning world started to take notice. In general, plank variations are best held for an extended period of time. Endurance strength of the core muscles helps minimize the risk of back pain in a large population of athletes and nonathletes alike (McGill 2015). However, since very few people enjoy holding a plank for 60 or 90 seconds, and since excessive endurance work might be detrimental to an explosive athlete, more challenging versions are outlined.

MUSCLES WORKED:

rectus abdominis

transversus abdominis

internal oblique

psoas

iliacus

rectus femoris

serratus anterior

latissimus dorsi

Hardstyle Plank

The hardstyle plank (also known as the RKC plank) increases muscle activation beyond a standard plank. In this version, the lats, glutes, and all four layers of the abdominals are engaged to create maximal muscle recruitment throughout the core.

◉ HOW TO DO IT

1. Start with your elbows resting directly below your shoulders and your body in a straight line from neck to ankles (see figure).
2. Brace your abs, squeeze your glutes, and then pull your elbows toward your knees. Your elbows won't move but you'll feel an intense contraction in your lats and abdominals.
3. Maintain the effort for as long as possible.

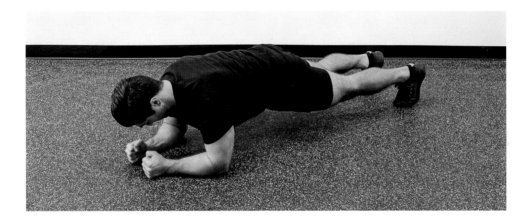

ADVANTAGE

This plank variation increases activation of the lats, glutes, hip flexors, and abdominal muscles.

COACHING CUES

- Don't let the hips elevate or sag.
- To make the exercise easier, rest your knees on the floor.

One-Leg Hardstyle Plank

The one-leg hardstyle plank progresses beyond the previous version. For this exercise, one leg is elevated to provide two benefits. First, the core's anti-rotation muscles are activated. Second, the glutes and hip flexors are more activated in the hip of the support leg.

HOW TO DO IT

1. Start with your elbows resting directly below your shoulders and your body in a straight line from neck to ankles, feet shoulder-width apart (see figure a).
2. Brace your abs, squeeze your glutes, and then pull your elbows toward your knees.
3. Next, lift your left leg about a foot (30 cm) off the ground without letting your torso shift or rotate (see figure b).
4. Maintain the position for the desired length of time, and then repeat with your right leg elevated.

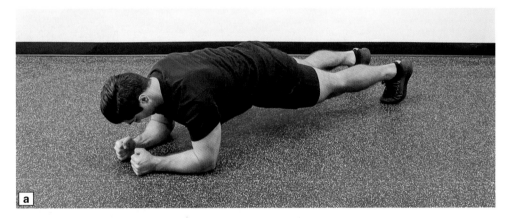

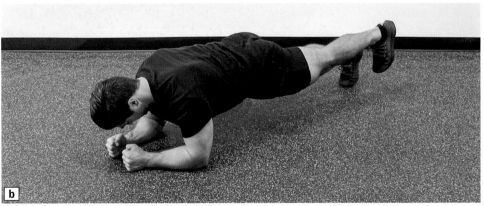

ADVANTAGE

The one-leg version increases activation of the core's anti-rotation muscles.

COACHING CUES

- Don't let the hips elevate or sag.
- The pelvis should remain parallel to the floor when one leg is elevated.

Swiss Ball Rollout

The Swiss ball rollout is technically not a plank exercise, but it requires a similar level of muscle activation throughout the core so it is included in this section. Once you become proficient at the plank variations, the next progression is a rollout. For this exercise you'll use a large Swiss ball, which requires greater activation of the anterior core muscles and lats compared with a standard plank. The dynamic nature of this exercise creates a unique challenge for the midsection.

HOW TO DO IT

1. Start on your knees with your forearms resting on a large Swiss ball, elbows bent and resting below your chin (see figure a).
2. Brace your abs, squeeze your glutes, and then shift your body forward as far as possible while you simultaneously extend your elbows, rolling the ball forward (see figure b).
3. Slowly reverse to the starting position and repeat.

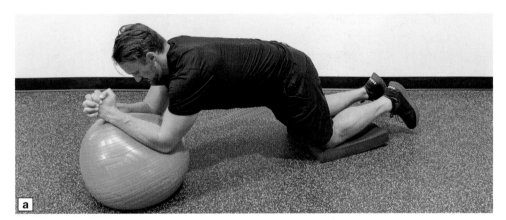

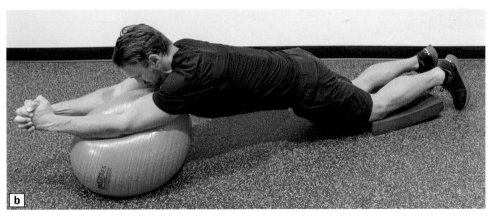

ADVANTAGE

The rollout increases activation of the lats and requires dynamic stability throughout the core.

COACHING CUES

- Maintain a double chin to avoid neck strain.
- To make the exercise more challenging, perform it with your legs straight and knees off the floor.

Hand Walkout

The hand walkout is technically not a plank exercise, but it requires a similar level of muscle activation throughout the core so it is included here.

▶ HOW TO DO IT

1. Start on all fours with your hands directly below your shoulders and your knees resting on the ground or a pad (see figure a).
2. Brace your abs, squeeze your glutes, and then reach your left hand a few inches (10 cm) in front without rotating your trunk (see figure b). Then reach your right hand about four inches in front of your left. Continue walking your hands forward until your stomach is a few inches off the ground, or as far as your strength allows.
3. Walk your hands back to the starting position and repeat.

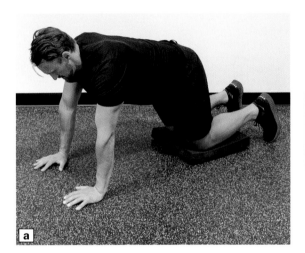
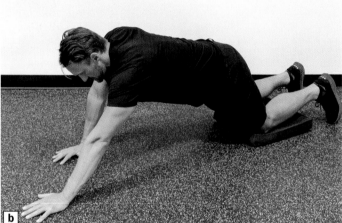

ADVANTAGES

- The walkout increases activation of the lats and requires dynamic stability throughout the core.
- It increases stability strength of the shoulders more than a rollout.

COACHING CUES

- Maintain a double chin to avoid neck strain.
- Walk your hands out into a V pattern, so they're wider as your stomach gets closer to the floor, to reduce shoulder strain.
- To make the exercise more challenging, perform it with your legs straight and knees off the floor.

SIDE PLANK VARIATIONS

The side plank strengthens muscles around the trunk and pelvis that maintain stability in the frontal plane. Research demonstrates that sufficient endurance strength in the side plank is an important component for preventing, or recovering from, low back injuries (McGill 2015).

MUSCLES WORKED:

internal and external obliques

quadratus lumborum

gluteus medius

serratus anterior

latissimus dorsi

Side Plank

Twenty years ago, most people had never seen a side plank. Thanks to McGill's research, it's a foundational exercise in any core training program. This exercise strengthens your lateral trunk and hips using nothing but your body weight for resistance.

HOW TO DO IT

1. Prop your body up on your right forearm, with your elbow resting directly below your shoulder. Your body is in a straight line from neck to ankles, with your left foot resting directly in front of your right (see figure).
2. Hold for the desired time, and then switch sides so your left forearm rests on the ground.

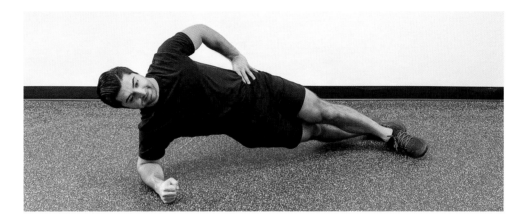

ADVANTAGE

Side planks strengthen the obliques, quadratus lumborum, and gluteus medius.

COACHING CUES

- Terminate the exercise as soon as the hips drop toward the floor.
- To make the exercise more challenging, attempt to pull your elbow toward your hip. The elbow won't move, but you'll feel greater activation of the latissimus dorsi and lateral trunk muscles.
- To make it easier, perform it with your knees bent and resting on the floor.

Stacked Side Plank

In this version of the plank, the feet are stacked so the outside of only one foot rests on the floor. This narrower base of support increases activation of the gluteus medius and lateral trunk musculature.

HOW TO DO IT

1. Prop your body up on your right forearm, with your elbow resting directly below your shoulder. Your body is in a straight line from neck to ankles, with your feet together (see figure).
2. Hold for the desired time, and then switch sides so your left forearm rests on the floor.

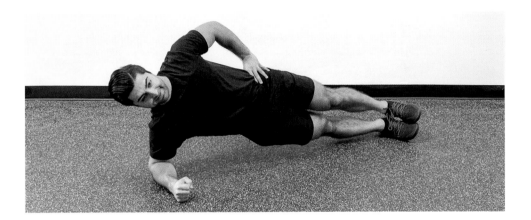

ADVANTAGE

The stacked variation increases activation of the gluteus medius more than a standard side plank.

COACHING CUES

- Terminate the exercise as soon as the hips drop toward the floor.
- To make the exercise more challenging, attempt to pull your elbow toward your hip. The elbow won't move, but you'll feel greater activation of the lats and lateral trunk muscles.

One-Leg Side Plank

This is the most advanced version of a side plank. Elevating the top leg creates a unique challenge for the gluteus medius muscles in both hips. The hip and ankle of the stance leg have to work harder, while the glutes of the other hip activate to hold the leg elevated.

HOW TO DO IT

1. Prop your body up on your right forearm, with your elbow resting directly below your shoulder. Your body is in a straight line from neck to ankles, with your feet together (see figure a).
2. Lift your left leg up about 12 inches (30 cm) while keeping your foot parallel to the floor (see figure b).
3. Hold the leg elevated for the desired length of time, or perform reps, and then switch sides so your left forearm rests on the floor.

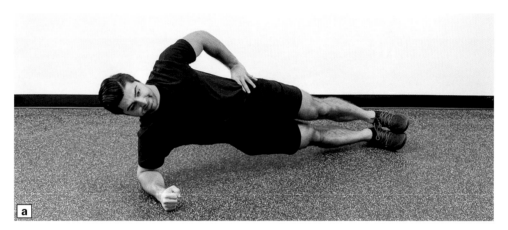

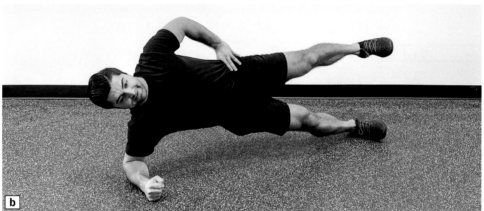

ADVANTAGE

The one-leg variation increases activation of the glutes in both hips.

COACHING CUES

- Terminate the exercise as soon as the hips drop toward the floor.
- To make the exercise more challenging, attempt to pull your elbow toward your hip. The elbow won't move, but you'll feel greater activation of the lats and lateral trunk muscles.
- Avoid any rotation of the trunk as the top leg elevates.

ANTI-ROTATION VARIATIONS

In order to throw a powerful punch or kick, or push your opponent, or hold a heavy object on one side of your body, your trunk must maintain stability. This is accomplished by developing strong anti-rotation muscles throughout the core to stiffen the trunk and reduce any "energy leaks," as Stuart McGill likes to call them. These core exercises are especially important because they strengthen the trunk and pelvis in a way that many compound exercises don't.

Stir the Pot

The stir the pot exercise is a simple way to strengthen the anti-rotation muscles using nothing but a Swiss ball. This exercise increases stability strength around the lumbar spine while minimizing stress on the spinal discs.

▸ HOW TO DO IT

1. Start in the plank position with your elbows directly below your shoulders and resting on a Swiss ball (see figure a).
2. Brace your abs, squeeze your glutes, and then slowly move your elbows clockwise using the largest arc of motion possible without moving your torso or hips (see figure b). Then slowly move your elbows counterclockwise through the largest range of motion.
3. Continue alternating between clockwise and counterclockwise movements.

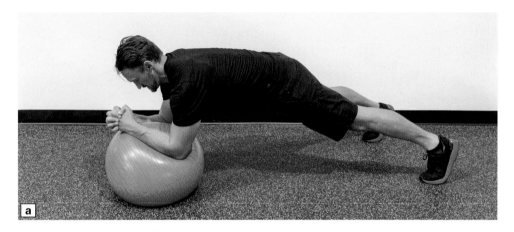

a

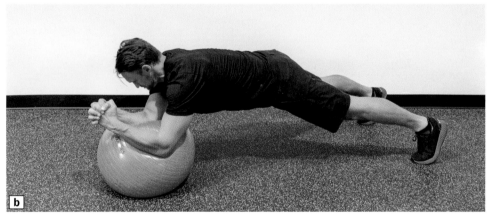

b

ADVANTAGE

This exercise strengthens the core's anti-rotation muscles while sparing the lumbar spine.

COACHING CUES

- Keep your chin tucked to reduce neck strain.
- The pelvis and trunk should not move during the exercise.
- To make it more challenging, make larger circles in each direction.

Pallof Press

The Pallof press, named after physical therapist John Pallof, has become a popular anti-rotation exercise over the last decade. Unlike the previous exercises, the Pallof press is performed while standing, which adds a unique stability challenge throughout the lower body.

HOW TO DO IT

1. Position a cable or band around chest height. Grab the handle of the cable or the band with both hands, fingers interlocked.
2. Step away from the cable or band so it's to your right and approximately parallel to the floor. Stand with your feet slightly wider than shoulder width, hands against your chest (see figure a).
3. Brace your abs, squeeze your glutes, and then slowly straighten your arms in front, parallel to the ground (see figure b). Maintain the position without rotating your trunk or pelvis.
4. Hold for the recommended time, then switch sides so the cable or band is to your left.

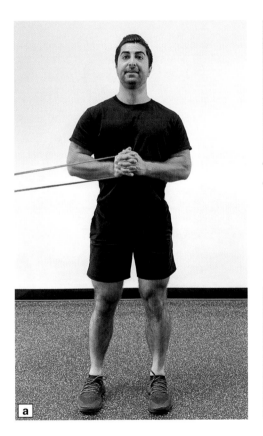
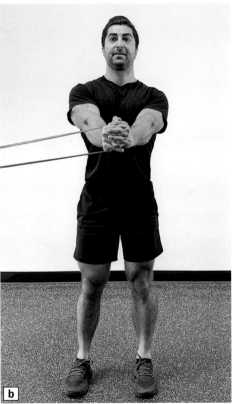

ADVANTAGE

The Pallof press engages the lower body musculature with the core to resist trunk rotation.

COACHING CUES

- Tuck the chin to avoid neck strain.
- Maintain a tall posture, with the shoulders parallel to the floor.

Half-Kneeling Pallof Press

The half-kneeling Pallof press is performed with one knee resting on the floor. This requires increased activation from the glutes in that hip while placing the hip flexors in a stretch position. This exercise is often considered a regression from the standing version, although many people find the half-kneeling position to be more challenging.

HOW TO DO IT

1. Position a cable or band around hip height. Grab the handle of the band or the cable with both hands, fingers interlocked.
2. Step away from the cable or band so it's to your right. Rest your left knee on a pad and your right foot on the floor, the knee bent to 90 degrees, with the cable or band parallel to the ground (see figure a). Get into a tall posture, hands against your chest.
3. Brace your abs, squeeze your left glutes, and then slowly straighten your arms in front, parallel to the ground (see figure b). Maintain the position without rotating your trunk or pelvis.
4. Hold for the recommended time, then switch sides so the cable or band is to your left.

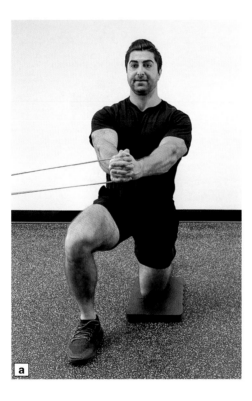 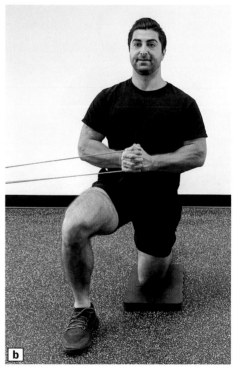

ADVANTAGE

The half-kneeling version requires greater gluteal activation of the hip when the knee is resting on the floor, and it helps improve mobility of the hip flexors.

COACHING CUES

- Tuck the chin to avoid neck strain.
- Maintain the tallest posture possible, with the shoulders parallel to the floor.

Tall-Kneeling Pallof Press

The tall-kneeling Pallof press is performed with both knees resting on the floor. This places a stretch on both hip flexors as you resist rotational movement from the band. The tall-kneeling position is often programmed first in Pallof progressions to teach people how to maximally engage their anti-rotation muscles without the help of a wide stance.

HOW TO DO IT

1. Position a cable or band around hip height. Grab the handle of the band or the cable with both hands, fingers interlocked.
2. Step away from the cable or band so it's to your right. Rest both knees on a pad, around hip-width apart, with your trunk upright and the cable or band parallel to the ground (see figure a). Get into a tall posture, hands against your chest.
3. Brace your abs, squeeze your glutes, and then slowly straighten your arms in front, parallel to the ground (see figure b). Maintain the position without rotating your trunk or pelvis.
4. Hold for the recommended time, then switch sides so the cable or band is to your left.

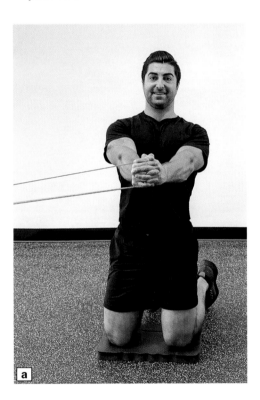
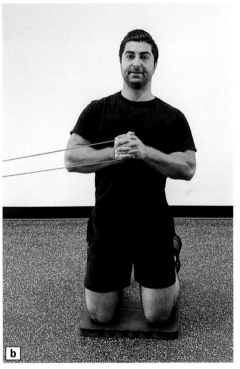

ADVANTAGE

The tall-kneeling version teaches people how to maximally engage the core's anti-rotation muscles while placing a stretch on the hip flexors.

COACHING CUES

- Tuck the chin to avoid neck strain.
- Maintain the tallest posture possible, with the shoulders parallel to the floor.
- For some, placing the knees wider than shoulder width is more comfortable and allows for greater resistance from the band.

Landmine Rotation

The landmine rotation exercise isn't purely anti-rotation since the thoracic spine rotates. However, it is anti-rotation for the lumbar spine. This exercise requires high-level activation from the shoulder stabilizers and helps improve mobility of the thoracic spine. It is also an effective exercise to strengthen the obliques.

▶ HOW TO DO IT

1. Stand with your feet wider than shoulder width, arms straight and held about four inches (10 cm) higher than your head, fingers interlocked around the barbell (see figure a).

2. Brace your midsection, squeeze your glutes, and then slowly rotate your arms down and to the right without any lumbar rotation (see figure b).

3. Slowly reverse to the starting position, and then rotate the arms down and to the left. Keep your arms straight throughout the movement. Repeat for the desired number of reps.

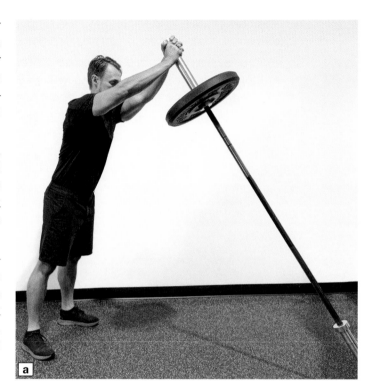

ADVANTAGE

This exercise recruits the shoulders, hips, and upper back while training the lumbar spine's anti-rotation muscles.

COACHING CUES

- Your feet should be wider than shoulder width for stability, but the feet can move closer together as you get stronger.

- Avoid any lumbar rotation; the rotation should be limited to the thoracic spine.

- You can also perform this exercise in a tall posture (i.e., tall-kneeling position), with both knees resting on the ground.

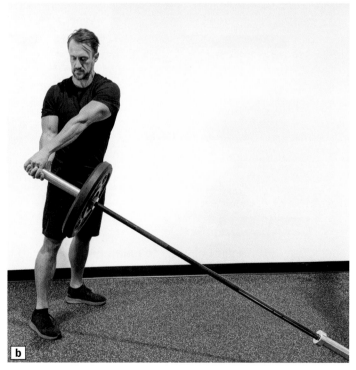

One-Arm Plank

The one-arm plank is an excellent anti-rotation progression using nothing but your body weight. With only one arm resting on the floor, it requires intense activation of the shoulder stabilizers to maintain the proper position.

◉ HOW TO DO IT

1. Start in the standard plank position, elbows resting directly below your shoulders and your body in a straight line from neck to ankles (see figure a).
2. Brace your abs, squeeze your glutes, and then lift your left arm straight in front without letting your torso rotate or shift (see figure b).
3. Maintain the position for the desired length of time, and then repeat with your right arm elevated.

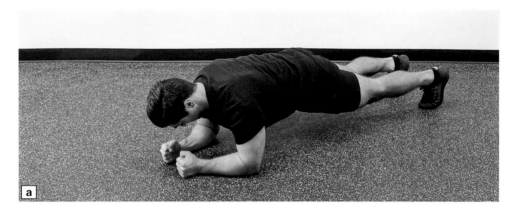

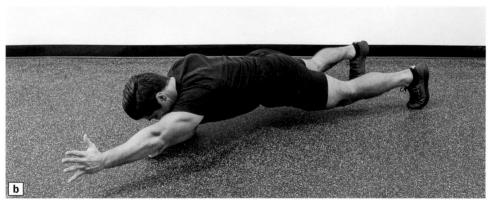

ADVANTAGE

The one-arm plank recruits the core's anti-rotation muscles as well as the shoulder stabilizers of the side that's resting on the floor.

COACHING CUES

- Your feet should be wider than shoulder width for stability, but the feet can move closer together as you get stronger.
- Avoid any rotation of the trunk while one arm is elevated.
- Avoid shifting the pelvis to the side, a common compensation for this exercise.

LEG RAISE VARIATIONS

Variations of the leg raise create novel stimuli to the core region. The action of lifting and lowering your legs builds strength in the hip flexors, developing your ability to throw more powerful kicks (Vagner et al. 2019). For any of the three versions, it's imperative to activate your lats to support your lumbar spine, offsetting low back strain that's common during these exercises.

Lying Leg Raise

The lying leg raise is popular with both athletes and bodybuilders. It's a simple move that can be performed anywhere since it requires no equipment. In many cases, a person performs this exercise with the arms crossed at the chest or resting on the floor. In this version, however, the arms are held straight over the chest with fingers interlocked to activate the lats, which supports the lumbar spine.

HOW TO DO IT

1. Lie on your back with your legs straight and feet together, arms extended over your chest and fingers interlocked (see figure a).

2. Squeeze your elbows toward each other to activate your lats, flatten your low back, and then slowly lift your legs until they reach about a 45-degree angle relative to the ground (see figure b).

3. Slowly lower your legs back to the starting position and repeat.

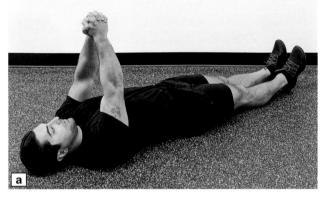

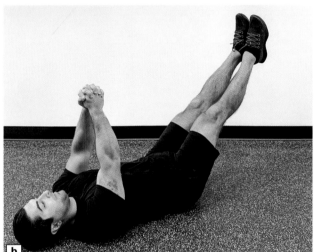

ADVANTAGE

The lying leg raise recruits the core's anti-rotation muscles as well as the shoulder stabilizers of the side that's resting on the floor.

COACHING CUES

- For some, it's more comfortable to rest the head on a pillow to avoid neck strain.

- Lifting your legs any higher than approximately 60 degrees decreases activation of the hip flexors and lower abdomen.

- To make the exercise easier, shorten the range of motion or slightly bend your knees.

Band Lying Leg Raise

In this version of a lying leg raise, a band is used to engage the lats to provide lumbar support. In most cases, the lat activation eliminates any low back strain, or at the very least allows you to lift and lower your legs through a greater range of motion without discomfort.

HOW TO DO IT

1. Attach a long resistance band to a secure structure about 24 inches (60 cm) from the floor. Grab the band, and then lie on your back with your legs straight and feet together.

2. With your hands wider than shoulder width and held over your chest, pull your palms toward your knees to activate your lats (see figure a).

3. Flatten your low back and then slowly lift your legs until they reach about a 45-degree angle relative to the ground (see figure b).

4. Slowly lower your legs back to the starting position and repeat.

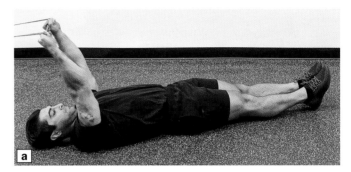

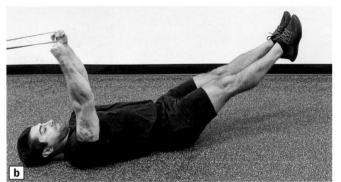

ADVANTAGE

This variation maximally activates the lats to provide lumbar support.

COACHING CUES

- Sometimes it's best not to lower the legs to the floor during the early stages. Use a range of motion that's free of any low back strain.
- Some people prefer to rest the head on a pillow to avoid neck strain.
- Avoid lifting the legs higher than approximately 60 degrees to keep tension on the working muscles.

Hanging Leg Raise

The hanging leg raise is a challenging progression beyond the lying leg raise. For this exercise, you'll need a strong grip. You'll also need a good base of strength in your hip flexors. Unlike a lying leg raise, which gets easier as your legs elevate, the hanging leg raise challenges your hip flexors through the entire range of motion.

HOW TO DO IT

1. Grab a pull-up bar with an overhand grip, using a grip width that's most comfortable for your shoulders. Hang with your legs straight and feet off the ground.
2. Pull yourself up an inch (2.5 cm) to activate that lats, and then lift your legs up, keeping them as straight as possible (see figure a).
3. Lift as high as your strength allows or until your legs are parallel to the ground (see figure b).
4. Slowly lower your legs back to the starting position and repeat.

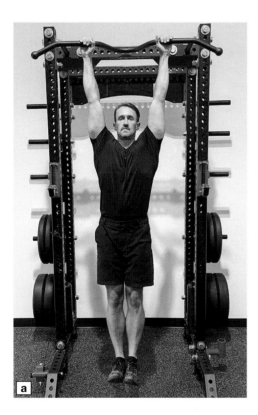
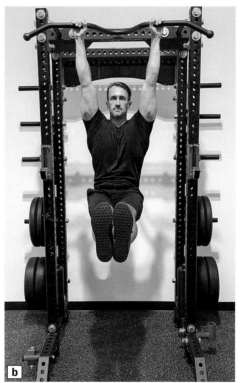

ADVANTAGE

This advanced variation strengthens the lats, shoulder stabilizers, and grip while challenging the abdominals and hip flexors.

COACHING CUES

- Avoid swinging your body or using leg momentum.
- To make the exercise easier, bend your knees a little or a lot, and pull them to your chest to shorten the lever arm.
- To make it more challenging, lift your legs until your shins touch the bar, or use ankle weights and lift your legs to parallel.

FULL-BODY CORE EXERCISES

The final exercises in this chapter—the Turkish get-up (TGU), popularized by Pavel Tsatsouline, and the loaded carries—stand alone. These "core exercises" actually build full-body strength. The TGU challenges the strength and motor control of all layers of the abdominal wall as well as stabilizers in your shoulder. Loaded carries are an effective way to strengthen your entire trunk, pelvic region, and grip (Butcher and Rusin 2016).

Loaded Carry

As covered back in chapter 1, the loaded carry, also known as the farmer's walk, requires high levels of stability strength throughout the trunk, pelvis, hips, and ankles. Walking while carrying a heavy load is one of the simplest ways to build full-body strength that carries over to virtually any sport or task.

HOW TO DO IT

1. Load a trap bar, or grab two dumbbells of equal weight and hold one in each hand.
2. Stand with a tall posture, tuck your chin (i.e., make a double chin), and keep your shoulders pulled back.
3. Walk slowly, striking your heel with each step (see figure), preferably in a figure-eight pattern.

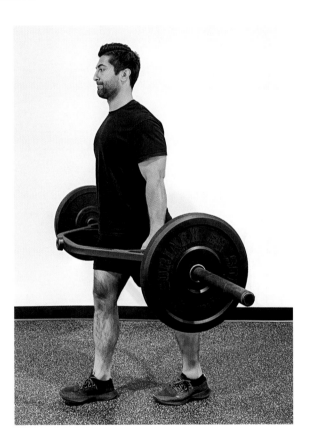

ADVANTAGES

- The loaded carry simultaneously strengthens the trunk, pelvis, ankles, and grip.
- It carries over to countless functional activities in life and sport.

COACHING CUES

- Maintain the tallest posture possible while walking.
- Maintain a level pelvis during each step.

One-Arm Loaded Carry

The one-arm loaded carry, also known as a suitcase carry, is a popular exercise in both sport and low back rehabilitation. Compared with a two-arm carry, holding a heavy weight in one hand requires greater activation of the obliques and quadratus lumborum muscles, which resist lateral flexion of the spine.

HOW TO DO IT

1. Hold a heavy dumbbell in your left hand.
2. Stand with a tall posture, tuck your chin (i.e., make a double chin), and keep your shoulders pulled back.
3. Walk slowly, striking your heel with each step (see figure), preferably in a figure-eight pattern.
4. Switch hands and repeat for the same time or distance.

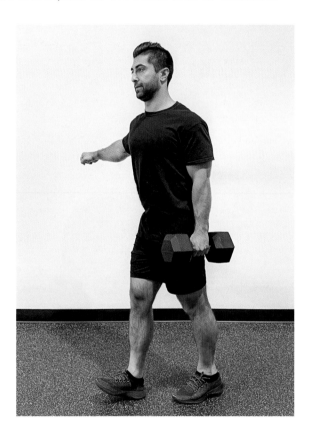

ADVANTAGES

- This one-arm variation strengthens the core muscles that resist lateral flexion of the spine (i.e., obliques and quadratus lumborum).
- It provides many of the benefits of a two-arm loaded carry when only one heavy weight is available.

COACHING CUES

- Maintain a perfectly vertical trunk during the exercise.
- Sometimes it's helpful to watch yourself in the mirror during the early stages of this exercise to ensure your trunk is vertical and your shoulders are level.

Turkish Get-Up

The Turkish get-up (TGU) is one of those exercises that, if you never saw it before, probably wouldn't strike you as a core exercise. That's because there are so many other things going on from head to toe. Unlike every other exercise in this chapter, the TGU improves full-body strength and mobility at the same time.

▷ HOW TO DO IT

1. Lie on your back with your left knee bent to 90 degrees and the left foot flat on the ground. Your right leg is straight, toes pointed up, and angled out slightly (see figure a). Hold a kettlebell in your left hand at arm's length, with your right arm flat on the ground and angled outward.

2. Drive through your left heel, and prop your trunk up on your right elbow as your right heel stays on the ground (see figure b). The left knee remains pointed upward, or the leg can shift slightly inward if you experience an impingement in the left hip.

3. Push through your right forearm to make the trunk more vertical as your left arm remains straight and perpendicular to the ground. Move your right hand back behind your body where it feels most comfortable (see figure c).

4. Push through your left foot to elevate your hips as high as possible, using your straightened right arm for support (see figure d).

5. With your hips held high, bend your right knee and place it on the ground directly below the kettlebell (see figure e).

6. Shift your torso to vertical as your left arm remains perpendicular to the ground, and then internally rotate your right hip until the right lower leg is perpendicular to the trunk, chin tucked and eyes facing forward (see figure f).

7. Stand up by pushing equally through both feet while keeping your left arm perpendicular to the ground, chin tucked and eyes facing forward (see figure g). Reverse the steps to return to the starting position and repeat for reps, then switch the kettlebell to the right hand and repeat the steps on the opposite side of the body.

(continued)

Turkish Get-Up *(continued)*

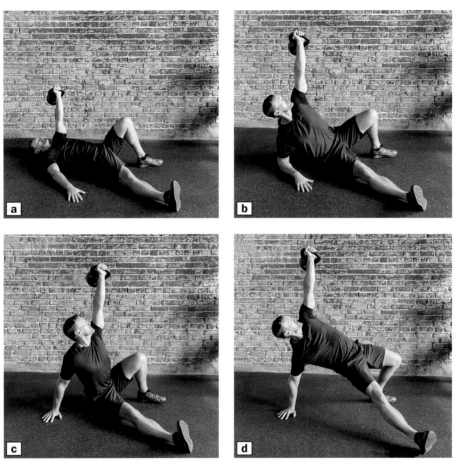

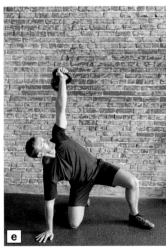

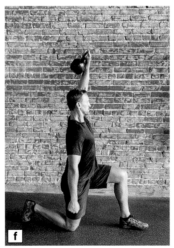

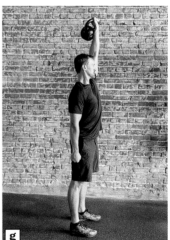

ADVANTAGE

The TGU strengthens all layers of the abdominal wall while building full-body strength.

COACHING CUES

- Maintain full lockout of the elbow that's holding the weight.
- Transition slowly between phases of the movement to improve the mind–muscle connection. The exercise should be a slow grind from start to finish.

CHAPTER 7

Upper Body Training

Here's one thing we can probably all agree on: Guys love training their upper body muscles. Especially the ones they can see in the mirror. Many weekend warriors will spend countless hours in the gym grunting and grinding through endless variations of the bench press and biceps curl. Far less likely is the chance they're putting as much effort into developing the muscles they can't see in the mirror.

Development of Upper Body Musculature

An essential aspect of building an impressive upper body physique is maintaining the health and integrity of your shoulder joints. These ball-and-socket joints rely heavily on the strength of many of the smaller muscles that attract less attention on the beach. Deep within your shoulder are four small muscles that work in concert to stabilize your humerus as you lift weights, throw, or punch. Of the four, two that are on the back of the shoulder—infraspinatus and teres minor—externally rotate the joint and hold the ball (head of humerus) in the center of its socket (glenoid cavity). This joint centration helps prevent wear and tear in your shoulders. You'll often see physical therapists prescribe external rotation exercises with five-pound (2.5 kg) dumbbells or light bands to strengthen those muscles.

The rhomboids and middle trapezius muscles attach the medial border of your scapulae to the spine. They're easy enough to activate—just squeeze your shoulder blades together without shrugging your shoulders—but difficult to sufficiently strengthen without devoting as much time to rows as you do to bench presses. The face pull exercise, performed with a strong resistance band or cable, will strengthen your external rotators as well as your rhomboids and middle trapezius muscles. And you already know the row builds the size and strength of those muscles. That's why you'll frequently see variations of the row and face pull in every program in chapters 8 and 9.

What you won't find in any program is the standard barbell bench press with a wider than shoulder-width grip. The reason is simple: There are better ways to strengthen your pectorals and triceps with less risk to your shoulders. (But you will see the more shoulder-friendly narrow-grip bench press.) That might not surprise you. However, I also avoid programming the bent-over barbell row. Now that might surprise you because it is, after all, a row. The problem is not in the basic movement pattern but in the faulty position of the load. Your knees get in the way of the ideal path of the barbell, forcing it excessively forward, which places undue strain on your lumbar spine. That's why you'll perform variations of the row that allow the load to be held closer to your body, reducing the likelihood of a low back injury.

If you choose to design your own plan with the exercises in this chapter, rotate between a horizontal pull and vertical pull from workout to workout. The same is true with a horizontal and vertical push. This helps ensure a balance of development of the pectorals, deltoids, serratus anterior in the front and rhomboids, trapezius, infraspinatus, supraspinatus, and teres minor in the back (see figure 7.1 for upper body musculature). Now let's cover all the upper body exercises you'll need to build high-performance muscle and strength while preserving the integrity of your joints.

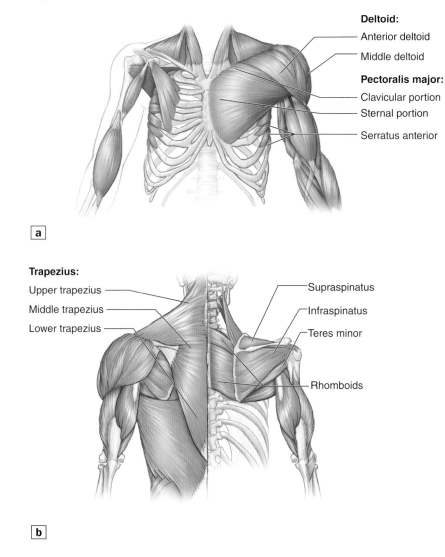

FIGURE 7.1   Upper body muscles : *(a)* front view and *(b)* rear view.

Upper Body Exercises

In this section we cover a myriad of exercises to strengthen and build every major muscle group in the upper body. The key to both performance and aesthetics is a balance of muscle size and strength around the shoulder complex. We include variations of upper body pulls and pushes from the vertical and horizontal planes, as well as isolation exercises to target your arms and shoulders.

HORIZONTAL PULL VARIATIONS

It is common for athletes to be able to push more weight than they can pull. This strength imbalance can negatively affect posture, joint health, and overall performance. Therefore, it's important to perform many different horizontal pull variations in order to build upper back strength and improve the integrity of your shoulder complex.

MUSCLES WORKED:

forearms

biceps

latissimus dorsi

rhomboid

middle trapezius

rear deltoid

spinal erectors

stabilizing muscles of the shoulder girdle

Inverted Row

The inverted row strengthens and builds the upper back, biceps, and forearms while challenging core stability. Using rings or straps allows the wrists to move freely, which reduces strain on the elbows and shoulders. This is also a low back–friendly exercise for people who suffer from low back pain.

HOW TO DO IT

1. Use rings or straps for this exercise, and start by getting the height correct. Lie on your back with your arms extended above your chest and fingers fully extended. Adjust the rings or straps so they hang at a height that's the same as the tips of your fingers.
2. Grab the handles and start with your arms fully extended, palms facing each other and shoulder blades separated (see figure a). Your body should make a straight line from neck to ankles.
3. Squeeze your glutes, make a double chin, and then pull your body as one unit while keeping your elbows close to your sides without shrugging your shoulders (see figure b).
4. Slowly reverse the motion and repeat.

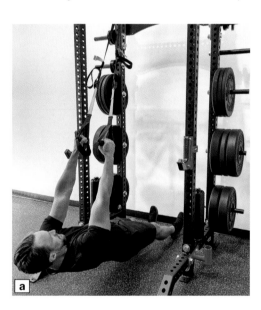 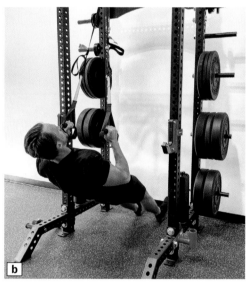

ADVANTAGES

- The inverted row allows the wrists to move freely, reducing strain on the elbows and shoulders.
- It is a low back–friendly option that increases core activation.

COACHING CUES

- For variety, hold your hands in different positions from workout to workout or month to month. Rotate between your palms facing in, facing up, or facing down.
- This exercise can also be performed with a straight bar resting on the hooks in a power rack.

Feet-Elevated Inverted Row

This version of the inverted row provides a simple body weight progression. By elevating your heels on a box or bench, you will pull a greater proportion of your body weight vertically. This exercise is also a great way to build your biceps.

HOW TO DO IT

1. Use rings or straps for this exercise, and start by getting the height correct. Lie on your back with your arms extended above your chest and fingers fully extended. Adjust the rings or straps so they hang at a height that's the same as the tips of your fingers.
2. Grab the handles and start with your arms fully extended, palms facing each other and shoulder blades separated. Rest your heels on a box or bench with your legs straight (see figure a). Your body should make a straight line from neck to ankles.
3. Squeeze your glutes, make a double chin, and then pull your body as one unit while keeping your elbows close to your sides without shrugging your shoulders (see figure b).
4. Slowly reverse the motion and repeat.

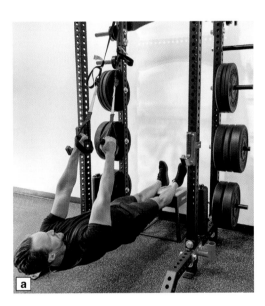 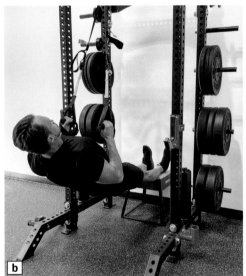

ADVANTAGE

Elevation provides a simple body weight loading progression for the inverted row.

COACHING CUES

- For variety, hold your hands in different positions from workout to workout or month to month. Rotate between your palms facing in, facing up, or facing down.
- This exercise can also be performed with a straight bar resting on the hooks in a power rack.

Split-Stance Row

A typical bent-over barbell row can place unnecessary stress on your low back. This variation of a bent-over row is performed with a split stance to reduce strain on your lumbar discs. Dumbbells or kettlebells are required since a barbell's path would not clear your front leg.

▶ HOW TO DO IT

1. Grab a dumbbell or kettlebell in each hand. Stand with your feet shoulder width, then step your right leg forward about a meter. Push your hips back and shift your trunk forward until it's around 45 degrees relative to the floor. Slightly arch your low back. The majority of your weight is on your right (front) leg. Your arms are straight and hanging down, palms facing each other (see figure a).

2. Bend your elbows and pull the weights up until your palms are near the side of your torso (see figure b).

3. Slowly reverse the motion and repeat.

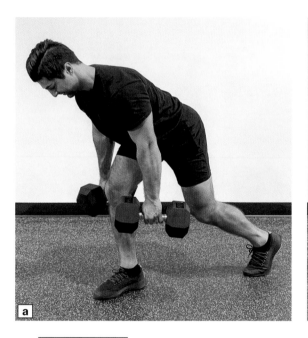
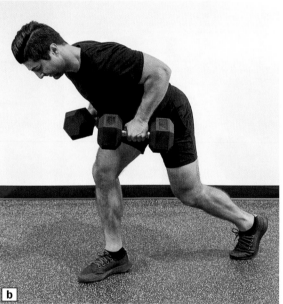

ADVANTAGE

The split stance drastically reduces strain on the low back compared with a standard bent-over row.

COACHING CUE

Switch which leg is forward with each set.

Yates Row

This version of a row was popularized by Dorian Yates, a former professional body-builder and six-time consecutive winner of the Mr. Olympia title. A wide underhand grip is used to emphasize the biceps, and the relatively vertical trunk angle reduces strain on the lumbar spine.

HOW TO DO IT

1. Grab the barbell with a wide underhand grip. Push your hips back and let your knees slightly bend until your torso is around 60 degrees relative to the floor (see figure a). Slightly arch your low back.
2. Bend your elbows and pull the barbell until it touches your abdomen, or just short of it (see figure b).
3. Slowly reverse the motion and repeat.

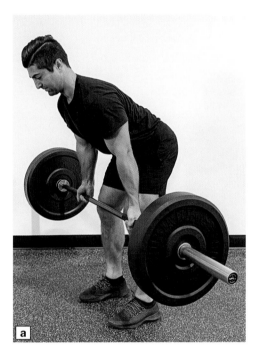 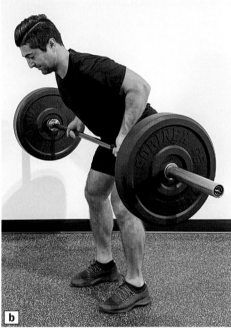

ADVANTAGE

This rowing variation can be used with heavy loads to target the biceps.

COACHING CUE

If you don't have the wrist mobility or low back strength for this exercise, perform the split-stance row instead.

One-Arm Row

The one-arm row is a foundational exercise for bodybuilders and athletes. The split-stance position, paired with trunk support from the nonworking arm, allows heavy loads to be used with minimal stress on the low back.

HOW TO DO IT

1. Grab a dumbbell or kettlebell in your left hand. Stand with your feet shoulder width, then step your right leg forward about a meter. Push your hips back and shift your trunk forward until it's around 45 degrees relative to the floor. The majority of your weight is on your right (front) leg. Your left arm is straight and hanging down, palm facing in (see figure a). Place your right hand on the top of your right thigh, and slightly arch your low back.

2. Bend your left elbow and pull the weight up until your left palm is near the side of your torso (see figure b).

3. Slowly reverse the motion. Switch the weight to your right hand with your left leg forward and repeat.

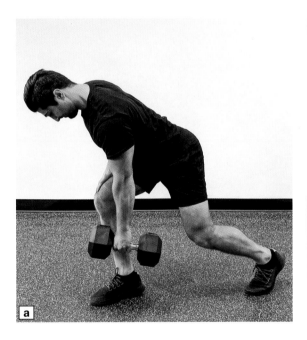
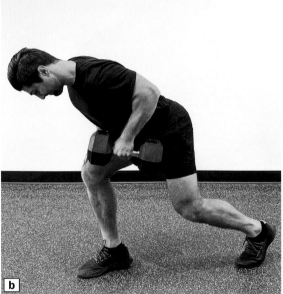

ADVANTAGE

This rowing variation can be used with heavy loads while minimally stressing the lumbar spine.

COACHING CUE

For variety, hold your rowing hand in different positions from workout to workout or month to month. Rotate between your palm facing in, facing forward, or facing back.

One-Arm Cable Row

The one-arm cable row is performed standing in a split stance, which provides two important benefits. First, there's no stress on the lumbar spine, making it an effective variation for those with low back pain. Second, the split stance allows you to pull a heavy load. It is common to see lifters perform this exercise with a band, but that is not recommended since the band has the highest tension where you're naturally weakest (hand close to the trunk) and lowest tension where you're strongest (arm extended in front of you).

HOW TO DO IT

1. Set the cable pulley at the height of your upper abdomen. Grab the handle with your right hand and get in a split stance with your left leg forward. Hold your right arm straight in front, parallel to the ground, palm facing in (see figure a). Place your left hand on your abdomen.

2. Bend your right elbow and row the handle until your right palm is close to the right side of your trunk (see figure b).

3. Slowly reverse the motion. Switch the handle to your left hand with your right leg forward and repeat.

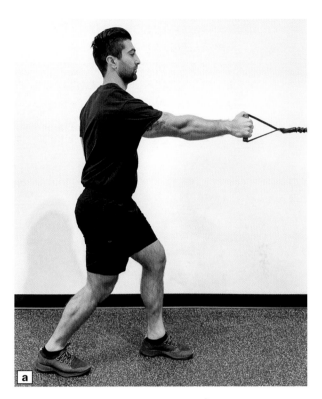
a

ADVANTAGE

This rowing variation allows for heavy loads without stressing the lumbar spine.

COACHING CUES

- For variety, hold your rowing hand in different positions from workout to workout or month to month. Rotate between your palm facing in, facing up, or facing down.

- Don't perform this exercise with a band because its tension is lowest where you're strongest (arm extended) and highest where you're weakest (hand close to torso). If you don't have a cable, perform a one-arm kettlebell or dumbbell row instead.

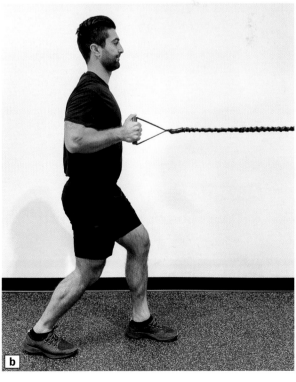
b

Face Pull

The face pull simultaneously strengthens and builds the rhomboids, middle traps, and external rotators. Sufficient strength of those muscles is crucial to shoulder health. This exercise should be part of any resistance training program, which is why you'll see it programmed so frequently in this book.

HOW TO DO IT

1. Stand tall with your arms held in front and parallel to the floor. Loop a long resistance band across the back of your wrists with your palms facing forward, fingers spread and pointing up (see figure a). Step back to generate tension on the band.

2. Perform a horizontal row, and then at the halfway point of the motion, externally rotate the shoulders until the upper arms are slightly below parallel to the floor (see figure b).

3. Slowly reverse the motion and repeat.

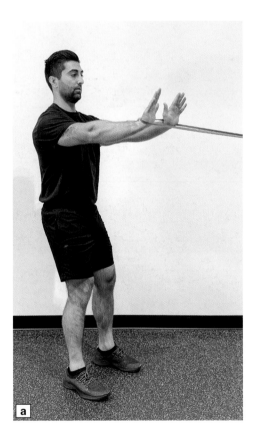
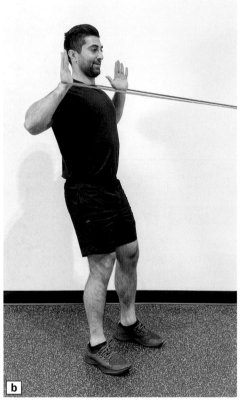

ADVANTAGE

The face pull improves shoulder integrity by simultaneously strengthening the external rotators and scapular retractors.

COACHING CUE

This exercise can also be performed by looping the band through the clip of a cable with the pulley set at a lower chest height. The cable will extend toward you as you pull the band closer to your body.

One-Arm Band Face Pull

This version of the face pull provides three important benefits. First, it's great for people who don't have access to a band that's strong enough to challenge them during the two-arm version. Second, it can be used as a rehabilitation exercise for one shoulder. Third, the one-arm version helps identify imbalances between the right and left shoulder complex.

HOW TO DO IT

1. Loop a long resistance band across the back of your right wrist with the palm facing forward, fingers spread and pointing up. Stand tall with your right arm held in front and parallel to the floor. Place your left palm on your abdomen (see figure a).

2. Perform a horizontal row, and then at the halfway point of the motion, externally rotate the right shoulder until the upper arm is slightly below parallel to the floor (see figure b).

3. Slowly reverse the motion for the desired reps, then switch to the left hand and repeat.

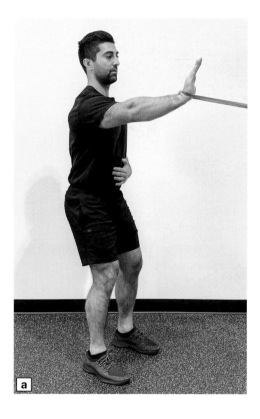
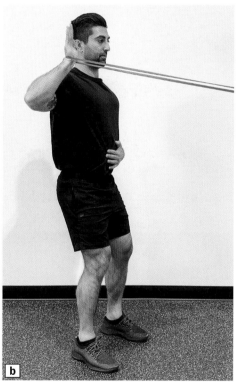

ADVANTAGES

- This variation allows you to work one shoulder at a time, which can be beneficial during rehabilitation or to identify imbalances between the right and left shoulder.
- It provides a loading progression when minimal bands are available.

COACHING CUE

This exercise can also be performed by gripping the handle of a cable with the pulley set at a lower chest height.

Kettlebell Bent-Over Row

The traditional bent-over row is usually performed with a barbell using an overhand grip. However, people often use excessive load and poor form, which places strain on the lumbar discs. Here you'll use a single kettlebell, providing three benefits. First, you pull it from between your legs instead of in front of the knees, decreasing stress on your low back. Second, since it's only one kettlebell, it's less likely to be too heavy to row with proper form. Third, holding the kettlebell by the horns is great for building your biceps.

▶ HOW TO DO IT

1. Stand with your feet slightly wider than shoulder width while holding a kettlebell by the horns, down in front at arm's length (see figure a). Push your hips back, slightly bend your knees, and shift your trunk forward until it's 45 degrees relative to the ground. Slightly arch your low back.

2. Squeeze your glutes, brace your abs, and then bend your elbows and pull the kettlebell, without shrugging your shoulders, until it touches your midsection (see figure b).

3. Lower under control and repeat.

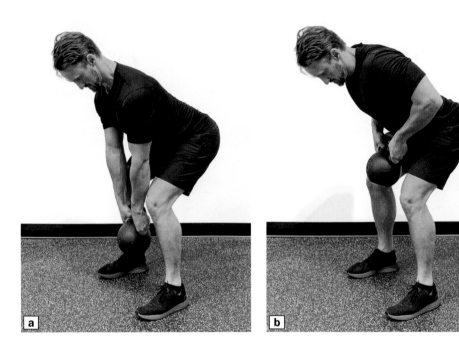

ADVANTAGES

- Using a kettlebell emphasizes development of the biceps while strengthening the upper back.
- This is a good row variation for people who don't have many kettlebells.

COACHING CUE

If you feel strain in your low back, elevate your trunk to a slightly more vertical position.

VERTICAL PULL VARIATIONS

The pull-up is a foundational strength exercise that helps balance strength and muscle development in the upper body. For decades, the pull-up has been an effective measure of upper body pulling strength for the military, gymnastics, and extreme fitness groups. To be clear, a pull-up is performed with an overhand or hammer grip. Conversely, the classic chin-up is performed with an underhand grip (i.e., palms facing you) on a straight bar. That exercise is purposely omitted from this section because of the stress it places on the elbows. The ideal way to perform a chin-up is with gymnastics rings that allow your wrists to move freely, thus reducing stress on your elbows.

MUSCLES WORKED:

forearms

biceps

latissimus dorsi

rear deltoid

rhomboid

middle trapezius

stabilizing muscles of the shoulder girdle and abdomen

Overhand-Grip Pull-Up

The pull-up has long been touted as the "king" of upper body exercise by athletes, bodybuilders, and military personnel. It simultaneously strengthens your grip, biceps, upper back, lats, and abdominals.

HOW TO DO IT

1. Use an overhand grip, with your hands slightly wider than shoulder width. Hang with your arms fully extended, but keep your shoulders pulled down, away from your ears (see figure a).
2. Bend your elbows and pull up until your chin clears the bar; squeeze your shoulder blades together (see figure b).
3. Slowly reverse the motion and repeat.

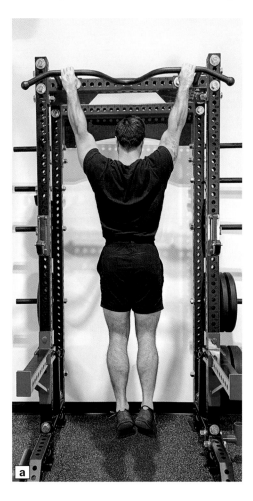 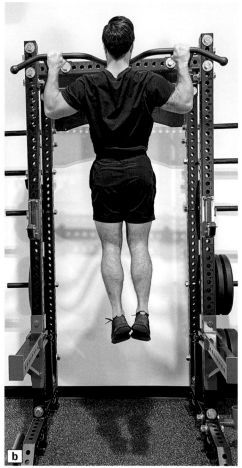

ADVANTAGE

The pull-up simultaneously strengthens and builds the grip, biceps, upper back, latissimus dorsi, and abdominals.

COACHING CUES

- To make it easier, place one foot on a chair in front of you to provide leg drive for assistance.
- To make it harder, add weight to a chin/dip belt or hold a dumbbell vertically between your feet.

Overhand-Grip Pull-Down

The overhand-grip pull-down is a good vertical pulling option for people who have access to a high pulley. It is also ideal for lifters who don't have the strength to perform a pull-up, even with assistance from leg drive.

HOW TO DO IT

1. Grab the bar with a slightly wider than shoulder-width grip, then sit on the seat with the pads resting against the top of your thighs. Extend your arms without shrugging your shoulders, and lean your torso back slightly (see figure a).
2. Pull the bar down until the tops of your knuckles are below your chin; squeeze your shoulder blades together (see figure b).
3. Slowly extend your arms back to the starting position and repeat.

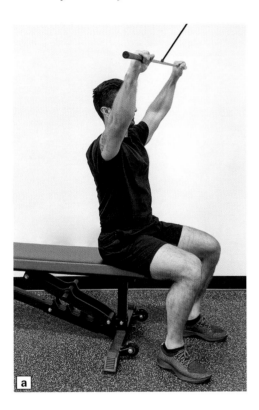
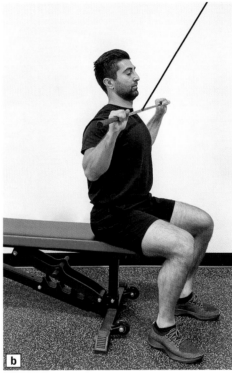

ADVANTAGE

The pull-down is a good vertical pulling option for people who don't have the strength to perform a pull-up.

COACHING CUES

- Avoid pulling the bar to your chest to reduce strain on the anterior shoulders.
- Never pull the bar behind your head since it places unnecessary stress on the shoulders.

Hammer-Grip Pull-Up

The hammer-grip pull-up is naturally the strongest vertical pulling variation for almost everyone, thanks to the ideal line of pull on the biceps when your palms are facing each other. This also means the hammer-grip version is excellent for biceps development.

HOW TO DO IT

1. Grip the handles with your palms facing each other and arms fully extended. Keep your shoulders pulled down, away from your ears (see figure a).
2. Bend your elbows and pull up until your chin clears your knuckles; squeeze your shoulder blades together (see figure b).
3. Slowly reverse the motion and repeat.

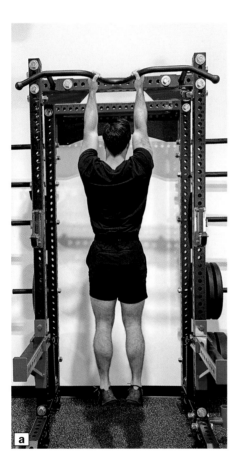
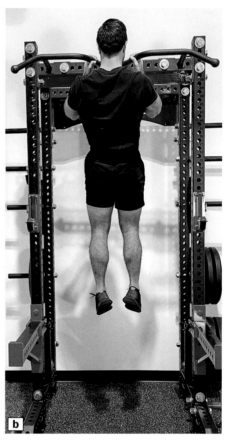

ADVANTAGES

- This grip provides the naturally strongest vertical pulling pattern.
- It activates the biceps more than an overhand grip.

COACHING CUES

- To make it easier, place one foot on a chair in front of you to provide leg drive for assistance.
- To make it harder, add weight to a chin/dip belt or hold a dumbbell vertically between your feet.
- Some pull-up devices have hammer handles that are wider or narrower than what's shown in the photos, which is perfectly fine.

Hammer-Grip Pull-Down

Performing a pull-down with a hammer grip provides three benefits. First, it increases activation of the biceps, making it an excellent arm builder. Second, it's less stressful on the shoulders than an overhand grip. Third, your arm position allows the lats to fully stretch, which is beneficial for shoulder mobility. This is the ideal vertical pulling exercise for people who lack the strength to perform a hammer-grip pull-up.

HOW TO DO IT

1. Attach the V-shaped handle to the highest pulley. Grip the handle with your palms facing each other, then sit on the seat with the pads resting against the top of your thighs. Extend your arms without shrugging your shoulders, and lean your torso back slightly (see figure a).
2. Pull the handle down until the tops of your knuckles are lower than your chin; squeeze your shoulder blades together (see figure b).
3. Slowly extend your arms back to the starting position and repeat.

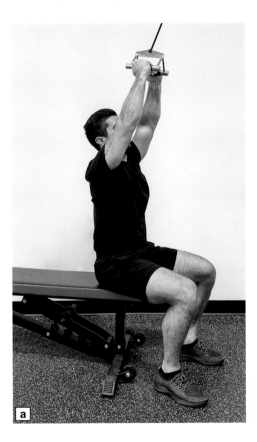
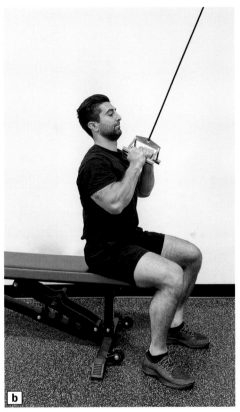

ADVANTAGES

- This variation increases activation of the biceps.
- It improves mobility of the lats.

COACHING CUE

Avoid pulling the handle to your chest to reduce strain on the anterior shoulders.

Rings Pull-Up

Using the rings for this exercise creates a shoulder- and elbow-friendly pull-up variation. Your wrists can move freely, which decreases strain on the elbows. That, in turn, decreases strain on the shoulder joints. Many of my athletes who suffer from elbow or shoulder pain with standard pull-ups can perform this version without pain.

HOW TO DO IT

1. Place the rings shoulder-width apart. Grip the handles with your palms facing each other and arms fully extended (see figure a). Keep your shoulders pulled down, away from your ears.
2. Bend your elbows and pull up until your chin clears your knuckles (see figure b).
3. Slowly reverse the motion and repeat.

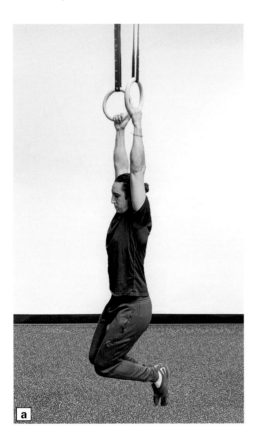
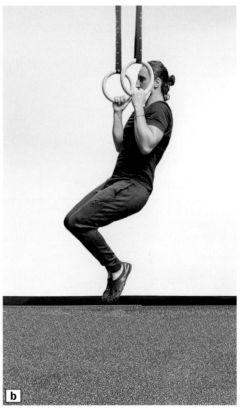

ADVANTAGE

The rings allow the wrists to move freely, decreasing strain on the elbows and shoulders.

COACHING CUES

- For variety, hold your hands in different positions from workout to workout or month to month. Rotate between your palms facing in, facing forward, or facing you.
- To increase the load, add weight to a chin/dip belt or hold a dumbbell vertically between your feet.

Rings L-Sit Pull-Up

This challenging exercise takes all the advantages of a rings pull-up and adds a few more. Lifting the legs to the L-sit position strengthens the hip flexors and lower abdominal region. The L-sit also requires greater activation of the lats and shoulder stabilizers to maintain proper posture.

HOW TO DO IT

1. Place the rings shoulder-width apart. Grip the handles with your palms facing each other and arms fully extended (see figure a). Keep your shoulders pulled down, away from your ears. Perform a straight leg raise until both legs are parallel to the ground.

2. Bend your elbows and pull up until your chin clears your knuckles (see figure b). The legs remain parallel to the ground throughout the movement.

3. Slowly reverse the motion and repeat.

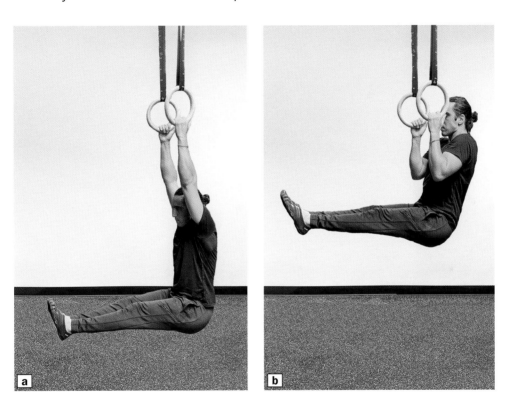

ADVANTAGE

This variation increases muscle activation of the hip flexors and lower abdominal region.

COACHING CUE

If this version is too difficult, lift your legs to parallel and then lower at the top position of the pull-up instead of holding them elevated throughout the set.

Straight-Arm Lat Pull-Down

The straight-arm lat pull-down is a shoulder-friendly way to increase the size and strength of your lats. It is also an excellent exercise to strengthen the anterior core. The combined lat and anterior core activation makes it an ideal exercise to perform before a deadlift since you'll be able to lift a heavier load with less stress on the lumbar spine.

HOW TO DO IT

1. Loop one end of a long resistance band over a secure structure higher than your head. Loop the other end under your palms, and stand with your feet slightly wider than shoulder-width apart. Push your hips back and bend your knees slightly to shift your trunk forward to around 70 degrees relative to the floor. Hold your arms parallel to the floor, slightly wider than shoulder width (see figure a).
2. Brace your abs, squeeze your glutes, and then pull your arms down until your palms are just outside your thighs (see figure b).
3. Slowly elevate your arms back to the starting position and repeat.

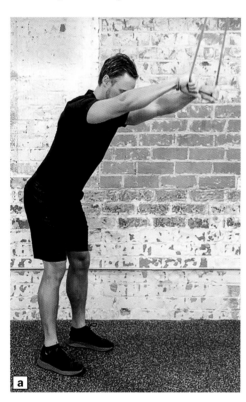 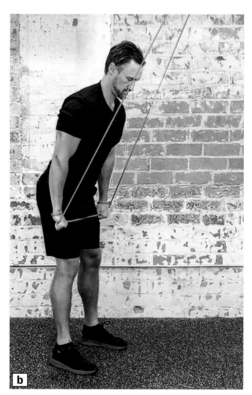

ADVANTAGES

- This is a shoulder-friendly way to build the lats.
- It strengthens the anterior core muscles.

COACHING CUES

- Keep your arms locked straight throughout the movement.
- A band is the preferable choice for this exercise since it accommodates resistance, meaning the resistance is lowest where you're weakest (top position) and highest where you're strongest (palms close to thighs).
- This exercise can be performed with a straight bar attached to a high cable, using the same technique.

Straight One-Arm Lat Pull-Down

This version of a straight-arm lat pull-down provides two benefits. First, you can emphasize one lat at a time to overcome any size or strength imbalances between the right and left side. Second, using one arm increases activation of the lateral core muscles. This exercise is also a good option when your band doesn't provide enough tension for the two-arm version.

HOW TO DO IT

1. Loop one end of a long resistance band over a secure structure higher than your head. Loop the other end under your right palm, and stand with your feet shoulder-width apart. Push your hips back and bend your knees slightly to shift your trunk forward to around 70 degrees relative to the floor. Place your left palm over your abdomen (see figure a).

2. Brace your abs, squeeze your glutes, and then pull your right arm down until your palm is just outside your left thigh (see figure b).

3. Slowly elevate your right arm back to the starting position and repeat for desired reps, then switch to your left arm.

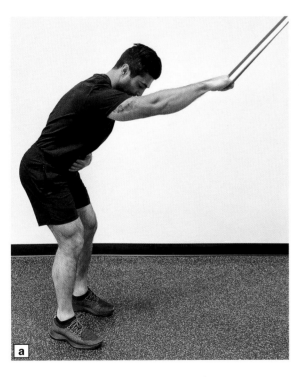
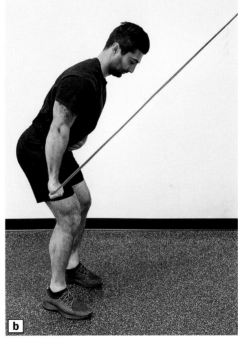

ADVANTAGES

- Using one arm allows you to overcome imbalances between the right and left side.
- It increases activation of the lateral core muscles.

COACHING CUES

- Keep your arm locked straight throughout the movement.
- This exercise can be performed with a cable handle attached to a high pulley.

HORIZONTAL PUSH VARIATIONS

In the classic push-up, you're lifting about two-thirds of your body's weight off the floor on each rep. Raise your feet 24 inches (60 cm) and you're working with 75 percent of your weight. On any push-up variation, you're allowing free movement of the shoulder blades. In many cases, it's optimal to focus on push-up variations to build the upper body horizontal pushing muscles since push-ups are typically less stressful to the shoulder complex, and they strengthen the abdominals to a greater extent than the bench press.

MUSCLES WORKED:

chest

front deltoid

serratus anterior

stabilizing muscles of the shoulder girdle and abdomen

triceps

Push-Up

A push-up has been a mainstay in athletic and military circles for eons. Unlike a standard barbell bench press, the push-up allows your shoulder blades to move freely, which reduces strain on the shoulder joints and increases muscle activation throughout the shoulder complex. Another benefit of a push-up over a bench press is that the anterior core has to work much harder to maintain rigidity from neck to ankles.

HOW TO DO IT

1. Place your hands on the floor slightly wider than your shoulders, arms extended, feet about hip-width apart, and body aligned from neck to ankles (see figure a).
2. Bend your elbows and lower your body as one unit until your chest is near the floor (see figure b).
3. Push back up and repeat.

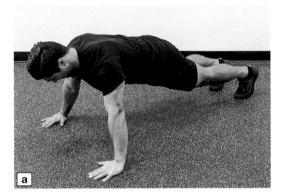
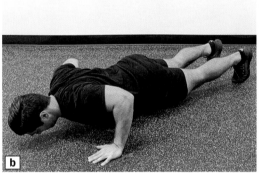

ADVANTAGES

- The push-up allows the shoulder blades to move freely, making it more joint-friendly than a bench press.
- It requires high levels of muscle activation in the anterior core.

COACHING CUE

To progress this exercise, use a long resistance band. Stretch it across your upper back, and loop each end around your palms (see figure c).

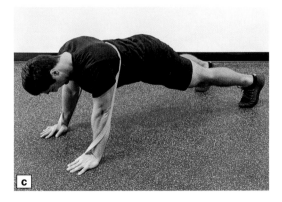

Feet-Elevated Push-Up

The feet-elevated push-up is the first progression from a standard push-up. In this version, your feet will rest on a box or bench, which shifts a greater percentage of your body weight through your shoulders and arms. This exercise also places a greater emphasis on the upper (i.e., clavicular) portion of the pectorals to increase muscle mass in that area.

HOW TO DO IT

1. Get into the top position of a push-up, with your hands on the floor slightly wider than shoulder-width apart (see figure a). Your feet are approximately hip-width apart and resting on a box or step that's up to 24 inches (60 cm) high. Your body is aligned from neck to ankles.
2. Bend your elbows and lower your body as one unit until your chest is near the floor (see figure b).
3. Push back up and repeat.

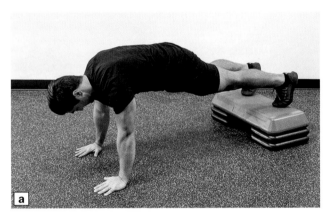

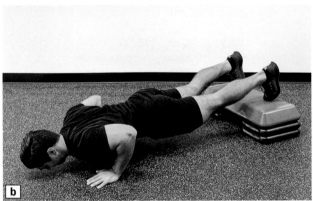

ADVANTAGES

- Elevation shifts a greater percentage of body weight to your chest and shoulders.
- It increases muscle activation of the upper portion of the pectorals.

COACHING CUE

It is common for people to lose stiffness throughout their anterior core. Maintain tension from neck to ankles to prevent any sagging of the midsection.

Dead-Stop Push-Up

A standard push-up starts with your arms fully extended. In this version, you'll start each repetition with your body weight resting on the floor. This eliminates the stretch reflex, causing your muscles to work harder as your body moves away from the floor. Another benefit: You can't cheat this exercise.

HOW TO DO IT

1. Lie face down, with your palms flat on the floor just outside your shoulders and your toes on the floor (see figure a). Your body weight is resting on the floor.
2. Squeeze your glutes, brace your abs, and then explosively push up until your elbows are locked straight (see figure b). Your hands will elevate from the ground if you're very strong.
3. Lower to the starting position of your body resting on the floor, and repeat.

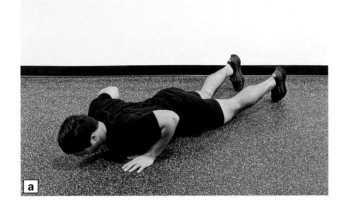

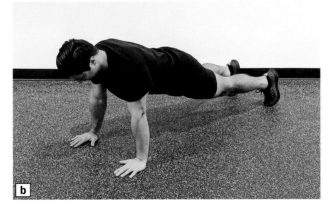

ADVANTAGE

This variation builds starting strength by eliminating the stretch reflex.

COACHING CUE

Maintain tension from neck to ankles while the body rests on the floor between repetitions.

Explosive Push-Up

The explosive push-up is a progression that increases motor unit recruitment throughout the chest, deltoids, and anterior core. It is a challenging exercise, even for the strongest athletes. The key is to push your body away from the floor with maximum effort to achieve the most air possible.

HOW TO DO IT

1. Get into the top position of a push-up, with your hands on the floor slightly wider than shoulder-width apart. Place your feet approximately hip-width apart, with your toes resting on the floor. Your body is aligned from neck to ankles (see figure a).
2. Bend your elbows and lower your body as one unit until your chest is near the floor (see figure b).
3. Squeeze your glutes, brace your abs, and then explosively push up until your elbows are locked straight to elevate your hands (see figure c).
4. Repeat as explosively as possible.

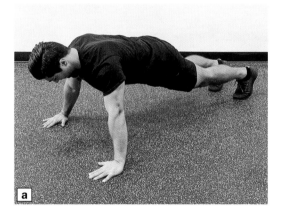
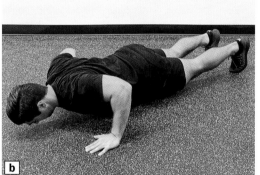

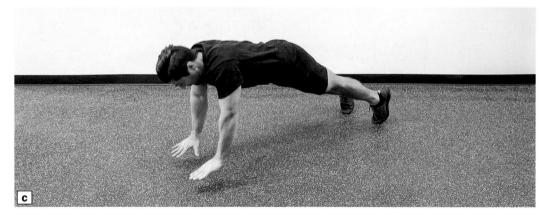

ADVANTAGE

This variation increases muscle activation throughout the chest, deltoids, and anterior core.

COACHING CUE

Some people prefer to perform a clap when their hands are elevated.

Hand Walk Push-Up

A standard push-up builds and strengthens your chest and anterior core, but the hand walk push-up goes far beyond that. Walking your hands from side to side between each push-up strengthens your rotator cuff and anti-rotation core muscles as well. This little-known push-up variation is a terrific progression from a standard push-up.

▶ HOW TO DO IT

1. Get into the top position of a push-up, with your hands on the floor slightly wider than shoulder-width apart. Place your feet approximately hip-width apart, with your toes resting on the floor. Your body is aligned from neck to ankles (see figure a).

2. Bend your elbows and lower your body as one unit until your chest is near the floor (see figure b), and then push up until your elbows are locked straight (see figure c).

3. Next, walk your hands a few feet to the left without rotating your pelvis (see figure d) and perform one push-up.

4. Walk your hands back to the right to the starting position in the center and perform one push-up. Walk your hands a few feet to the right and perform one push-up.

5. Finally, walk your hands a few feet back to the left to the starting position in the center and perform one push-up.

6. This entire cycle is one repetition. Repeat for as many reps as possible, which is usually two to four for most people.

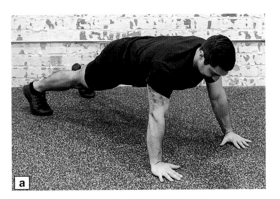

a

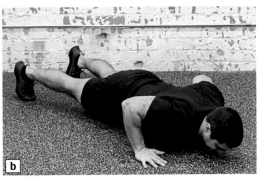

b

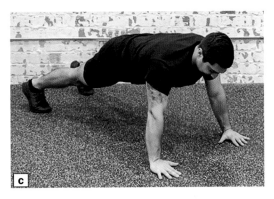

c

ADVANTAGES

- The hand walk increases muscle activation of the rotator cuff and anti-rotation core muscles.
- It builds stability strength throughout the shoulder complex.

COACHING CUE

To increase the difficulty, perform an explosive push-up in each position.

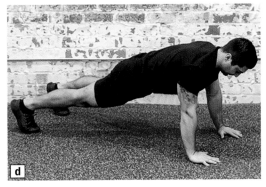

d

165

Rings or Straps Push-Up

Using rings or straps provides an excellent progression for the push-up. The instability of the rings or straps increases muscle activation throughout the core and shoulder complex. And since your wrists can move freely, this variation is more shoulder-friendly than a barbell bench press.

HOW TO DO IT

1. Place rings or straps so the handles are four inches (10 cm) from the floor.
2. Get into the top position of a push-up, with your hands slightly wider than shoulder width and gripping the handles, palms facing your feet (see figure a). Your feet are approximately hip-width apart, with your toes resting on the floor. Your body is aligned from neck to ankles.
3. Squeeze your glutes, brace your abs, and then bend your elbows and lower your body as far as your strength allows (see figure b).
4. Push up until your elbows are locked straight and repeat.

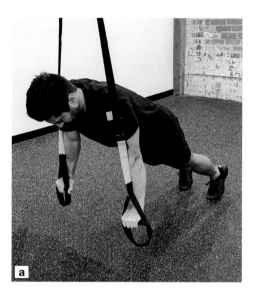 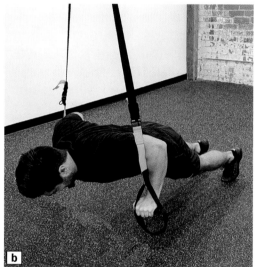

ADVANTAGES

- This variation increases muscle activation throughout the anterior core and shoulder stabilizers.
- The wrists can move freely, which reduces strain on the elbows and shoulders.

COACHING CUE

There is no perfect position for the shoulders and elbows. Perform the motion that feels most natural and stable to your shoulders.

Swiss Ball Push-Up

Performing a push-up from a Swiss ball creates a unique challenge. The instability from the ball requires increased muscle activation throughout the core and shoulder complex. This exercise is also an excellent way to build the triceps when minimal equipment is available.

HOW TO DO IT

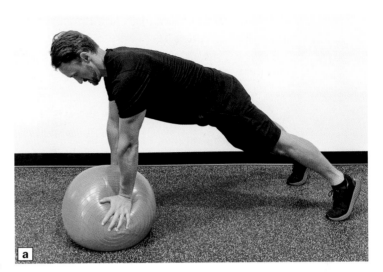

1. Place your hands shoulder-width apart on a large Swiss ball, fingers angled slightly outward. Get into the top position of a push-up with your feet approximately hip-width apart and your toes resting on the floor (see figure a). Your body is aligned from neck to ankles.

2. Squeeze your glutes, brace your abs, and then lower your body until your chest touches the ball, or as far as your strength allows (see figure b).

3. Push up until your elbows are locked straight and repeat.

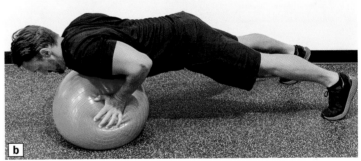

ADVANTAGES

- Performing a push-up on a Swiss ball increases muscle activation throughout the anterior core and shoulder stabilizers.
- This variation emphasizes development of the triceps when free weights aren't available.

COACHING CUE

In the early stages, start with a large, fully inflated ball. As your strength increases, progress to a smaller ball with less air in it.

Dumbbell or Kettlebell Bench Press

Most of us have asymmetries between our left and right shoulders. This means each arm prefers to move in a slightly different pattern during a bench press. With a standard barbell bench press, your wrists are locked into one position, forcing your shoulders to move in a pattern that might not be ideal. Therefore, dumbbells or kettlebells are a more shoulder-friendly option.

HOW TO DO IT

1. Lie on your back on a flat bench with your feet on the floor, shoulder-width apart. Hold the dumbbells or kettlebells shoulder-width apart directly above your chest, palms facing each other, with your elbows locked straight (see figure a).
2. Lower the weights under control to your maximum range of pain-free motion (see figure b).
3. Press the weights back to the starting position and repeat.

ADVANTAGE

The hands can move freely, reducing strain on the wrists, elbows, and shoulders.

COACHING CUES

- Press and lower in a pattern that feels most natural to your shoulders.
- Avoid bringing your hands closer together as you press to maintain tension on the pectorals.

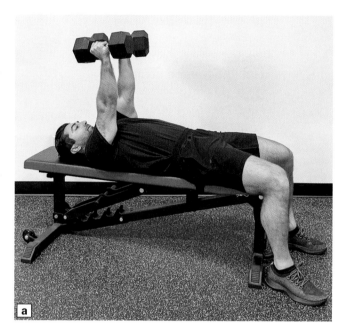
a

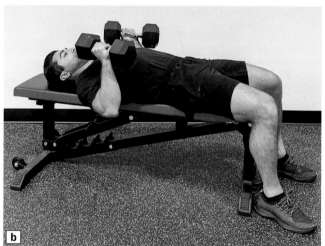
b

Narrow-Grip Bench Press

The narrow-grip bench press is a foundational exercise used by bodybuilders and powerlifters for eons. It is one of the most effective ways to increase the size and strength of your triceps because it can be used with a very heavy load.

HOW TO DO IT

1. Lie on your back on a flat bench, with your feet wide and low back arched. Grip the barbell so your thumbs are the same width as your torso.

2. Unrack the barbell and hold it directly above your chest, with your elbows locked (see figure a).

3. Brace your abs, squeeze your glutes, and lower the barbell until it touches your lower chest (see figure b).

4. Press the barbell back to the starting position, while pushing through your feet as much as possible, and repeat.

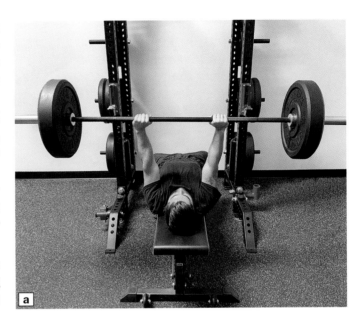

a

ADVANTAGE

You can use a very heavy load, which is excellent for size and strength development of the triceps.

COACHING CUE

Don't use a grip that's narrower than your torso to eliminate unnecessary strain on your wrists.

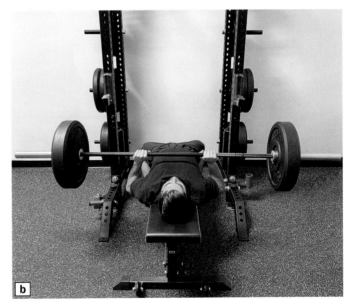

b

Incline Bench Press

The incline bench press adds variety to the horizontal push options. Furthermore, it emphasizes the clavicular portion of the pectorals, which builds the muscle fibers in your upper chest. The key is to use a minimal incline to avoid unnecessary strain on the shoulders.

HOW TO DO IT

1. Adjust the bench to 20 to 30 degrees above parallel, and lie on your back with your feet on the floor, shoulder-width apart. Hold the dumbbells or kettlebells shoulder-width apart directly above your chest, palms facing each other, with your elbows locked straight (see figure a).
2. Lower the weights under control to your maximum range of pain-free motion (see figure b).
3. Press the weights back to the starting position and repeat.

ADVANTAGE

This exercise emphasizes the clavicular portion of the pectorals.

COACHING CUES

- Adhere to the movement pattern that feels most natural to your shoulders.
- For variety, use slightly different incline angles from workout to workout, such as 20 degrees one week and 40 degrees the next week. Avoid incline angles greater than 45 degrees to spare the shoulders.

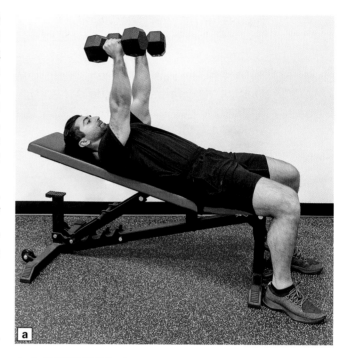

a

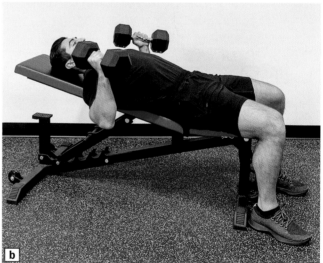

b

One-Arm Cable or Band Chest Press

This shoulder-friendly version of a bench press can be performed with a cable or band. The band works especially well since it accommodates resistance, meaning the band has the most tension where you're naturally strongest and the least where you're naturally weakest.

HOW TO DO IT

1. Adjust the pulley or secure a band at chest height. Grip the pulley or band with your left hand, then step forward with your right leg to get in a split stance (see figure a).
2. Squeeze your glutes, brace your abs, and then press forward until your left elbow is locked straight (see figure b). Repeat for target reps.
3. Switch the cable or band to your right hand, with your left leg forward, and repeat.

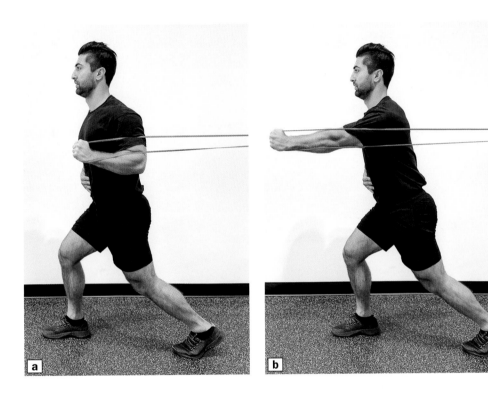

ADVANTAGES

- This variation is less stressful on the shoulders than a barbell bench press.
- It increases activation of the core's anti-rotation muscles.

COACHING CUE

Adhere to the pressing pattern that feels most natural to your shoulder. For some, that means the elbow is close to the torso throughout the pressing pattern.

One-Arm Floor Press

The one-arm floor press is easier on the shoulders than a standard barbell bench press. The floor limits the range of motion you can lower the weight, preventing the most stressful shoulder position of a bench press.

▶ HOW TO DO IT

1. Lie on your back with your knees bent and feet flat on the floor, wider than shoulder width. Hold a dumbbell or kettlebell in your right hand directly above your right shoulder, with your elbow locked straight. Place your left arm on the floor, angled out slightly from your body (see figure a).

2. Squeeze your glutes, brace your abs, and then bend your right elbow and lower the weight until your elbow is resting on the floor (see figure b). Press the weight until your elbow is locked straight. Repeat for target reps.

3. Switch to your left hand and repeat.

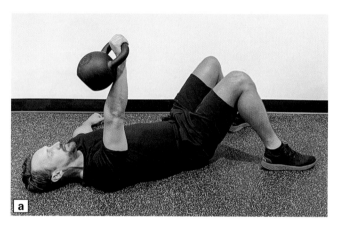

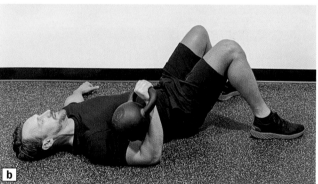

ADVANTAGES

- This variation is less stressful on the shoulders than a barbell bench press.
- It increases activation of the core's anti-rotation muscles.

COACHING CUE

Adhere to the pressing pattern that feels most natural to your shoulder. For some, that means the elbow is close to the torso in the bottom position.

Dip

The dip is often thought of as a triceps exercise since it targets that muscle group with a heavy load. But it's also an effective way to build your chest. The shoulder angle places an emphasis on the sternal portion of the pectorals, which increases the size of the lower half of the chest.

HOW TO DO IT

1. Grip the handles with your hands shoulder-width apart, or slightly wider, palms facing each other. Your arms are fully extended and your traps are as far from your ears as possible (see figure a).

2. Bend your elbows and lower your body through tension in your triceps as your trunk shifts forward. Slowly lower as far as your mobility and strength allow (see figure b).

3. Press up until your elbows are fully locked and repeat.

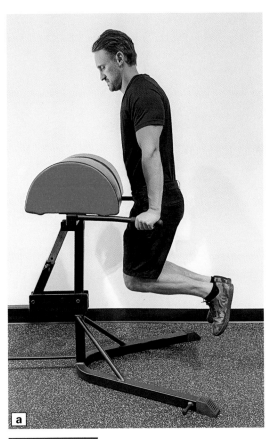 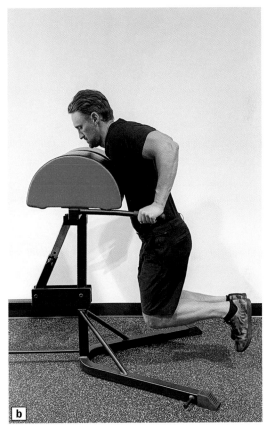

ADVANTAGE

The dip simultaneously increases the size and strength of the triceps and chest.

COACHING CUE

To increase the load, add weight to a chin/dip belt or hold a dumbbell vertically between your feet.

Rings Dip

Using the rings to perform a dip provides two big benefits. First, it allows your wrists to rotate freely, which reduces stress on the elbows and shoulders. Second, the instability of the rings requires greater muscle activation of the lats and shoulder stabilizers.

HOW TO DO IT

1. Set the rings the width of your shoulders. Grip the handles with your hands shoulder-width apart, palms facing each other. Your arms are fully extended and your traps are as far from your ears as possible (see figure a).
2. Bend your elbows and lower your body as your trunk shifts forward. Lower as far as your mobility and strength allow (see figure b).
3. Press up until your elbows are fully locked and repeat.

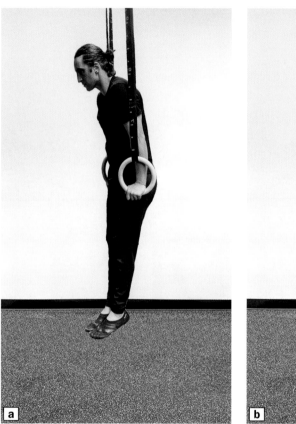 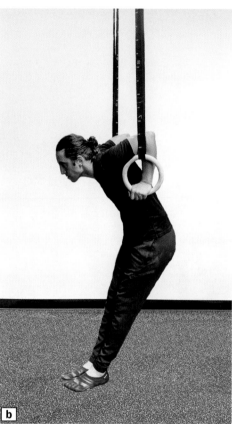

ADVANTAGES

- The wrists can move freely, reducing stress on the elbows and shoulders.
- This variation increases muscle activation of the lats and shoulder stabilizers.

COACHING CUE

To increase the load, add weight to a chin/dip belt.

Rings Dip to L-Sit

This challenging variation of the rings dip is popular among gymnasts who perform the rings event. At the top of the dip you'll lift your legs to parallel, which increases muscle activation throughout the abdomen and shoulder complex.

HOW TO DO IT

1. Set the rings the width of your shoulders. Grip the handles with your hands shoulder-width apart, palms facing each other. Your arms are fully extended and your traps are as far from your ears as possible (see figure a).
2. Bend your elbows and lower your body as your trunk shifts forward. Lower as far as your mobility and strength allow (see figure b).
3. Press up until your elbows are fully locked, and then lift both legs to parallel (see figure c).
4. Lower your legs and repeat.

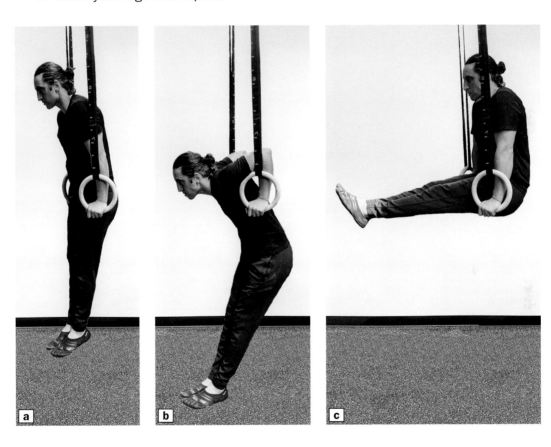

ADVANTAGE

This variation increases activation of the abdominals, hip flexors, and shoulder stabilizers.

COACHING CUES

- In the early stages it's fine to lift your legs as far as your strength allows; increase to the parallel position as your strength increases.
- Move slowly to minimize swinging of your body.
- This exercise can also be performed on a standard dip bar.

175

VERTICAL PUSH VARIATIONS

Lifting weights overhead, with one or two hands, has probably been a part of strength sports for as long as they've existed. The barbell clean and press was part of Olympic weightlifting back in 1928. Since overhead barbell presses can be stressful on your shoulders, many one-arm variations with a dumbbell or kettlebell are recommended.

MUSCLES WORKED:

front and middle deltoids

upper trapezius

stabilizing muscles of the shoulder girdle and abdomen

triceps

Overhead Press

This version of the overhead press—a movement associated with shoulder impingement—is performed with dumbbells or kettlebells. Holding a weight in each hand, instead of a barbell, allows each shoulder to move in its most natural pattern while maintaining integrity of the joints. And using a split stance reduces strain on the low back.

HOW TO DO IT

1. Hold dumbbells or kettlebells against the front of your shoulders, palms facing each other (see figure a). Step your right leg forward about a meter. Bend both knees slightly, and evenly distribute your weight between both feet to create a split stance.
2. Push the weights overhead until the elbows are fully locked (see figure b).
3. Lower under control and repeat for target reps.

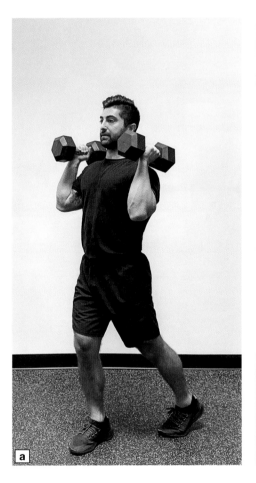
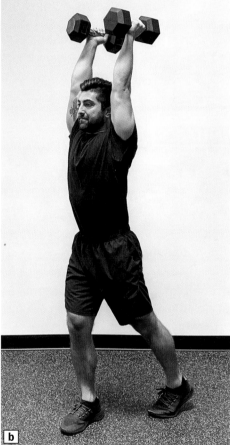

ADVANTAGE

Using dumbbells or kettlebells allows the wrists and arms to move freely, reducing strain on the elbows and shoulders.

COACHING CUE

Avoid any backward lean of the trunk when pressing overhead.

One-Arm Overhead Press

This version of the overhead press also uses dumbbells or kettlebells to reduce strain on the elbows and shoulders. The split stance reduces strain on the low back.

HOW TO DO IT

1. Hold a kettlebell or dumbbell in your left hand at the side of your shoulder, palm facing in (see figure a). Take a step forward with your right foot to get in a split stance, with your toes forward and both knees bent slightly. Extend your right arm to the side for balance.
2. Press the weight straight up until full lockout of the left elbow (see figure b).
3. Lower it and repeat for target reps.
4. Switch the weight to the right hand, put your left foot forward, and repeat.

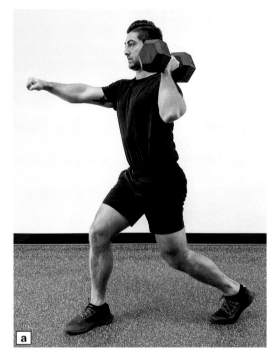

a

ADVANTAGES

- This exercise works more upper back muscles than the back squat, and it also works the biceps.
- It is a good choice for people who lack the wrist mobility necessary for a front squat.
- The Zercher barbell position can be used for a wide variety of exercises including the split squat and lunge variations.

COACHING CUES

- For most lifters, the goal is to lower until the elbows touch the tops of the thighs.
- Keep your chest high, knees wide, and shoulder blades pulled together.

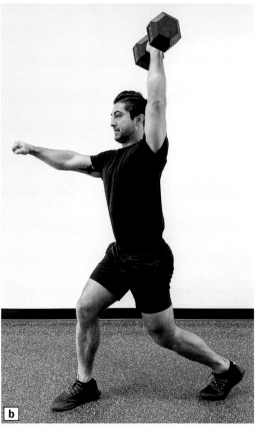

b

One-Arm Overhead Push Press

This version of a one-arm overhead press uses leg drive, which provides two benefits. First, it allows a heavier load to be used. Second, driving from the legs improves full-body strength since you work the legs and upper body simultaneously. This exercise is a favorite among old-school strongman competitors.

▶ HOW TO DO IT

1. Hold a kettlebell or dumbbell in your left hand at the side of your shoulder, palm facing in and elbow tucked tightly to your side. Take a step forward with your right foot to get in a split stance, with your toes forward and both knees bent slightly. Extend your right arm to the side for balance (see figure a).
2. Bend your knees to lower your body four to six inches (10-15 cm) to prepare for the leg drive (see figure b).
3. Push through the center of your feet to straighten both legs as you simultaneously press the weight overhead until your elbow is locked straight (see figure c).
4. Lower under control and repeat for target reps.
5. Switch the weight to the right hand, put your left foot forward, and repeat.

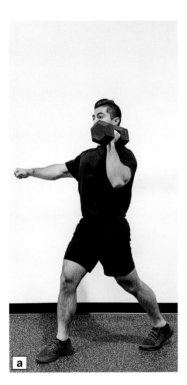
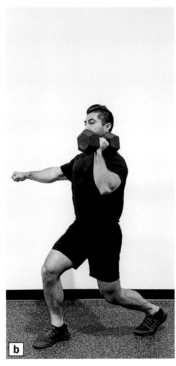
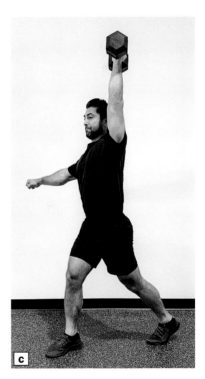

ADVANTAGES

- This exercise builds full-body strength due to simultaneous activation of the upper and lower body.
- It allows for heavier loads than a standard one-arm overhead press.

COACHING CUE

Don't turn this exercise into a split squat. You need to lower your body just a few inches (10-15 cm) to get plenty of leg drive.

Half-Kneeling One-Arm Overhead Press

This variation is performed with one knee resting on the floor, creating a half-kneeling posture. Placing one knee on the floor creates a unique stability challenge for the hip on that side, as well as the abdominals. This variation is also good for people recovering from an ankle or foot injury.

▶ HOW TO DO IT

1. Hold a dumbbell or kettlebell in your left hand in front of your left shoulder, elbow tucked to your side and palm facing in (see figure a). Rest your left knee on a pad, with your right foot forward and knee bent to 90 degrees.
2. Press the weight straight up until full lockout of the elbow (see figure b).
3. Lower under control and repeat for target reps.
4. Switch the weight to your right hand, with the right knee down and your left foot forward, and repeat.

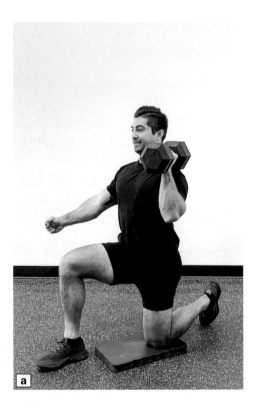
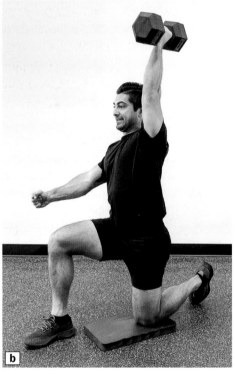

ADVANTAGE

This variation increases muscle activation in the hips and core.

COACHING CUES

- Ninety percent of your weight should be resting on the knee that's down.
- Avoid any lateral shifting of the trunk while pressing overhead.

Ahrens Press

This variation of an overhead press places a greater emphasis on the middle deltoid, which is often neglected during upper body exercises. It was popularized by the late Chuck Ahrens, a Muscle Beach strongman from the 1950s and '60s who had extraordinary shoulder width and was known for displaying incredible feats of strength.

▶ HOW TO DO IT

1. Stand while holding a relatively light dumbbell in each hand. Elevate your arms out to the sides so they're parallel to the ground, elbows bent to 90 degrees and palms facing forward (see figure a).
2. Press the weights up and out at a 45-degree angle until your elbows are locked straight, basically in a V position (see figure b).
3. Lower under control and repeat.

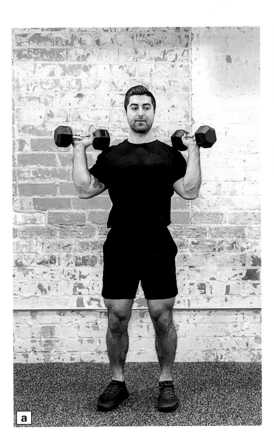
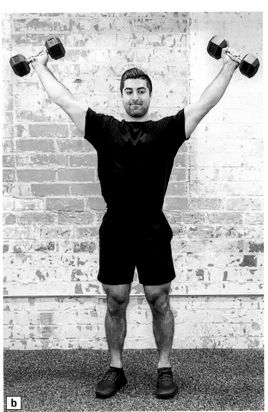

ADVANTAGE

This press variation emphasizes the often neglected middle deltoid.

COACHING CUE

The palms stay facing forward throughout the movement, but allow your wrists to slightly rotate in a pattern that feels most natural.

Inverted Push-Up

The inverted push-up is a body weight exercise that builds and strengthens your vertical pushing muscles. This exercise is good alternative for people who don't have the strength or coordination to do a traditional handstand push-up. Another benefit is the emphasis placed on the triceps, which helps build that muscle group faster than many standard overhead press variations.

▶ HOW TO DO IT

1. Start in the push-up position but with your hips raised as high as possible, hands on the floor wider than shoulder-width apart (see figure a).

2. Bend your elbows and slowly lower your torso down and forward until the top of your head touches the floor (see figure b).

3. Press back to the starting position and repeat.

ADVANTAGE

This push-up variation builds and strengthens the vertical pushing muscles using nothing but your body weight.

COACHING CUES

- Allow your elbows to flare outward during the lowering phase during the early stages of training.

- To increase the difficulty, don't flare your elbows.

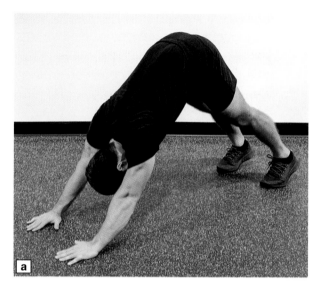

a

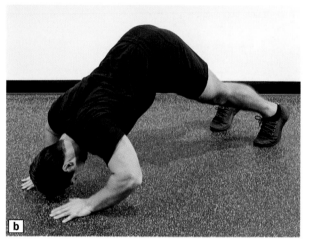

b

Inverted Narrow Push-Up

This version of the inverted push-up provides two benefits. First, it's a simple way to make the inverted push-up more challenging. Second, a narrower hand position puts a greater emphasis on the triceps. A common mistake with this exercise is to perform it with your hands together, which places unnecessary strain on the wrists and elbows.

HOW TO DO IT

1. Start in the push-up position but with your hips raised as high as possible, hands on the floor shoulder-width apart (see figure a).

2. Bend your elbows and slowly lower your torso down and forward until the top of your head touches the floor (see figure b).

3. Press back to the starting position and repeat.

ADVANTAGE

This variation places a greater emphasis on the triceps than a standard inverted push-up.

COACHING CUE

- Avoid flaring your elbows outward during the lowering phase.

- Don't place your hands together in order to minimize strain on your wrists and elbows.

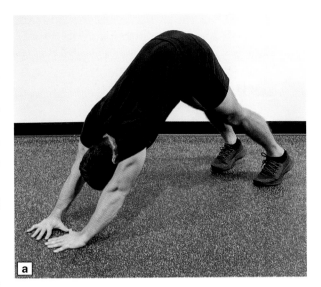
a

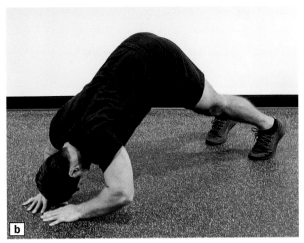
b

Feet-Elevated Inverted Push-Up

The feet-elevated inverted push-up shifts a greater percentage of your body weight to your hands. This makes it an effective body weight progression that builds your deltoids and triceps. Over time, place your feet on a higher box to make it even more challenging.

HOW TO DO IT

1. Start in the push-up position but with your hips raised as high as possible, hands on the floor wider than shoulder-width apart (see figure a). Rest the balls of your feet on a box or step that's up to 24 inches (60 cm) high.
2. Bend your elbows to slowly lower your torso down and forward until the top of your head touches the floor (see figure b).
3. Press back to the starting position and repeat.

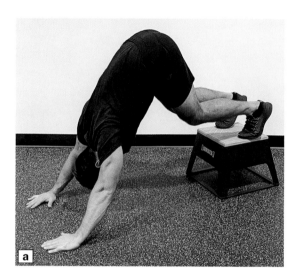 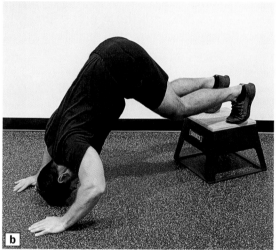

ADVANTAGE

This is a simple body weight progression for the inverted push-up.

COACHING CUE

To increase the difficulty, place your hands closer together and don't flare your elbows.

Rings or Straps Inverted Push-Up

This variation of the inverted push-up uses rings or straps, which provides two benefits. First, your wrists can move freely, reducing strain on your elbows and shoulders. Second, the instability of the rings or straps increases activation of the rotator cuff muscles to stabilize the movement.

HOW TO DO IT

1. Place rings or straps so the handles are four inches (10 cm) from the floor. Grip the handles with palms facing each other, hands slightly wider than shoulder-width apart. Get into the top position of a push-up with your hips held as high as possible (see figure a). Your feet are approximately hip-width apart, toes resting on the floor.
2. Squeeze your glutes, brace your abs, and then bend your elbows to lower your body as far as your strength allows (see figure b).
3. Push up until your elbows are locked straight and repeat.

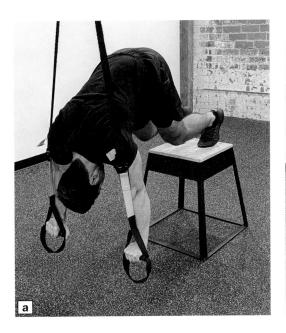
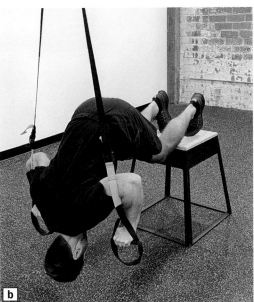

ADVANTAGE

Rings or straps allow your wrists to move freely, reducing strain on your elbows and shoulders.

COACHING CUE

To increase the difficulty, place your feet on a box or step that's up to 24 inches (60 cm) high.

ISOLATION VARIATIONS

The exercises in this section isolate and develop key muscle groups to build a more impressive physique. Some of the exercises are part of your full-body workouts, and others are intended for your targeted HFT plans (more about these in chapter 10).

Biceps Iso-Hold

Guys love to show off their biceps, which is why they'll try countless arm workouts to make them bigger. Furthermore, you would be hard-pressed to find many weekend warriors who are 100 percent satisfied with the size of their guns. You would be just as unlikely to find guys who have put much effort into training their biceps isometrically. But you need only look at gymnasts who perform the rings event to see some powerful empirical evidence that isometric contractions can lead to substantial biceps development. Another benefit of isometrics is their high level of motor unit recruitment.

❯ HOW TO DO IT

1. Grab a kettlebell by the horns and hold it against your chest, elbows bent and tucked to your sides (see figure a). Stand with your feet shoulder-width apart.

2. Brace your abs, squeeze your glutes, and then lower the kettlebell halfway down; hold it in this midposition, with your elbows against the side of your torso (see figure b).

3. Once you reach momentary muscular failure, slowly straighten your arms to end the set.

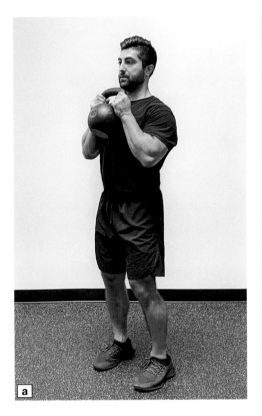
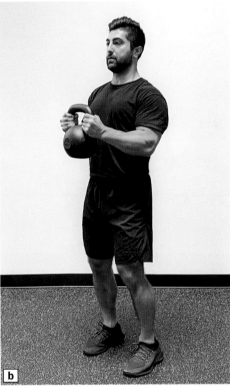

ADVANTAGE

Isometric muscle actions provide a novel stimulus to the biceps through maximum motor unit recruitment.

COACHING CUE

Maintain a chin tuck during the hold to reduce neck strain.

Biceps Curl

It's safe to say that virtually every guy on earth over the age of 16 has performed a biceps curl, often with atrocious form. The key with the biceps curl is to maintain a wrist position that feels as natural as possible to reduce unnecessary stress on the elbows. That is why this version of the curl is performed with dumbbells or kettlebells instead of a standard barbell, which sometimes locks the wrists into a position that stresses the elbow joints.

HOW TO DO IT

1. Stand with a dumbbell or kettlebell in each hand, palms facing forward and elbows against the side of your torso (see figure a).
2. Brace your abs, squeeze your glutes, and then bend your elbows until your palms are six inches (15 cm) in front of your shoulders (see figure b).
3. Slowly straighten your arms while keeping your elbows against your sides and repeat.

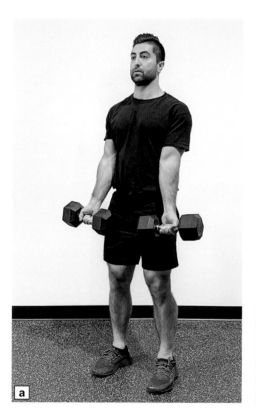 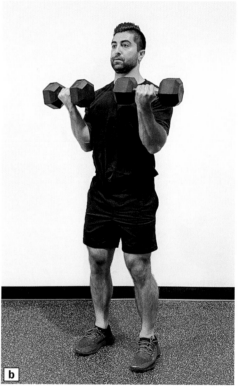

ADVANTAGE

Using dumbbells or kettlebells allows the wrists to maintain a more natural position.

COACHING CUES

- Avoid curling the weights to the highest position to keep tension on the biceps.
- For some, it's better to let the palms slightly rotate inward in the bottom position to reduce strain on the elbows.

Biceps Hammer Curl

The biceps hammer curl is a favorite exercise among many bodybuilders and strongman competitors. This variation of the curl provides two benefits. First, it almost always places less stress on the elbows than a standard curl. Second, most people can use a heavier load. The hammer curl also has great carryover to the pull-up.

HOW TO DO IT

1. Stand with a dumbbell or kettlebell in each hand, palms facing inward and elbows against the side of your torso (see figure a).
2. Brace your abs, squeeze your glutes, and then bend your elbows until your palms are six inches (15 cm) in front of your shoulders (see figure b).
3. Slowly straighten your arms while keeping your elbows against your sides and repeat.

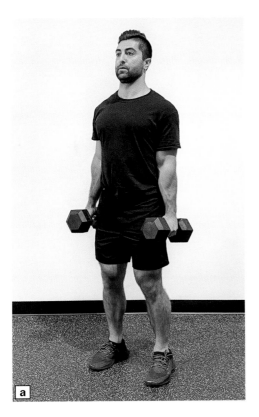 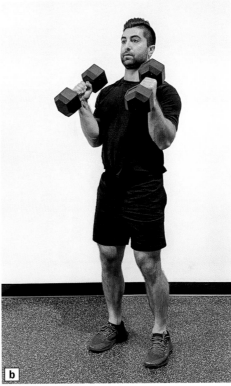

ADVANTAGES

- This is a more elbow-friendly curl variation.
- It has great carryover to the pull-up.

COACHING CUE

Avoid any flaring or forward shifting of the elbows.

Biceps Reverse Curl

Most people train their biceps using a curl with their palms facing up (i.e., standard curl) or facing each other (i.e., hammer curl). However, performing an arm curl with the palms facing down provides two benefits. First, it increases activation of the wrist extensors, which get neglected by traditional presses and pulls. Second, the reverse curl targets the brachialis that sits under the biceps. Taken together, the reverse curl helps you increase the size of your forearms and upper arms.

HOW TO DO IT

1. Stand with a dumbbell or kettlebell in each hand, palms facing behind you and elbows against the side of your torso (see figure a).
2. Brace your abs, squeeze your glutes, and then bend your elbows until your forearms are six inches (15 cm) in front of your shoulders (see figure b).
3. Slowly straighten your arms while keeping your elbows against your sides and repeat.

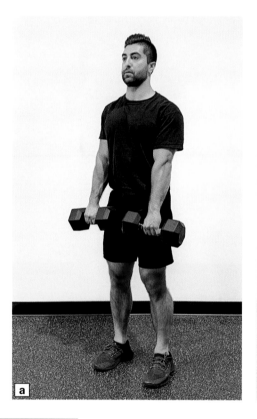
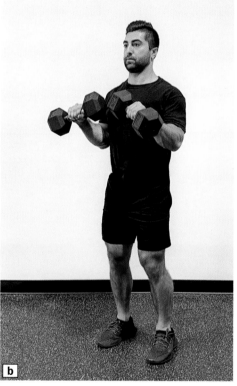

ADVANTAGE

This variation targets the wrist extensors and brachialis muscles.

COACHING CUES

- Avoid any flaring or forward shifting of the elbows.
- This exercise can also be performed with an EZ-curl bar.

One-Arm Band Biceps Curl

For eons, professional bodybuilders have extolled the virtues of training their biceps one arm at a time. It helps them improve the mind–muscle connection between the brain and biceps, which in turn can lead to greater motor unit recruitment and growth. Using a band provides a simple way to perform this exercise almost anywhere, plus it allows people to focus on just one biceps, if it happens to be asymmetrical to the other arm.

◉ HOW TO DO IT

1. Hold one end of a long resistance band in your left palm, and loop the other end under your right foot. Stand with your feet hip-width apart, with the band under your left foot. Hold your left arm down at your side, palm facing forward (see figure a). Place your right palm on your abdomen.

2. Bend your left elbow as far as possible, while holding it against your side, and squeeze your biceps when your left arm is in front of your left shoulder (see figure b).

3. Slowly return to the starting position and repeat for target reps.

4. Switch the band to your right hand with it looped around your left foot and repeat.

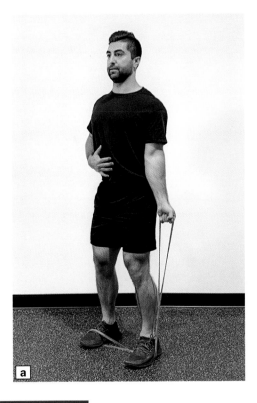
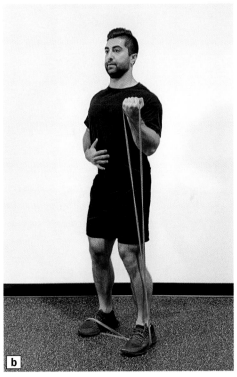

ADVANTAGES

- Using a band increases the mind–muscle connection between the brain and biceps.
- It can be performed anywhere.

COACHING CUES

- The band tension should be sufficient to induce momentary muscular failure by the last repetition.
- Avoid flaring the elbow or allowing it to move forward as the elbow flexes.

Lying Triceps Extension

The lying triceps extension has long been a staple strength move for powerlifters. That's because this exercise strengthens the triceps in a way that has great carryover to the bench press. The problem is that many lifters butcher the form because they're trying to lift an excessively heavy load.

HOW TO DO IT

1. Lie on your back on the floor or a flat bench. Hold a dumbbell or kettlebell in each hand, with your arms fully extended above your chest, palms facing each other (see figure a).
2. Bend your elbows without letting them flare outward, and slowly lower the weights (see figure b).
3. Straighten your elbows until they're locked straight and repeat.

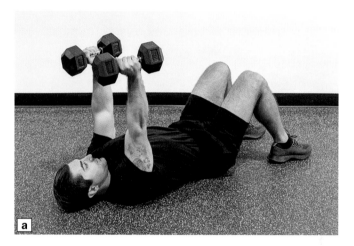

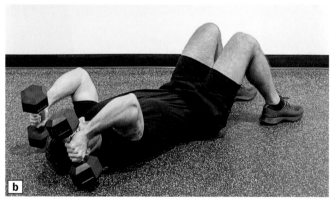

ADVANTAGE

The lying triceps extension has great carryover to pushing exercises.

COACHING CUES

- Avoid any flaring of the elbows during the movement.
- This exercise can also be performed with an EZ-curl bar or by gripping the horns of a single kettlebell.

Overhead Triceps Extension

The overhead triceps extension is beneficial for overall development of the triceps because it trains that muscle group in its fully stretched position. This provides a novel stimulus to the muscle. Another benefit of this exercise is the emphasis it puts on the long medial head of the triceps.

HOW TO DO IT

1. Stand and hold a dumbbell upright and overhead with both hands, with your arms fully extended (see figure a).
2. Bend your elbows while keeping them close to the sides of your head to lower the weight under control (see figure b).
3. Straighten your arms and repeat.

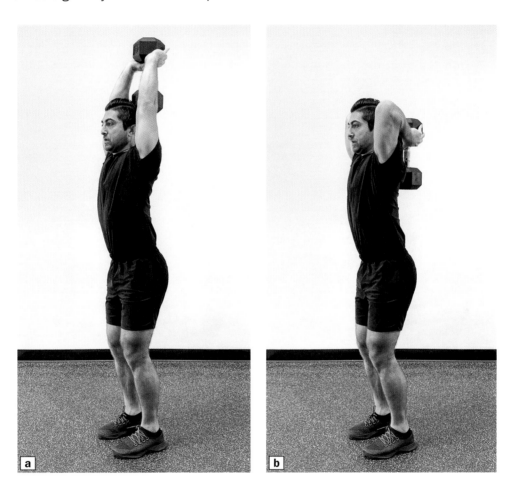

ADVANTAGE

This exercise emphasizes the long (i.e., inner) head of the triceps.

COACHING CUE

This exercise can also be performed with an EZ-curl bar or by gripping the horns of a single kettlebell.

Triceps Press-Down

The triceps press-down trains all three heads of the triceps muscle but emphasizes the lateral head, which helps give the "horseshoe" look when viewed from the side. Performing this exercise with a cable set on the high pulley position is a good option, but a band is even better. Using a band matches the strength curve of the movement, meaning the band has the most tension where you're naturally strongest (i.e., arms straight) and the least tension where you're naturally weakest (i.e., elbows flexed).

HOW TO DO IT

1. Loop one end of a long resistance band over a secure structure higher than your head. Loop the other end under your palms. Stand 12 inches (30 cm) away from the overhead attachment, push your hips back, and slightly bend your knees. Start with your elbows fully bent, next to the sides of your trunk, and your palms facing down (see figure a).
2. Straighten your elbows until full lockout, and squeeze the triceps (see figure b).
3. Slowly return to the starting position, keeping your elbows against the sides of your torso, and repeat.

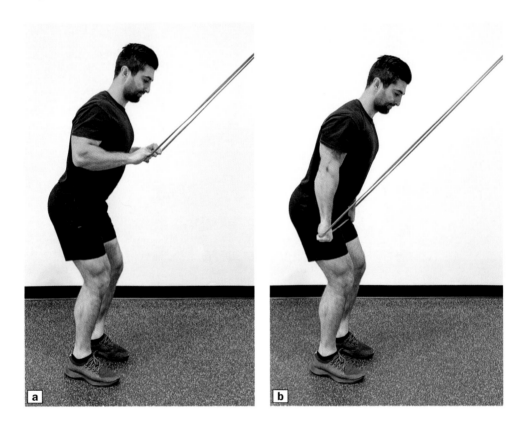

ADVANTAGE

This exercise emphasizes the lateral head of the triceps, which helps create a "horseshoe" shape.

COACHING CUE

Keep your elbows against the side of your trunk throughout the movement. People will often let their elbows shift forward when the arms are bent.

One-Arm Band Triceps Press-Down

It is common for people to have imbalanced development between the right and left arm. Performing the triceps press-down one arm at a time allows you to target the side that's smaller, if that's an issue. For those with equal development, the one-arm version helps increase the mind–muscle connection.

HOW TO DO IT

1. Loop one end of a long resistance band over a secure structure higher than your head. Loop the other end under your right palm (see figure a). Stand 12 inches (30 cm) away from the overhead attachment with your feet hip-width, push your hips back slightly, and place your left hand on your abdomen.
2. Straighten your right elbow to lockout, and squeeze the triceps (see figure b).
3. Slowly return to the starting position and repeat for target reps.
4. Switch the band to your left hand, place your right hand on your abdomen, and repeat.

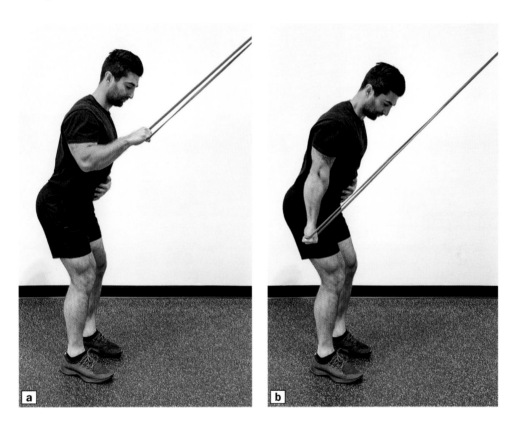

ADVANTAGE

This variation improves the mind–muscle connection with the triceps.

COACHING CUE

Keep your elbow against the side of your trunk throughout the movement.

One-Arm Band Fly

The one-arm band fly is an excellent way to build your chest for three reasons. First, it overloads the pectorals with minimal strain on the shoulder joint. Second, the exercise matches the strength curve of that movement, meaning the band tension is highest where you're naturally strongest (i.e., arm in front of the torso). Third, it can be performed anywhere, as long as you find a secure place to wrap the band.

HOW TO DO IT

1. Loop one end of a long resistance band around a secure structure at chest height. Loop the other end around your left palm. Stand to the side of the band with your right leg in front, your weight equally distributed through both feet. Hold your left arm out to the side, parallel to the floor (see figure a). Place your right palm on your abdomen.

2. Brace your abs, squeeze your glutes, and then pull your left arm across the front of your body until it's perpendicular to your torso (see figure b).

3. Slowly return your arm to the starting position, keeping it straight, and repeat for target reps.

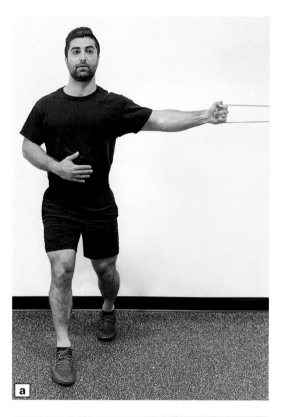

a

ADVANTAGES

- This shoulder joint–friendly variation builds the pectorals.
- It can be performed almost anywhere.

COACHING CUES

- For some, a little elbow flexion in the working arm helps them develop more tension in the chest.
- Focus on achieving an intense peak contraction when the working arm is in front of the torso.

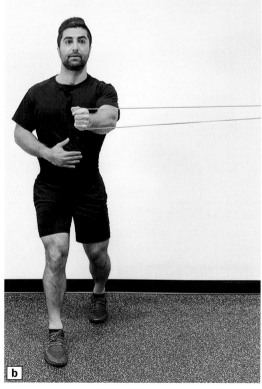

b

Lateral Raise

The deltoid muscle wraps from the front to the back of your shoulder. Traditional upper body pushing exercises target the anterior fibers, while upper body pulls work the posterior fibers. What is missing, however, is an exercise that builds the middle fibers. The lateral raise is the ideal solution since it's one of the few exercises that target those middle fibers, which in turn helps widen your shoulders.

HOW TO DO IT

1. Stand tall with a light dumbbell or kettlebell in each hand, arms hanging down at your sides. Turn your palms so they face inward, and hold your hands 12 inches (30 cm) away from your thighs (see figure a).
2. Make a double chin and slowly elevate your arms until they're parallel to the floor (see figure b).
3. Slowly lower to the starting position and repeat.

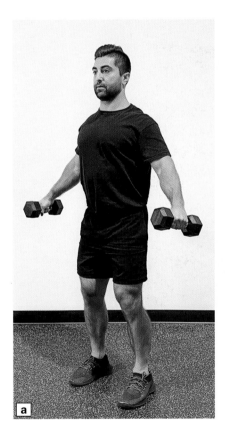
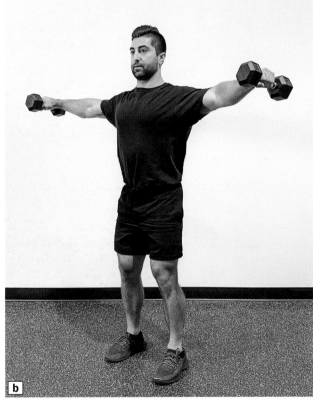

ADVANTAGE

This exercise targets the middle deltoid to help widen your shoulders.

COACHING CUES

- Lower your arms no farther than 12 inches (30 cm) from your thighs to maintain tension on your deltoids.
- Avoid performing this exercise with a band because its tension is highest where you're weakest (i.e., arms parallel to floor).
- It's essential to maintain a double chin (i.e., chin tuck) to avoid neck strain.

One-Arm Lateral Raise

ISOLATION

The one-arm lateral raise targets the middle deltoid. Performing the exercise one arm at a time is often a better option for people who get neck strain from the two-arm version. This variation is also harder to cheat, which is beneficial for building the mind–muscle connection.

▶ HOW TO DO IT

1. Stand tall with a light dumbbell or kettlebell in your left hand, arm hanging down at your sides. Hold your hand 12 inches (30 cm) away from the outside of your left thigh with your palm facing your outer thigh (see figure a). Place your right hand on your abdomen.
2. Make a double chin and slowly elevate your left arm until it's parallel to the floor (see figure b). Slowly lower to the starting and repeat for target reps.
3. Switch the weight to your right hand and repeat.

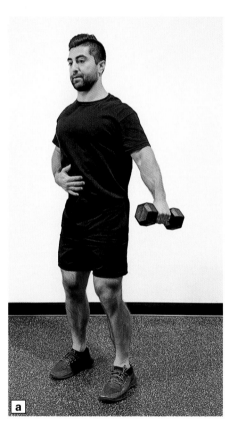
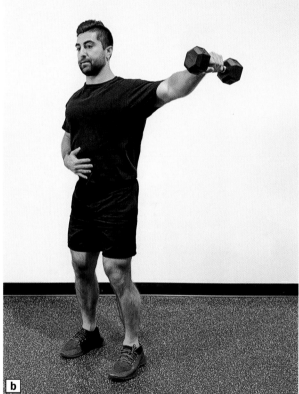

ADVANTAGES

- This is a neck-friendly variation for strengthening and building the middle deltoids.
- It is more difficult to cheat, compared with the two-arm version.

COACHING CUES

- Lower your arm no farther than 12 inches (30 cm) from your thigh to maintain tension on your deltoid.
- Avoid performing this exercise with a band because its tension is highest where you're weakest (i.e., arm parallel to floor).

One-Arm Band Shrug

A standing shrug with a barbell or heavy dumbbells has been a staple exercise for athletes and bodybuilders who seek bigger traps. But guys often perform the exercise with too much load, causing poor technique that can lead to neck pain. This version uses a band, and focuses on one side a time, to induce maximal muscle activation with minimal strain on your neck.

► HOW TO DO IT

1. Hold one end of a long resistance band in your left palm, and loop the other end under your right foot. Stand with your feet hip-width apart, with the band under your left foot. Hold your left arm down at your side, palm facing in (see figure a). Push your hips back and slightly bend your knees to angle your trunk slightly forward. Place your right palm on your abdomen.
2. Slowly shrug your left shoulder toward the back of your left ear (see figure b).
3. Slowly return to the starting position and repeat for target reps.
4. Switch the band to your right hand, with it looped around your left foot, and repeat.

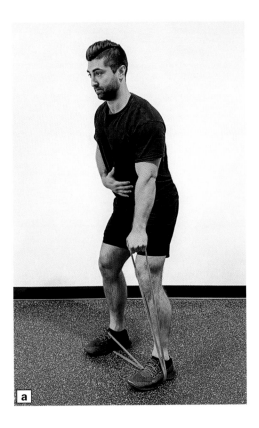
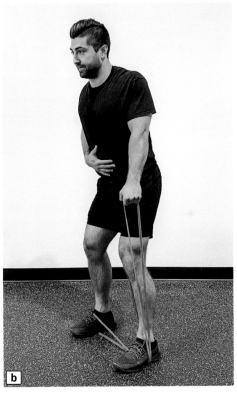

ADVANTAGE

This is a neck-friendly variation for strengthening and building the upper trapezius.

COACHING CUES

- If your band has light tension, perform the exercise with each end of the band looped around your palms and under your feet. Use the same stance, with your hips back and knees slightly bent.
- A band is recommended for convenience, but holding a dumbbell works just as well, if not better.

One-Arm Wrist Extension and Flexion

Almost every guy wants bigger, stronger forearms. There are countless exercises in the gym that challenge your grip, including the pull-up, deadlift, and loaded carry. The problem is that all those exercises challenge your grip exactly the same way: isometrically. And none of them work the wrist extensors, a collection of muscles that pull your knuckles closer to your biceps. Therefore, the wrist extension and flexion movements need to be trained to develop those forearm fibers that other exercises miss. Even the strongest guys can use a relatively light dumbbell for this exercise.

▶ HOW TO DO IT

1. Hold a light dumbbell in your right hand and sit in a chair. Rest your right forearm on the top of your right thigh Lift your knuckles as high as possible while the forearm remains on the armrest (see figure a).

2. Lower your knuckles as far as possible, limiting all motion to the wrist (see figure b), and repeat through a full range of motion until you reach momentary muscular failure.

3. Next, rest the top of your right forearm on the top of your right thigh. Lift your knuckles as high as possible (see figure c).

4. Lower your knuckles as far as possible, limiting all motion to the wrist (see figure d), and repeat through a full range of motion until you reach momentary muscular failure.

5. Switch the dumbbell to your left hand and repeat the sequence.

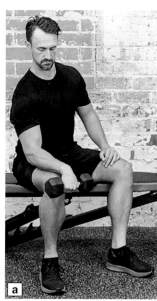
a

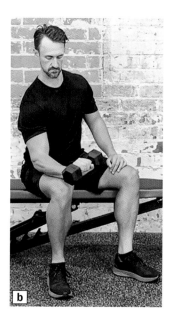
b

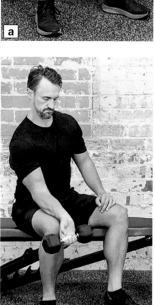
c

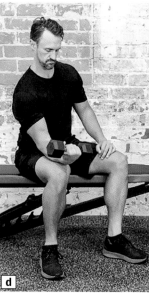
d

ADVANTAGE

These exercises strengthen and build the forearm fibers that upper body pulls, deadlifts, and loaded carries neglect.

COACHING CUES

- Use a load that's light enough to work through a full range of motion.
- When training the wrist flexors with the palm up, some people prefer to let their fingers open as the hand moves closer to the floor in order to achieve a greater range of motion.
- For some, it's more comfortable to perform these exercises with your forearm in front of your torso, resting at an inward angle on a table.

PART III

MUSCLE PROGRAMMING

CHAPTER 8

Muscle-Building Programs

In chapter 3 we cover the rules for building muscle. Those principles and other important factors help you get the most out of the following muscle-building programs. This chapter covers the components of designing workouts that maximize the principles for muscle and strength development. It also discusses ways to perform your sets; how to structure those sets; and how to choose the right exercises, loads, and frequency.

Structuring Your Workout to Build Muscle

As mentioned throughout this book, full-body training is the preferred workout structure because it stimulates the greatest amount of muscle building. It is also the most efficient, meaning it requires the fewest workouts per week to achieve the greatest frequency per muscle group. Perform a dynamic warm-up (see chapter 3) before any of the workouts in this chapter. When your body is ready, perform the first exercise.

Exercise Movement Patterns

It is generally accepted that an upper body pull (e.g., row) is less stressful on the shoulder joint than an upper body push (e.g., bench press). Therefore, your first exercise in these workouts will be an upper body pull, which increases blood flow to the shoulder joint and better prepares it for the upper body push that follows. After the upper body push you'll perform a lower body–dominant exercise. This makes up the three necessary movement patterns for a full-body workout:

- Upper body pull movement
- Upper body push movement
- Lower body–dominant movement

You can, and often should, add more exercises that stimulate other muscle groups you're trying to build—those lagging body parts that could use some extra volume. We cover that later in this chapter. For now, let's continue with the basic full-body workout structure.

Circuit or Straight Sets

Let's say you perform four sets for each of the three aforementioned movements. You could perform straight sets, which means you perform all four sets of the upper body pull before all four sets of the upper body push and then finish with the lower body movement. On the other hand, you could perform those sets in a circuit: one set of the upper body pull, then one set of the upper body push, and then one set of the lower body movement. You would perform that circuit for four rounds, equaling four sets of each exercise.

Research demonstrates that at least 3 minutes of rest before repeating an exercise is recommended to maximize strength and muscle development (Schoenfeld et al. 2016). Therefore, if you performed straight sets you would need to rest at least 3 minutes between each of the four sets to achieve a complete rest period (i.e., complete recovery). Let's say your first exercise is a pull-up that takes 20 seconds to complete for each set. That means you'll perform no activity for 9 minutes just to finish those four sets, as shown in table 8.1.

TABLE 8.1   Time Spent on an Upper Body Pull Exercise With Straight Sets

Movement	Duration (min)
Upper body pull	00:20
Rest	03:00
Upper body pull	00:20
Rest	03:00
Upper body pull	00:20
Rest	03:00
Upper body pull	00:20
Rest: move to upper body push	01:00
Time spent resting	*09:00*
Time spent lifting	*00:80*
Total duration	*10:20*

The problem of inactivity gets even worse when you look at the entire workout. Let's say you need 60 seconds to move to the next exercise. That means the entire workout, from the first set of the upper body pull to the last set of the lower body movement, will take 33 minutes, with 29 of those minutes being *inactivity*, as shown in table 8.2. Put another way: Your workout lasts around a half hour, but only 4 minutes are spent lifting. That might be good for your social life in the gym, but it would be bad for your time management. Indeed, straight sets with complete rest periods are a very inefficient and time-consuming way to train.

TABLE 8.2   Time to Completion for a Full-Body Workout With Straight Sets

Movement	Duration (min)
Upper body pull: 4 sets × 20 sec × 3 min rest	10:20
Rest: move to upper body push	01:00
Upper body push: 4 sets × 20 sec × 3 min rest	10:20
Rest: move to lower body movement	01:00
Lower body movement: 4 sets × 20 sec × 3 min rest	10:20
Time spent resting	*29:00*
Time spent lifting	*04:00*
Total workout duration	*33:00*

With a circuit format you choose rest periods that allow at least 3 minutes before repeating an exercise, just like the example with straight sets. That means you need approximately 50 seconds' rest between each movement to get 3 minutes of rest before repeating it the following circuit. Let's stay with the example that each set takes 20 seconds to complete, meaning the total time spent lifting will be the same: 4 minutes. But using a circuit structure, now the workout takes just over 13 minutes to complete, with just over 9 minutes being rest, as shown in table 8.3. This means your workout duration is now less than half of what it was with straight sets while still resting 3 minutes before repeating an exercise. That is efficient training.

TABLE 8.3   Time to Completion for a Full-Body Workout With a Circuit Structure

Movement	Duration (min)
1a: Upper body pull	00:20
Rest: move to upper body push	00:50
1b: Upper body push	00:20
Rest: move to lower body movement	00:50
1c: Lower body movement	00:20
Rest: move to upper body pull, repeating exercises a-c for 4 rounds	00:50
Time spent resting	*09:10*
Time spent lifting	*04:00*
Total workout duration	*13:10*

There are benefits of a circuit structure beyond efficiency. Even though you're training other muscle groups during the 3 minutes, you can achieve the same strength and muscle gains as if you rested passively using straight sets (Alcaraz et al. 2011). Indeed, research demonstrates you can work other muscle groups during a rest period without negatively affecting your strength for that exercise (Muñoz-Martínez et al. 2017).

Rest periods of 3 minutes are used because that is the minimum recommended duration before repeating an exercise (Schoenfeld et al. 2016). However, in many cases even longer rest periods are better. Regaining your full maximal strength after a set of squats or deadlifts can take 5 to 7 minutes, the time it takes the ATP-PC energy system, which fuels your muscle contractions, to recover. Here are two factors that determine whether you'll need to rest more than 3 minutes:

- The number of muscle groups recruited in an exercise (i.e., a squat requires more recovery than a row)
- The intensity of the set (i.e., performing a pull-up to failure requires more recovery than a set stopped two reps short of failure)

As a general rule, training for maximal strength requires more rest between sets than does training for hypertrophy. Furthermore, experienced strength athletes require longer rest periods than novice athletes do. Experienced lifters can recruit a greater number of motor units and expend energy more quickly, both of which are more taxing on their physiology, thus requiring a longer recovery. Therefore, when the goal is hypertrophy and strength, the recommended rest period before repeating an exercise in a circuit is 5 minutes. Seven minutes of rest before repeating an exercise is recommended in the following circumstances:

- Maximal strength development is the primary goal.
- All sets of multijoint exercises are taken close to momentary muscular failure.
- An advanced athlete is very strong.
- You have the available time to perform the recommended number of sets using 7 minutes of rest (i.e., more rest will only benefit your performance when strength and hypertrophy are the goals).

One simple way to program more rest before repeating an exercise is to place isolation exercises within the circuit. This can also preserve the efficiency of a workout, which means the rest periods between exercises remain 50 seconds in our example. The key is to use isolation exercises that don't compromise your performance in the multijoint exercises you're trying to build. For example, a biceps exercise before a pull-up will decrease your pull-up strength since it relies so heavily on that muscle group. The same is true with placing a triceps exercise before a dip or a quadriceps exercise before a squat. However, you can reverse the order and place a biceps exercise after a pull-up or a triceps exercise after a bench press, as two examples. Exercises that activate the abdominals are beneficial before a lower body exercise to maximize spinal stability (McGill 2015). And the lateral raise, which targets the deltoid's middle fibers to help widen the shoulders, is a good addition to any full-body workout since that area isn't directly overloaded with pulls and presses. Adding two isolation exercises (e.g., lateral raise and stir the pot) to our original full-body circuit increases the rest to 5 minutes and 50 seconds before any exercise is repeated, as shown in table 8.4.

During any rest period it's beneficial to perform light, easy movements. For example, you can walk around the gym while performing a few low-intensity arm circles or front kicks for 15 to 20 seconds. This example of active rest, first researched in 1903 by Russian physiologist Ivan Sechenov, promotes recovery

TABLE 8.4   Time to Completion for a Full-Body Workout Plus Two Isolation Exercises With a Circuit Structure

Movement	Duration (min)
1a: Upper body pull	00:20
Rest: move to lateral raise	00:50
1b: Lateral raise	00:20
Rest: move to upper body push	00:50
1c: Upper body push	00:20
Rest: move to stir the pot	00:50
1d: Stir the pot	00:20
Rest: move to lower body movement	00:50
1e: Lower body movement	00:20
Rest: move to upper body pull, repeat exercises a-e for 4 rounds	00:50
Duration before repeating an exercise	*05:50*

better than passively sitting. With all those points in mind, the recommended rest periods for maximal strength and hypertrophy are as follows:

- *Maximal strength and hypertrophy:* 5 to 7 minutes before repeating an exercise
- *Hypertrophy:* 3 to 5 minutes before repeating an exercise

Drop Sets

The aforementioned examples show how much more efficient a circuit structure is compared with straight sets for a given amount of exercise. So it will surely seem strange that one of the times I program straight sets with my athletes is when they're short on time. Let me explain.

For each movement pattern I program drop sets, which are three or more sets of the same exercise performed with 30 seconds' rest, or less, between each set. Since 30 seconds is well short of what's necessary for full recovery of the ATP-PC system, it is an *incomplete* rest period. In the drop set method, each set is taken to momentary muscular failure in order to elicit muscle damage, and the incomplete rest periods create metabolic stress. This accomplishes two of the three key mechanisms for hypertrophy. Indeed, drop sets have been shown to be an effective muscle builder when you're short on time (Fink et al. 2018). We continue with the aforementioned example of four sets of each movement pattern, with each set lasting 20 seconds. The drop set workout takes 10 minutes and 30 seconds to complete compared with 13 minutes and 10 seconds for the full-body circuit, as shown in table 8.5.

At this point you might think that drop sets are an ideal way to train all the time. But this method has two shortcomings. First, it is very taxing on your system because all three sets are taken to momentary muscular failure. That is fine once every two or three weeks, but it's not an ideal way to manage fatigue and maintain optimal hormonal levels over the course of months (Fry and Kraemer 1997). Second, drop sets require you to decrease the load or the repetitions with

The Many-Named System

The phosphagen system, which fuels your high-intensity muscle contractions, is sometimes referred to as the ATP-PC system, where *PC* stands for *phosphocreatine*. Some textbooks refer to it as the ATP-PCr system, where the *r* is added to indicate that the *C* stands for *creatine*. Some scientists don't even use the word *phosphocreatine*; they call the molecule *creatine phosphate*, using the letters *ATP-CP* to describe the system. And here's yet another: the anaerobic alactic system, a name devised to distinguish it from the anaerobic lactic system, aka anaerobic glycolysis. (*Lactic* means it produces lactic acid, while *alactic* means it doesn't).

TABLE 8.5 Time to Completion for a Full-Body Workout Using the Drop Set Method

Movement	Duration (min)
Upper body pull: 4 sets × 20 sec × 30 sec rest	02:50
Rest: move to upper body push	01:00
Upper body push: 4 sets × 20 sec × 30 sec rest	02:50
Rest: move to lower body movement	01:00
Lower body movement: 4 sets × 20 sec × 30 sec rest	02:50
Time spent resting	*06:30*
Time spent lifting	*04:00*
Total workout duration	*10:30*

each subsequent set because of incomplete replenishment of the ATP-PC system, which fuels your intense muscle contractions. Therefore, you get less volume per exercise per workout, which is not ideal for muscle growth (Schoenfeld, Ogborn, and Krieger 2017). For the majority of your training time, it's recommended to rest at least 3 minutes before repeating an exercise so you can maintain the load and repetitions. Longer rest periods are probably better, especially when you want maximal strength development to accompany your hypertrophy. Therefore, you'll often see longer than 3 minutes of rest for the programs in this chapter.

Repetitions and Sets

Now we discuss how many repetitions and sets are recommended. With regard to repetitions, anywhere from 3 to 30 per set have been shown to be equally effective for muscle growth (Morton et al. 2016). However, 3 repetitions per set are better for gaining maximal strength with the hypertrophy (Schoenfeld et al. 2017). Building strength early in a program helps you generate more muscular force to recruit more motor units. Then, when higher-repetition sets are added later in the program, you can lift a heavier load than if you had skipped the earlier strength training. In any case, sets with repetitions that range from 3 to 30 per set are programmed to get maximal stimulation of all motor units.

For optimal hypertrophy, the minimum number of sets per major muscle group per week appears to be 10 (Schoenfeld, Ogborn, and Krieger 2017). We consider 10 sets to be the minimum effective dose, with more sets likely being even better for short periods given the empirical evidence from bodybuilders. More total sets per week per muscle group will also add variety to your training.

The number of sets is most often inversely related to repetitions, with 2 sets being the minimum per muscle group per workout for hypertrophy (Krieger 2010). Put another way, 2 sets of 30 repetitions is effective for muscle growth if the sets are taken to momentary muscular failure, while 2 sets of 3 repetitions is not sufficient. From a practical standpoint, lower repetitions with heavy loads (e.g., 3-5 repetitions with 85 percent of 1RM) work well for the core of your full-body circuit. Sets of 30 repetitions serve as an intense finisher for lagging muscle

What Exercises and Programs Are Best for Your Experience Level?

Many fitness experts classify lifters as beginner, intermediate, or advanced. And if there are beginner and advanced lifters, there must also be exercises and programs that are appropriate for one but not the other. For example, some say beginners should perform more repetitions per set because they have a harder time recruiting motor units.

After 25 years in this industry, I've realized those terms are too arbitrary, and it makes little sense to design programs around them. In my experience, 3 to 5 repetitions per set is optimal for building maximal strength, regardless of the person's experience. And 6 to 12 repetitions work well to stimulate hypertrophy for virtually anyone.

One seemingly logical difference between the two is the number of sets per exercise. Beginners can often do more sets and still manage fatigue because it's harder for them to recruit the largest motor units. An inexperienced lifter might need four or five sets to reach the same level of fatigue an advanced lifter could achieve with two or three. If that experienced lifter knows they're doing five sets, they'll strategically manage their fatigue by holding back on the first few and pushing themselves on the final ones. Thus, it probably makes more sense to designate those opening sets as warm-ups, with the goal of conserving the advanced lifter's strength for maximal efforts on the others.

Another genuine difference is that beginners quickly increase their muscular fitness in their first few months of training. They can often add repetitions or load to every set of every exercise from one workout to the next. Meanwhile, the most experienced trainees have to fight for every additional rep or plate.

But that doesn't necessarily change things from a programming perspective. It just means the least experienced lifters can increase their load or repetitions faster than the most experienced. To me, the primary differences between beginner and advanced programs come down to two factors:

- *The technical skill required for a given movement.* For example, a one-leg deadlift is usually much more difficult for a beginner than an advanced lifter.

- *The speed of movement.* Most trainees can jump or do a push-up, but jump squats and clap push-ups are best reserved for advanced athletes.

This goes back to the movement progression covered in chapter 3: First develop movement competence, then build strength, then build power. If an exercise requires relatively high skill or speed, save it for the later stages of a program. But if it's a more basic movement for strength or hypertrophy, you can use it at any and every stage. The exercise may look the same from the outside. What changes is the training effect the individual lifter derives from it, based on motor unit recruitment, the amount of tension on the muscles, and the accumulated level of fatigue.

groups at the end of the workout, or at the beginning if it doesn't compromise your performance in the full-body circuit (e.g., standing calf raise for 2×30 before the circuit).

For maximal strength, the recommended parameters are 3 to 5 sets of 3 to 5 repetitions. Since hypertrophy is the goal, we often use the upper end of those parameters to get a higher volume (i.e., 5×5). Indeed, the strength- and muscle-building benefits of 5×5 with approximately 80 to 85 percent of 1RM was popularized by the late Bill Starr, former strength and conditioning coach of the Baltimore Colts, in his classic text *The Strongest Shall Survive*. For variety, 8 sets of 3 repetitions with 80 to 85 of 1RM, similar to the volume Starr popularized, is programmed. And sometimes we go as high as 10 sets per exercise (i.e., 10 rounds of a circuit) to achieve a very high training volume per workout.

With those points in mind, here are the general recommendations for sets and repetitions per major muscle group per workout:

- *Maximal strength and hypertrophy:* 3 to 10 sets of 3 to 5 repetitions
- *Hypertrophy and strength:* 3 to 6 sets of 6 to 12 repetitions
- *Hypertrophy and endurance strength:* 2 to 4 sets of 13 to 30 repetitions taken to momentary muscular failure

Maximizing Muscle Growth

Virtually any form of resistance training can cause some muscle growth, provided you apply a decent level of effort. The key, however, is to stimulate the most growth as quickly and efficiently as possible. That is why most of the programs in this chapter prioritize full-body workouts and compound (i.e., multijoint) exercises. Single-joint exercises that target specific muscle growth also have their place, as discussed earlier.

After an intense full-body workout, your muscles need sufficient time for recovery, which is 48 to 72 hours for most people. Three workouts per week, such as Monday, Wednesday, and Friday or Tuesday, Thursday, and Saturday, works well (more about this later). This structure is a tried and tested way to build muscle, dating back to old-school bodybuilders such as Roy "Reg" Park, star of the Hercules movies from the 1960s and mentor to Arnold Schwarzenegger. Back before heavy steroid use became rampant, full-body training was a popular way to stimulate strength and hypertrophy.

The final step is to provide your body with sufficient nutrients to build new muscle, which we cover in chapter 11. For now, let's focus on what you can do in the gym to maximize your results.

Apply Hypertrophy Mechanisms When Training

In chapter 4 we discuss the three mechanisms of hypertrophy outlined by Brad Schoenfeld (2010)—mechanical tension, muscle damage, and metabolic stress (see figure 8.1). It is often simplest to think of each mechanism as it applies to what you do in the weight room. For example, to achieve high levels of mechanical tension, it's best to work with heavy loads, which is typically defined as a load you can't lift for more than five repetitions (i.e., maximal strength training). Muscle damage can occur either by performing a sufficient volume with a heavy load (e.g., eight sets of three repetitions of the squat) or by lifting a lighter load

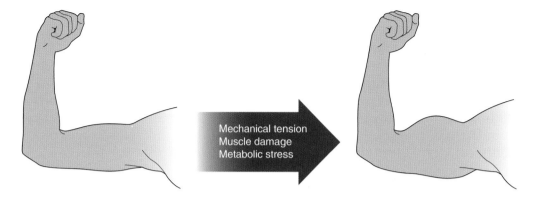

FIGURE 8.1 Three mechanisms of hypertrophy.

to failure. Metabolic stress occurs when a lighter load is taken to failure (or close to it) or when the rest periods are incomplete. Importantly, the three aforementioned mechanisms are not mutually exclusive. They can occur at the same time, which you will see in the programming in this chapter. More detail about the three mechanisms is as follows:

- *Mechanical tension:* There are two types of tension generated in your muscles during resistance training. One is active tension, which occurs when muscle is shortening (i.e., concentric action). The other is passive tension, which occurs when muscle is lengthening (i.e., eccentric action). The combination of these "force" and "stretch" tensions appears to have a compounding effect on hypertrophy (Hornberger and Chien 2006).

- *Application:* Train with heavy loads (i.e., three to five repetitions per set).

- *Muscle damage:* Resistance training with sufficient volume or intensity creates microtears within the trained muscles. This microtrauma causes various growth factors to release in order to help your muscles grow (Vierck et al. 2000).

- *Application:* Perform a high volume of work with heavy loads (e.g., 8 to 10 sets of three to five repetitions), or push one or more of your sets close to failure or to failure when the load is submaximal.

- *Metabolic stress:* When you perform a set of high repetitions to failure, or perform multiple sets of the same exercise with minimal rest, you feel a burn in your muscles. This stress is due to a buildup of metabolites, most notably hydrogen ions (H+), which are associated with high acidity (Takada et al. 2012). A lack of oxygen (i.e., muscle hypoxia) is another potential stressor; it can be induced either by performing a set of high repetitions (e.g., 30) with a fast tempo to failure or by applying a cuff that restricts blood flow to the working muscles. Blood flow restriction has been shown to be promising for hypertrophy; however, it's often impractical for the typical gym-goer (Patterson 2019).

- *Application:* Perform sets of the same exercise with incomplete rest periods, or take your sets to momentary muscular failure.

A note about momentary muscular failure: Limit training to momentary muscular failure to single-joint and body weight exercises that are performed for a high number of repetitions (i.e., >13). Training to failure over the course of months with compound, multijoint exercises has been shown to reduce levels of IGF-1, a key muscle-building hormone (Izquierdo, Ibañez, González-Badillo, et al. 2006). In this same study, participants who avoided failure reduced cortisol and increased testosterone. However, when light loads are used with less taxing exercises, such as a biceps curl or push-up, training to failure has been shown to be a potent stimulus for muscle growth (Mitchell CJ, Churchward-Venne TA, West DW, et al. 2012).

Incorporate Progressions

Programming a progression, such as adding a repetition to each set or increasing the load by 2 to 3 percent every few weeks, is a tricky endeavor. For a variety of reasons, each lifter progresses at a different pace. The aforementioned programs have parameters that change every four weeks. Indeed, you'll rarely be on any phase long enough to worry about programming a significant increase in load. Nevertheless, training volume and muscle growth are positively correlated (Schoenfeld et al. 2019). Therefore, the recommended progression for these plans is to first focus on adding two repetitions to your first few sets over the course of a few weeks. If you can add two repetitions to every set before the phase ends, increase the load to the point where you're near failure on the last repetition of the last round with regard to the recommended repetitions.

Increase Load for More Challenge

At first glance, some of you might think these workouts look too challenging, especially if you're accustomed to body part splits. Others might think they look pretty easy, given there are fewer exercises per workout than they might normally perform. But looks can be deceiving. In either case, the programs are designed to maximize muscle and strength gains while managing fatigue, which is a key to long-term progress. Therefore, first perform the program for two weeks, making sure the loads are challenging. If at that point you want to make them more challenging, you have several options:

- Take the last two or three sets of each circuit to momentary muscular failure, instead of just the final set as originally recommended.
- Perform each repetition as explosively as possible while maintaining perfect form.
- Perform an additional round of the circuit, and push all sets close to momentary muscular failure.
- Add one or two more isolation exercises within the circuit while keeping the same basic rest periods between exercises. Perform 6 to 12 repetitions for the assistance exercises. Avoid placing an isolation exercise before a multijoint exercise that works the same muscle groups (e.g., biceps curl before a pull-up).
- Maximally squeeze the peak contraction of all upper body exercises for 4 to 5 seconds on the final repetition of each set.
- Accommodate resistance for any horizontal push, squat, or deadlift variation by using resistance bands with those movements as shown in chapters 5 and 7.

Time-Tested Ways to Build Strength

I do my best to surround myself with the best minds in strength and conditioning. I'll call up these guys or gals and offer to buy them lunch, coffee, or a beer (depending on what phase of dieting they're in). Pavel Tsatsouline, founder of StrongFirst and the reason kettlebells are now so popular, has shared an immense amount of knowledge with me. During one of our hangouts, he explained two ways to vary your loading: cycle loading and step loading. Russian endocrinologists have determined that two weeks of very heavy lifting per month is basically the limit for what anyone with training experience can handle. To be clear, very heavy lifting consists of pushing to your repetition maximum during sets of fewer than six repetitions (i.e., maximal strength training). Therefore, two loading protocols he recommended—cycle loading and step loading—work up to very heavy loads, but only for a few weeks before backing off. We'll use the deadlift as an example for each loading plan.

Cycle Loading

In this plan you will steadily increase your training load of the deadlift over the course of four weeks. The following protocol was popularized by Marty Gallagher, winner of six straight titles across three different weight classes in the United States Powerlifting Federation. You will break up your training into three four-week cycles:

- *Weeks 1-4:* eight repetitions per set
- *Weeks 5-8:* five repetitions per set
- *Weeks 9-12:* three repetitions per set

Each of those four-week cycles follows the same intensity (i.e., loading) progression. What you need to know before you start the first cycle is your 8RM for the deadlift. Let's say it's 250 pounds (113 kg). This is how the loading progression will work:

- *Week 1:* Perform eight repetitions with a relatively easy load (6/10 effort), which might be around 200 pounds (91 kg).
- *Week 2:* Perform eight repetitions with a moderate load (8/10 effort), which we'll call 225 pounds (102 kg).
- *Week 3:* Perform eight repetitions with your original 8RM, which in this case is 250 pounds (113 kg).
- *Week 4:* Try to beat the 8RM you performed in week 3, such as 260 pounds (118 kg) for eight repetitions.

This same loading and intensity pattern repeats for two more cycles, but instead of performing eight repetitions per set you'll perform five repetitions per set (weeks 5-8) and three repetitions per set (weeks 9-12). Then you will start the 12-week cycle over, using your new 8RM as your guide for the first four weeks.

Step Loading

In this plan you will choose a challenging load (9/10 effort) for a specific number of repetitions. Let's say you rate five repetitions of the deadlift with 300 pounds (136 kg) as 9/10 effort. You will continue with that same load and repetitions for weeks, or months, until it feels relatively easy (6/10 effort). At that point, you'll increase the load until you're back to 9/10 effort, which might be 340 pounds (154 kg) in this case, and then continue with five repetitions. For variety, you could switch to three or four repetitions for your next cycle or choose a new variation of the movement. In any case, start with a challenging load and stick with it until it becomes relatively easy, then bump up the load until it's challenging again.

Designing Your Own Muscle-Building Program

One of the challenges of creating training programs for the masses is guessing which training equipment they'll have access to. That is why I try to program workouts using the least equipment possible. But some pieces of equipment, such as a pull-up apparatus, are invaluable. Notwithstanding, there are plenty of people who don't have access to equipment. Therefore, in this section we outline how you can create your own training program around what you have available. Here are the six steps:

1. Program two to four full-body workouts per "week" based on what fits your schedule. Ideally, four full-body workouts would span over eight days instead of seven to allow 48 hours' rest between each workout.

2. Program an upper body push, an upper body pull, a lower body exercise, and up to three isolation exercises within a circuit.

3. Program rest periods that allow 3 to 7 minutes before repeating an exercise, with 7 minutes being better for strength gains and 5 minutes being the sweet spot for most people.

4. Program using the guidelines for sets and repetitions covered earlier in this chapter, and avoid programming more than two workouts per week using maximal strength and hypertrophy parameters.

5. Avoid lifting heavy loads close to momentary muscular failure more than two weeks per month.

6. Rest at least 48 hours between training with maximal strength and hypertrophy parameters. If two workouts need to be programmed 24 hours apart, the first workout should be maximal strength and hypertrophy parameters and the second hypertrophy and endurance strength parameters, followed by at least one day of rest (i.e., day 1 is heavy, day 2 is light, day 3 is off).

Note that steps 3 to 6 apply to any training program. The recommended minimum training frequency for hypertrophy and strength is twice per week per major muscle group (Schoenfeld, Ogborn, and Krieger 2016). If you decide to split your training, the only viable option is an upper and lower split. One benefit of this split is it allows you to prioritize the upper or lower body musculature if you naturally have an imbalance. For example, a guy who has naturally large musculature in his lower body could program two upper body workouts per week and one lower body workout. That being said, most people will benefit from a balance of upper and lower body training. Within a seven-day span, you can program two or three upper and lower body workouts. However, if you choose three of each, an eight-day cycle is recommended since it's very difficult for most people to intensely train four days in a row. A sample cycle for three upper and lower workouts is shown in table 8.6.

TABLE 8.6 Eight-Day Cycle for Three Upper and Lower Body Workouts

Day 1	Day 2	Day 3	Day 4	Day 5	Day 6	Day 7	Day 8
LB	UB	LB	Rest	UB	LB	UB	Rest

LB = lower body; UB = upper body

If you choose an upper and lower split, training each twice throughout a seven-day cycle, you have a few options. Since a lower body workout is more taxing than an upper body workout, plan your rest days after the lower body workout. If you prefer to have the weekends off, plan your schedule as shown in table 8.7. Beyond that, any structure will work well as long as the lower body workout is followed by a day or two of rest.

TABLE 8.7   Seven-Day Cycle for Two Upper and Lower Body Workouts

Day 1	Day 2	Day 3	Day 4	Day 5	Day 6	Day 7
UB	LB	Rest	UB	LB	Rest	Rest

UB = upper body; LB = lower body

The general programming structure for full-body training that I've found most beneficial for managing fatigue is to alternate between upper body movement planes and hip- or quad-emphasis exercises from workout to workout. For example, if I program a bench press and deadlift on Monday, I'll program an overhead press and squat or lunge variation on Wednesday. For an upper and lower split, you can program horizontal and vertical plane upper body movements in the same workout, and hip- and quad-emphasis exercises in the lower body workouts. To manage fatigue and build structural balance, adhere to these two programming guidelines:

- Have an equal number of sets and repetitions for all upper body vertical plane movements and an equal number between horizontal plane movements at the end of the seven- or eight-day cycle. The solution here is as simple as programming the same parameters for the horizontal plane and the same parameters for the vertical. For example, Monday's upper body workout could be 5 × 5 for the bench press and row and 4 × 6 for the pull-up and overhead press.

- Avoid programming double-leg hip- and quad-emphasis exercises in the same workout. For example, on Tuesday you could program a sumo deadlift and a lunge or a front squat and a one-leg deadlift.

Sample Muscle-Building Programs

The following programs use a wide variety of equipment from an elaborate gym to a single kettlebell and are designed to build a balance of strength and muscle throughout the body without emphasizing any specific area. High frequency training (HFT) for developing specific muscle groups that are lagging behind, which will be added into these programs, is covered in chapter 10. There are three 12-week muscle-building programs presented here: Muscle Builder 1 (MB1), Muscle Builder 2 (MB2), and Muscle Builder 3 (MB3). These three programs are not arranged in any particular order. The purpose of three different plans is to give you a variety of choices based on your available equipment. They are all equally effective for building muscle and strength.

These three muscle-building programs follow a daily undulating periodization (DUP) structure, one I have used for most of my career. There is no doubt that your muscles and nervous system like variety in the gym, and this is especially true for more advanced lifters who are more easily overtrained. So, simply put, when following a DUP structure, your exercises, volume, and intensity fluctuate with each workout throughout the week. The DUP structure has been shown to be superior for building muscle and strength, compared with linear periodization structures that don't change parameters as often (Miranda et al. 2011; Simao et al. 2012). Regardless of the research, most people prefer some level of variety in their training throughout the week.

The programs should be done three times per week and completed within a seven-day cycle in the following recommended order:

1. Workout A
2. Workout B after 48 to 72 hours
3. Workout C after 48 to 72 hours

However, research does indicate that you can change the order of these DUP workouts and achieve the same results (Colquhoun et al. 2017). Also, we know life is unpredictable. So, let's say you did workout A on Monday and workout B on Wednesday. You were scheduled to perform workout C on Friday, but a family emergency happened that will keep you from training until the following Monday. When that happens, simply pick up where you left off in the program and continue. In other words, perform workout C on Monday and then workout A on Wednesday. Finally, if you prefer to take no more than one day off between each workout, that works perfectly well and will allow you to fit more workouts in each month.

As a general rule, avoid reaching momentary muscular failure, except on the final set. For the sake of convenience and simplicity, the workouts are intended to have you train with a constant load for all sets. Therefore, it is best to underestimate the load in the early stages of a plan and then adjust accordingly. There is nothing wrong with the first few sets being moderately easy, as long as the last set or two are challenging. In other words, the ideal load is one that allows you to perform all the recommended repetitions with perfect form, and then when fatigue accumulates toward the end of the workout, is challenging enough to push you close to, or to, momentary muscular failure on the last set.

Muscle Builder 1 (MB1)

The MB1 program is designed around a large selection of training equipment. It is intended for a commercial gym or an elaborate home gym. Whenever appropriate, alternatives are mentioned in parentheses in case you're missing that piece of equipment. For example, in workout A, a hammer-grip pull-up is one recommended exercise, but it can be performed as a hammer-grip pull-down instead, so it is written as hammer-grip pull-up or pull-down.

Each workout in this program starts with a circuit of four exercises (1a-1d) for five rounds, then finishes with a triple drop set for the calves, biceps, or triceps. For the drop set, start with a load that's your repetition maximum for the first set (e.g., a 12RM if the first set calls for 12 repetitions). Then you'll rest briefly, perform another set for as many repetitions as possible (AMRAP), rest briefly, and finish with AMRAP. Your repetitions will drastically decrease in the last two sets of the drop set, which is intended to create muscle damage and metabolic stress. The drop set is intended to maintain your strength of that muscle, while a targeted HFT plan will increase its size (if you choose to add an HFT plan into this program).

Importantly, when you see repetitions for a pull-up or dip that are significantly less than you can perform (e.g., three reps per set), be sure to add load to a chin/dip belt, which will also be necessary for belt squats. Also, for exercises that work one arm or one leg at a time, there is no recommended rest period before switching sides. Take as much or as little time as you want. Always start with your weakest side first.

EQUIPMENT NEEDED

Pull-up/dip station
Cable station with adjustable pulley
Long resistance band
Heavy and moderately heavy dumbbells or large selection of pairs of kettlebells
Trap bar
Chin/dip belt

MB1 WORKOUT A

Exercise or *rest*	Reps	Page
1a. Hammer-grip pull-up or pull-down	4	154, 155
Rest 45 sec		
1b. Face pull	8	148
Rest 30 sec		
1c. Dip	4	173
Rest 45 sec		
1d. Trap bar deadlift or regular bar	4	94, 91
Rest 60 sec; perform exercises 1a-1d for 5 rounds		
2. One-leg calf raise	20 (AMRAP in rounds 2 and 3)	107
Rest 30 sec; perform exercise 2 for 2 more rounds, then repeat on other side		

AMRAP = as many repetitions as possible

MB1 WORKOUT B

Exercise or *rest*	Reps	Page
1a. One-arm cable or dumbbell row	5 each side	147, 146
Rest 45 sec		
1b. One-arm cable or band chest press or one-arm floor press	5 each side	171, 172
Rest 45 sec		
1c. Split squat	5 each side	78
Rest 60 sec		
1d. Hip thrust	10	101
Rest 60 sec; perform exercises 1a-1d for 5 rounds		
2. Triceps press-down	15 (AMRAP in rounds 2 and 3)	194
Rest 20 sec; perform exercise 2 for 2 more rounds		

AMRAP = as many repetitions as possible

MB1 WORKOUT C

Exercise or *rest*	Reps	Page
1a. Overhand-grip pull-up or pull-down	5	152, 153
Rest 45 sec		
1b. Lateral raise	10	197
Rest 30 sec		
1c. One-arm overhead press	5 each side	178
Rest 45 sec		
1d. Belt squat	10	74
Rest 60 sec; perform exercises 1a-1d for 5 rounds		
2. Biceps curl	12 (AMRAP in rounds 2 and 3)	188
Rest 15 sec; perform exercise 2 for 2 more rounds		

AMRAP = as many repetitions as possible

MB1 WORKOUT A

Exercise or *rest*	Reps	Page
1a. Yates row	6	145
Rest 45 sec		
1b. Face pull	12	148
Rest 30 sec		
1c. Narrow-grip bench press	6	169
Rest 45 sec		
1d. Reverse lunge	6 each side	82
Rest 60 sec; perform exercises 1a-1d for 5 rounds		
2. One-leg calf raise	15 (AMRAP in rounds 2 and 3)	107
Rest 20 sec; perform exercise 2 for 2 more rounds, then repeat on other side		

AMRAP = as many repetitions as possible

MB1 WORKOUT B

Exercise or *rest*	Reps	Page
1a. Overhand-grip pull-up or pull-down	3	152, 153
Rest 45 sec		
1b. Incline bench press	6	170
Rest 45 sec		
1c. Straight-arm lat pull-down	12	158
Rest 60 sec		
1d. Sumo deadlift	3	93
Rest 60 sec; perform exercises 1a-1d for 5 rounds		
2. Lying triceps extension	12 (AMRAP in rounds 2 and 3)	192
Rest 15 sec; perform exercise 2 for 2 more rounds		

AMRAP = as many repetitions as possible

MB1 WORKOUT C

Exercise or *rest*	Reps	Page
1a. One-arm row	10 each side	146
Rest 45 sec		
1b. One-arm cable chest press or one-arm floor press	10 each side	171, 172
Rest 45 sec		
1c. Half-kneeling one-arm overhead press	5 each side	180
Rest 45 sec		
1d. Bulgarian split squat	5 each side	79
Rest 60 sec; perform exercises 1a-1d for 5 rounds		
2. Biceps hammer curl	20 (AMRAP in rounds 2 and 3)	189
Rest 30 sec; perform exercise 2 for 2 more rounds		

AMRAP = as many repetitions as possible

MB1 WORKOUT A

Exercise or *rest*	Reps	Page
1a. Hammer-grip pull-up or pull-down	8	154, 155
Rest 45 sec		
1b. Face pull	18	148
Rest 30 sec		
1c. Dip	8	173
Rest 45 sec		
1d. Barbell back squat or front squat	5	69, 71
Rest 90 sec; perform exercises 1a-1d for 5 rounds		
2. One-leg calf raise	12 (AMRAP in rounds 2 and 3)	107
Rest 15 sec; perform exercise 2 for 2 more rounds, then repeat on other side		

AMRAP = as many repetitions as possible

MB1 WORKOUT B

Exercise or *rest*	Reps	Page
1a. One-arm cable row	12 each side	147
Rest 45 sec		
1b. One-arm cable chest press	12 each side	171
Rest 45 sec		
1c. Forward lunge	6 each side	84
Rest 60 sec		
1d. Kettlebell swing	10	99
Rest 60 sec; perform exercises 1a-1d for 5 rounds		
2. Overhead triceps extension	20 (AMRAP in rounds 2 and 3)	193
Rest 30 sec; perform exercise 2 for 2 more rounds		

AMRAP = as many repetitions as possible

MB1 WORKOUT C

Exercise or *rest*	Reps	Page
1a. Overhand-grip pull-up or pull-down	5	152, 153
Rest 45 sec		
1b. Lateral raise	10	197
Rest 30 sec		
1c. One-arm overhead press	12 each side	178
Rest 45 sec		
1d. Belt squat	18	74
Rest 90 sec; perform exercises 1a-1d for 5 rounds		
2. Biceps reverse curl	15 (AMRAP in rounds 2 and 3)	190
Rest 20 sec; perform exercise 2 for 2 more rounds		

AMRAP = as many repetitions as possible

Muscle Builder 2 (MB2)

The MB2 program uses a combination of equipment you can easily have at home. Gymnastics rings, in particular, are one of the most beneficial and least expensive training tools. In the following plan, only one rings exercise is programmed per workout. This is intentional so you don't have to adjust the height of the rings between exercises, as you would if a pull-up and dip were programmed in the same workout.

In this program you will perform five rounds of a circuit of four exercises (1a-1d) and then a pairing of isolation exercises (2a-2b), using incomplete rest periods to create muscle damage and metabolic stress. You will use a constant load for each exercise during the pairing (e.g., 12RM for the first set) and then continue with that load. Your repetitions will decrease in the second and third rounds because of fatigue, as they should.

Importantly, when you see repetitions for a pull-up or dip that are significantly less than you can perform (e.g., three reps per set) be sure to add load to a chin/dip belt, which will also be necessary for belt squats. Also, for exercises that work one arm or one leg at a time, there is no recommended rest period before switching sides. Take as much or as little time as you want. Always start with your weakest side first.

EQUIPMENT NEEDED

Gymnastics rings

Moderate to heavy dumbbells or kettlebells

Long resistance band

Barbell

Chin/dip belt

Swiss ball

Sliders

MB2 WORKOUT A

Exercise or *rest*	Reps	Page
1a. Face pull	10	148
Rest 30 sec		
1b. Rings dip	5	174
Rest 45 sec		
1c. Stir the pot	3 each direction, slow	124
Rest 30 sec		
1d. Deadlift	3	91
Rest 60 sec; perform exercises 1a-1d for 5 rounds		
2a. Biceps hammer curl	12 (AMRAP in rounds 2 and 3)	189
Rest 30 sec		
2b. Lateral raise	12 (AMRAP in rounds 2 and 3)	197
Rest 30 sec; perform exercises 2a-2b for 3 rounds		

AMRAP = as many repetitions as possible

MB2 WORKOUT B

Exercise or *rest*	Reps	Page
1a. Rings pull-up	3	156
Rest 30 sec		
1b. Overhead press	6	177
Rest 45 sec		
1c. Elevated one-leg calf raise (hold dumbbell on opposite side)	5 each side	109
Rest 30 sec		
1d. Bulgarian split squat or split squat	6 each side	79, 78
Rest 60 sec; perform exercises 1a-1d for 5 rounds		
2a. Triceps press-down	15 (AMRAP in rounds 2 and 3)	194
Rest 30 sec		
2b. Slider leg curl	15 (AMRAP in rounds 2 and 3)	103
Rest 30 sec; perform exercises 2a-2b for 3 rounds		

AMRAP = as many repetitions as possible

MB2 WORKOUT C

Exercise or *rest*	Reps	Page
1a. One-arm row	3 each side	146
Rest 30 sec		
1b. Rings or straps push-up	AMRAP	166
Rest 45 sec		
1c. Step-up	5 each side	88
Rest 30 sec		
1d. Kettlebell swing	8	99
Rest 60 sec; perform exercises 1a-1d for 5 rounds		
2a. Landmine rotation	20 each side	128
Rest 30 sec		
2b. One-leg hop	20 each side (AMRAP in rounds 2 and 3)	110
Rest 30 sec; perform exercises 2a-2b for 3 rounds		

AMRAP = as many repetitions as possible

MB2 WORKOUT A

Exercise or *rest*	Reps	Page
1a. Face pull	14	148
Rest 30 sec		
1b. Rings dip	AMRAP	174
Rest 45 sec		
1c. Stir the pot	4 each direction, slow	124
Rest 30 sec		
1d. Staggered-stance Romanian deadlift	5 each side	96
Rest 60 sec; perform exercises 1a-1d for 5 rounds		
2a. Biceps curl	15 (AMRAP in rounds 2 and 3)	188
Rest 30 sec		
2b. Lateral raise	15 (AMRAP in rounds 2 and 3)	197
Rest 30 sec; perform exercises 2a-2b for 3 rounds		

AMRAP = as many repetitions as possible

MB2 WORKOUT B

Exercise or *rest*	Reps	Page
1a. Rings pull-up	AMRAP	156
Rest 30 sec		
1b. Ahrens press	8	181
Rest 45 sec		
1c. One-leg calf raise	15 each side	107
Rest 30 sec		
1d. Forward lunge	8 each side	84
Rest 60 sec; perform exercises 1a-1d for 5 rounds		
2a. Lying triceps extension	12 (AMRAP in rounds 2 and 3)	192
Rest 30 sec		
2b. One-arm band or dumbbell shrug	12 (AMRAP in rounds 2 and 3)	199
Rest 30 sec; perform exercises 2a-2b for 3 rounds		

AMRAP = as many repetitions as possible

MB2 WORKOUT C

Exercise or *rest*	Reps	Page
1a. Yates row	8	145
Rest 30 sec		
1b. Rings or straps inverted push-up	AMRAP	185
Rest 45 sec		
1c. Straight-arm lat pull-down	10	158
Rest 30 sec		
1d. Belt squat	12	74
Rest 60 sec; perform exercises 1a-1d for 5 rounds		
2a. Hanging leg raise	AMRAP, slow	133
Rest 30 sec		
2b. Slider one-leg curl	6 each side (AMRAP in rounds 2 and 3)	104
Rest 30 sec; perform exercises 2a-2b for 3 rounds		

AMRAP = as many repetitions as possible

MB2 WORKOUT A

Exercise or *rest*	Reps	Page
1a. Face pull	18	148
Rest 30 sec		
1b. Rings dip to L-sit	AMRAP	175
Rest 45 sec		
1c. Stir the pot	5 each direction, slow	124
Rest 30 sec		
1d. Sumo deadlift	5	93
Rest 60 sec; perform exercises 1a-1d for 5 rounds		
2a. Biceps curl	15 (AMRAP in rounds 2 and 3)	188
Rest 30 sec		
2b. Lateral raise	15 (AMRAP in rounds 2 and 3)	197
Rest 30 sec; perform exercises 2a-2b for 3 rounds		

AMRAP = as many repetitions as possible

MB2 WORKOUT B

Exercise or *rest*	Reps/time	Page
1a. Rings L-sit pull-up	AMRAP	157
Rest 30 sec		
1b. Overhead press	12	177
Rest 45 sec		
1c. One-leg Romanian deadlift	5 each side	97
Rest 45 sec		
1d. Goblet squat	12	68
Rest 60 sec; perform exercises 1a-1d for 5 rounds		
2a. Loaded carry (walk in figure-eight pattern)	30 sec	135
Rest 45 sec		
2b. Explosive push-up	3	164
Rest 45 sec; perform exercises 2a-2b for 3 rounds		

AMRAP = as many repetitions as possible

MB2 WORKOUT C

Exercise or *rest*	Reps	Page
1a. One-arm row	5 each side	146
Rest 30 sec		
1b. One-arm band fly	12 each side	196
Rest 45 sec		
1c. One-arm overhead press	10 each side	178
Rest 45 sec		
1d. Reverse lunge	6 each side	82
Rest 60 sec; perform exercises 1a-1d for 5 rounds		
2a. One-leg calf raise	12 each side (AMRAP in rounds 2 and 3)	107
Rest 30 sec		
2b. Overhead triceps extension	12 (AMRAP in rounds 2 and 3)	193
Rest 30 sec; perform exercises 2a-2b for 3 rounds		

AMRAP = as many repetitions as possible

Muscle Builder 3 (MB3)

The MB3 program requires the least equipment in this chapter, prioritizing your body weight. Body weight training can be an excellent way to build size and strength in virtually any major muscle group, and this program will progress through more challenging variations over the course of 12 weeks. The only aspect that body weight training misses is an exercise to strengthen your posterior chain (i.e., low back). Therefore, a kettlebell is necessary to perform swings and variations of a one-leg deadlift. You will see some unusual exercises, such as a kettlebell bent-over row to build your biceps, and push-ups off a Swiss ball to build your triceps. And a band is necessary to strengthen the rotator cuff and add variety to the program, as well as a Swiss ball to strengthen the abdominals and hamstrings. Since a range of loads isn't possible, most of the sets are performed for as many repetitions as possible (AMRAP). For the appropriate exercises you will see progressions that require you to hold the peak contraction of each repetition to increase muscle stimulation.

This workout will likely require some creativity, based on how heavy your kettlebell is (or dumbbells if you prefer). For example, a kettlebell you're using might be too heavy to perform certain exercises through a full range of motion. Ideally, you will be able to perform at least five repetitions where you see AMRAP programmed. If necessary, perform repetitions through a partial range of motion for more challenging exercises to fulfill that recommendation.

For exercises that work one arm or one leg at a time, there is no recommended rest period before switching sides. Take as much or as little time as you want. Always start with your weakest side first.

EQUIPMENT NEEDED

One moderately heavy kettlebell (or dumbbells)

Long resistance band

Swiss ball

MB3 WORKOUT A

Exercise or *rest*	Reps/time	Page
1a. One-arm row	AMRAP	146
Rest 45 sec		
1b. Inverted push-up	AMRAP	182
Rest 45 sec		
1c. Pallof press	20 sec each side	125
Rest 30 sec		
1d. Lateral lunge	AMRAP each side	86
Rest 60 sec; perform exercises 1a-1d for 5 rounds		
2a. One-leg calf raise	AMRAP each side	107
Rest 30 sec		
2b. Hand walkout	AMRAP	118
Rest 45 sec; perform exercises 2a-2b for 3 rounds		

AMRAP = as many repetitions as possible

MB3 WORKOUT B

Exercise or *rest*	Reps/time	Page
1a. Face pull	AMRAP	148
Rest 45 sec		
1b. Dead-stop push-up	AMRAP	163
Rest 45 sec		
1c. Side plank	Up to 30 sec each side	120
Rest 30 sec		
1d. Step-up	AMRAP each side	88
Rest 60 sec; perform exercises 1a-1d for 5 rounds		
2a. One-arm band fly	12 each side	196
Rest 30 sec		
2b. Kettlebell bent-over row	AMRAP	150
Rest 45 sec; perform exercises 2a-2b for 3 rounds		

AMRAP = as many repetitions as possible

MB3 WORKOUT C

Exercise or *rest*	Reps	Page
1a. Straight-arm lat pull-down	AMRAP	158
Rest 45 sec		
1b. One-arm overhead push press	AMRAP each side	179
Rest 45 sec		
1c. Swiss ball rollout	AMRAP	117
Rest 30 sec		
1d. One-leg Romanian deadlift	AMRAP each side	97
Rest 60 sec; perform exercises 1a-1d for 5 rounds		
2a. Hand walk push-up	AMRAP	165
Rest 30 sec		
2b. Biceps iso-hold	Max time	187
Rest 60 sec; perform exercise 2a-2b for 3 rounds		

AMRAP = as many repetitions as possible

MB3 WORKOUT A

Exercise or *rest*	Reps/time	Page
1a. One-arm row	AMRAP each side	146
Rest 45 sec		
1b. Feet-elevated inverted push-up	AMRAP	184
Rest 45 sec		
1c. Half-kneeling Pallof press	20 sec each side	126
Rest 30 sec		
1d. Alternating kettlebell swing	12 each side	100
Rest 60 sec; perform exercises 1a-1d for 5 rounds		
2a. Elevated one-leg calf raise	AMRAP each side	109
Rest 30 sec		
2b. Swiss ball push-up	AMRAP	167
Rest 45 sec; perform exercises 2a-2b for 3 rounds		

AMRAP = as many repetitions as possible

MB3 WORKOUT B

Exercise or *rest*	Reps/time	Page
1a. Face pull	AMRAP	148
Rest 45 sec		
1b. Explosive push-up	AMRAP	164
Rest 45 sec		
1c. Stacked side plank	Up to 30 sec each side	121
Rest 30 sec		
1d. Split jump squat	3 each side	80
Rest 90 sec; perform exercises 1a-1d for 5 rounds		
2a. One-arm band fly	AMRAP; hold peak contraction for 2 sec each rep	196
Rest 30 sec		
2b. Kettlebell bent-over row	AMRAP; hold peak contraction for 2 sec each rep	150
Rest 60 sec; perform exercises 2a-2b for 3 rounds		

AMRAP = as many repetitions as possible

MB3 WORKOUT C

Exercise or rest	Reps/time	Page
1a. Straight-arm lat pull-down	AMRAP; hold peak contraction for 2 sec each rep	158
Rest 45 sec		
1b. Hand walk push-up	AMRAP; hold bottom position or 2 sec each rep	165
Rest 45 sec		
1c. One-arm plank	Up to 5 sec each side	129
Rest 30 sec		
1d. Goblet squat	AMRAP	68
Rest 60 sec; perform exercises 1a-1d for 5 rounds		
2a. Stir the pot	AMRAP each direction, slow	124
Rest 30 sec		
2b. Biceps iso-hold	3 partial reps then hold for max time	187
Rest 60 sec; perform exercises 2a-2b for 3 rounds		

AMRAP = as many repetitions as possible

MB3 WORKOUT A

Exercise or rest	Reps	Page
1a. One-arm row	AMRAP each side	146
Rest 45 sec		
1b. Push-up with band	AMRAP each side	161
Rest 45 sec		
1c. Lying leg raise	AMRAP, slow	131
Rest 30 sec		
1d. One-leg squat	AMRAP each side	75
Rest 60 sec; perform exercises 1a-1d for 5 rounds		
2a. One-leg hop	AMRAP each side	110
Rest 30 sec		
2b. One-arm overhead push press	AMRAP each side	179
Rest 45 sec; perform exercises 2a-2b for 3 rounds		

AMRAP = as many repetitions as possible

MB3 WORKOUT B

Exercise or *rest*	Reps/time	Page
1a. Face pull	AMRAP	148
Rest 45 sec		
1b. Dead-stop push-up	AMRAP	163
Rest 45 sec		
1c. One-leg side plank	Up to 5 sec each side	122
Rest 30 sec		
1d. Step-through lunge	AMRAP each side	85
Rest 60 sec; perform exercises 1a-1d for 5 rounds		
2a. One-arm band fly	AMRAP; hold peak contraction for 3 sec each rep	196
Rest 30 sec		
2b. Kettlebell bent-over row	AMRAP; hold peak contraction for 3 sec each rep	150
Rest 60 sec; perform exercises 2a-2b for 3 rounds		

AMRAP = as many repetitions as possible

MB3 WORKOUT C

Exercise or *rest*	Reps/time	Page
1a. Straight-arm lat pull-down	AMRAP; hold peak contraction for 3 sec each rep	158
Rest 45 sec		
1b. Jump squat with kettlebell	3	73
Rest 45 sec		
1c. One-leg Romanian deadlift	AMRAP, slow	97
Rest 30 sec		
1d. Inverted narrow push-up	AMRAP	183
Rest 60 sec; perform exercises 1a-1d for 5 rounds		
2a. Stir the pot	AMRAP each direction, slow	124
Rest 30 sec		
2b. Biceps iso-hold	5 partial reps then hold for max time	187
Rest 30 sec; perform exercises 2a-2b for 3 rounds		

AMRAP = as many repetitions as possible

Final Thoughts

Building muscle and strength requires hard work, fatigue management, and patience. In this chapter we cover a variety of ways to structure your training to fit your schedule, equipment needs, and goals in order to promote variety. There will be times when you feel run down, and if it continues for a few days, don't push yourself to work harder. Give your body a break from any training for three to five days so you can recover from residual fatigue. After a long period of hard training, a break for up to a week can sometimes increase your strength and muscle mass.

CHAPTER 9

Fat-Burning Programs

At this point we've talked a lot about the principles for gaining muscle and strength. In this chapter we modify those strategies to help you retain your gains while you shift your focus to burning fat. We then cover energy systems training, which consists of both low- and high-intensity activity to maximize physique and performance benefits. Finally, we end with three different programs that will help you get the lean, strong body you desire.

Modifying Your Training for Fat Loss

In the last chapter we covered the principles of muscle building, and you saw my programs for achieving that goal. Everything I said there still applies when your primary goal is fat loss. The biggest difference is how much food you eat, a subject we cover in chapter 11. It surely won't surprise you to learn that successful fat loss requires eating fewer calories, just as hypertrophy requires a caloric surplus.

The simplest approach would be to follow any of the programs in chapter 8 while eating less. If you can undershoot your maintenance level by a couple hundred calories a day, you'll lose fat. And for the first few weeks, it should work exactly like you expect. It won't be easy, but it certainly is straightforward. However, problems begin after the first month or so. Sooner or later, you'll feel the effects of that calorie deficit. You'll have less strength during your workouts and slower recovery between them. With less total work in the weight room, you'll burn fewer calories than you did when you were eating more. You didn't do a lot of low-intensity cardio or high-intensity energy systems work when you were trying to build muscle, since those additional exercise sessions would burn calories you want to use for growth and repair. But in a fat-loss program, you need more ways to burn calories. High-intensity intervals, used strategically, are a great way to accelerate fat loss in relatively little time. Longer, slower physical activity not only burns calories but also improves recovery.

Thus, you need these program modifications when training for fat loss:

- Perform fewer rounds of a circuit, or the same number of rounds with fewer exercises in the circuit.

- Don't train to momentary muscular failure, except for the final set of body weight exercises.
- Supplement strength training with a broad spectrum of energy systems work.

These key changes, combined with a calorie deficit, will ensure that you lose fat while maintaining muscle and strength. And you'll build endurance that translates to virtually any sport. In the end, you'll emerge with a leaner, more athletic physique—exactly what you expected when you bought this book.

Utilizing Energy Systems Training for Fat Loss

Your body relies on three different systems to produce energy. First is the ATP-PC system, which uses phosphocreatine to fuel high-intensity muscle contractions for seconds at a time. Second is anaerobic glycolysis, a process where your body breaks down glucose without the help of oxygen. Third is aerobic metabolism, which breaks down glucose and fatty acids with oxygen. It also uses ketones when you're following a low-carbohydrate diet (Volek, Noakes, and Phinney 2015). These three systems constantly overlap to provide the energy you need during exercise, as shown in figure 9.1. Of the three systems, aerobic metabolism can directly burn fat for energy, which is why it should be part of any fat-burning program. The other two systems, ATP-PC and anaerobic glycolysis, are trained to build more muscle and mitochondria, which in turn increases your metabolic rate.

Importantly, each system does not make an equal contribution at any given level of intensity. During maximal activity, ATP-PC and anaerobic glycolysis are the primary drivers. Conversely, low-intensity activity is dominated by aerobic metabolism. For example, an MMA fighter could practice boxing at a low intensity for 30 minutes to develop his aerobic base, or strike with maximal intensity for 10 seconds and then rest a bit to build powerful endurance. Same activity, different energy systems.

There are two primary types of energy systems training (i.e., endurance training):

- *Continuous training*, which is performed at a relatively low intensity from start to finish without stopping, such as a 30-minute jog or 45 minutes on a bike.
- *Interval training*, which consists of two or more bouts of high-intensity exercise with a period of rest between each. For example, a swimmer might perform eight 50-meter sprints with 90 seconds' rest between each; a boxer might perform 12 20-second bouts of punching with 60-second rest intervals.

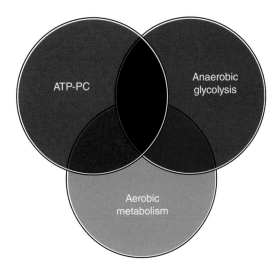

FIGURE 9.1 Overlap of the three energy systems.

Both types of energy systems training are beneficial for burning fat, developing endurance, and improving cardiovascular health (Ismail et al. 2012; Murawska-Cialowicz et al. 2020). However, different athletes require different types of endurance training. Cyclists, rowers, and marathon runners depend on continuous activity of their type I muscle fibers to sustain low force output for hours at a time. Conversely, football and ice hockey players must recruit their type IIx muscle fibers to produce explosive power for seconds at a time. For them,

Why Explosive Athletes Benefit From Building an Aerobic Base

Athletes used to spend considerable time performing LISS in the off-season to build their aerobic base. When research demonstrated that as little as 4 minutes of HIIT improved both aerobic and anaerobic capacity (Tabata et al. 1996), it sparked a fundamental shift in the application of endurance training.

Athletes, weekend warriors, and housewives were soon rushing to the gym to perform their "Tabata" workouts. Indeed, many athletes and fitness enthusiasts began to forego LISS training in favor of HIIT protocols that could be completed in a small fraction of the time. The idea was simple: HIIT gives people all the endurance training they need to develop both anaerobic and aerobic endurance.

To be clear, HIIT is not new, having been successfully used by athletes since the 1930s (Tabata 2019). But what is new is the shift away from LISS in favor of HIIT. Both have their unique place in anyone's program, especially athletes.

Most athletes benefit from periods of LISS to build their aerobic base, even athletes who compete in sports that rely heavily on anaerobic power. The only time aerobic metabolism will not play a significant role is when competition lasts less than 10 seconds followed by 7 minutes or more of rest. Very few popular sports fit that category except for powerlifting, Olympic lifting, and shot put.

Another benefit of a well-developed aerobic base is an increase in heart rate variability (HRV), a measure of the balance between sympathetic and parasympathetic nervous system activity. A high HRV helps athletes recover from the stressors of training and competition.

Mental fatigue can cause poor cognition and faulty movement patterns. One cause of mental fatigue is an excessive reliance on glucose (i.e., glycolysis) instead of fat for energy. Developing an aerobic base helps athletes better utilize fat for energy and improve oxygen delivery to the brain.

In summary, athletes benefit six different ways when they develop their aerobic base. It helps them

- recover more quickly between bouts of high-intensity activity;
- recover more quickly between competitions;
- better handle glycolytic stress during training and competition;
- better utilize fat for fuel, which minimizes or prevents acidosis and provides a virtually endless supply of energy;
- increase heart rate variability; and
- avoid mental fatigue.

A well-developed aerobic base generally requires 10 to 12 weeks of training, with more being better. In fact, it is recommended that athletes begin performing LISS as soon as possible after the competition or season ends. Finally, LISS doesn't have to be a boring jog on the treadmill. Athletes can perform drills that mimic movements in their sport, but at a much lower intensity and for a longer time.

and other explosive athletes, endurance is the ability to repeat their high force output throughout a game or competition.

There are countless ways to develop endurance, ranging from a brisk walk to pushing a heavy sled. Continuous low-intensity activities are programmed to develop an athlete's type I muscle fibers and aerobic base, which accelerates recovery and burns fat. This type of training is also known as low-intensity steady state (LISS) exercise. Conversely, interval training with high-intensity activities is programmed to develop your anaerobic systems and add mitochondria, your muscle's fat-burning furnaces, to your type II muscle fibers. Interval training, known as high-intensity interval training (HIIT) in the United States, usually consists of sprints, sled work, and other high-intensity activities that can create excessive fatigue if programmed improperly. Therefore, smart programming is crucial to manage your fatigue and improve performance. In summary, LISS exercise directly burns fat while HIIT builds more mitochondria, which makes your muscles able to burn more fat in the future.

Programming Energy Systems Training for Fat Loss

As mentioned, both LISS and HIIT are beneficial to your fat-burning program. Of the two, LISS is easiest to program. Think of 30 minutes of cycling or a 60-minute hike. For fitness enthusiasts or athletes in the off-season, it is difficult to get too much of it.

For years it was believed that performing strength and endurance training concurrently would reduce size and strength gains. This interference effect was first proposed over 40 years ago by Robert Hickson (1980). He demonstrated that adding leg-strengthening exercises to a predominantly aerobic program impaired strength gains compared with performing the same strength program without aerobic exercise. If you're not an athlete, that might be irrelevant. But for high-level athletes who need every possible advantage, many coaches took note. However, research indicates that the interference effect is probably not an issue for people with years of lifting experience (Petré, Löfving, and Psilander 2018). The simplest solution here is to program LISS on days when you don't lift weights whenever possible. As a general rule, 30 to 60 minutes of LISS exercise performed three days per week covers your bases. In the following programs you'll rotate between three distinctly different durations to promote variability, which we discuss later.

Regarding HIIT, the goal is to use a work:rest ratio that allows you to maintain your high-intensity performance. Think of HIIT as speed training: Once you start slowing down, the training effect diminishes. These days it's common to see HIIT protocols with extremely brief rest periods, resulting in high levels of acidosis and nausea. That is not necessary, and maybe even detrimental in the long run. In the programs in this chapter you'll see longer rest periods between bouts for HIIT than you'll typically find in YouTube videos or other places vying for your attention. That is by design. There will be times when you'll probably feel like you can perform these HIIT protocols with significantly less rest, but it's not recommended. As the saying goes, just because you can doesn't mean you should.

Programming Intensity

The intensity of HIIT training is straightforward: Exert maximum effort during each bout of activity. As Pavel Tsatsouline, kettlebell savant and creator of Strong

Endurance training, likes to say, there's no such thing as low-intensity interval training. With LISS, however, there are a few different ways to determine the correct intensity, and any of them can work. They are as follows:

- Start at a level of intensity you think you can maintain for 30 minutes.
- Be able to carry on a conversation, meaning you can complete a sentence without gasping for air (commonly referred to as the "talk test").
- Monitor your heart rate to determine your maximum aerobic heart rate (MAHR).

The third option here stems from Dr. Philip Maffetone, author of *The Big Book of Endurance Training and Racing*. His formula for LISS is simple: Subtract your age from 180 to determine your maximum aerobic heart rate (MAHR) in beats per minute (bpm) using this formula:

180 – age = maximum aerobic heart rate (MAHR)

The formula helps you determine the heart rate you don't want to exceed while performing LISS. For example, a typical 42-year-old man has an MAHR of 138 bpm And since it's impossible to maintain a specific heart rate during exercise, the MAHR range drops 10 bpm below that, which in this example is 128 to 138 bpm. Maintaining the MAHR range helps you train at an intensity high enough to improve aerobic power but low enough to avoid the anaerobic threshold, when your body starts burning more glucose for fuel and becomes more acidic (Maffetone 2010). Over the course of weeks and months you'll develop more mitochondria, capillaries, and myoglobin within the hypertrophied type I muscle fibers (Qaisar, Bhaskaran, and Van Remmen 2016). Low-intensity activity also increase your heart's stroke volume, allowing more blood to be ejected with each heartbeat (Hellsten and Nyberg 2015). This means your cardiovascular system can maintain your performance with fewer beats per minute. The MAHR calculation works well for most, with a few exceptions. It will probably not be accurate for someone who is severely deconditioned, is recovering from an injury, or has a very low resting heart rate. In those cases, stick to a level of intensity you can maintain for 30 minutes or follow the talk test.

Programming Variability

The goal of your endurance training is to make you a healthier, leaner athlete. Variability is a key principle for developing strength and endurance. The more distinct each training stimulus is from the next, the greater the adaptation that has to occur. Endurance training often gets programmed with no variability. A guy jogs for 30 minutes three times per week ad nauseum. This greatly diminishes the training stimulus, which impairs the physiological adaptations you're training for in the first place. As a general rule, there should be at least a 20 percent change in volume, either higher or lower, between endurance sessions (Tsatsouline 2018). That's why you'll see discrete changes in programming for endurance instead of a slow, linear progression.

For example, instead of programming LISS for 30 minutes in week 1, 35 minutes in week 2, and 40 minutes in week 3, you'll vary the times throughout the week. One LISS session is 30 minutes; another is 45 minutes; and another is 60 minutes. This not only promotes variability but is easier to schedule as well. You might choose to have your 60-minute session on a Saturday or Sunday when you're off work and have extra time to hike or take a long, brisk walk outside. During the week you could perform the 30-minute session on your busiest day, leaving you one 45-minute session to squeeze in. The options are endless, and any variation will work as long as you get the three sessions in each week.

For your LISS, choose an activity you will enjoy doing for 30 to 60 minutes straight. Avoid performing a cyclic activity, such as walking on a treadmill or pedaling a recumbent bike if those activities bore you. Instead, try some low-intensity boxing, basketball, or soccer drills. Any activity will work as long as you stay within the MAHR range. The key is to mix things up as much as possible.

This variability also applies to your HIIT sessions. You will perform three distinctly different HIIT protocols and change the exercise as often as possible from workout to workout. Basically, any exercise you can perform quickly that challenges most of your muscle groups will work. Here are some excellent options:

Kettlebell swings	Elliptical machine
Kettlebell snatches	Rower
Sprints	Assault bike
Stair stepper	Roundhouse kicks to a bag
Sled push or pull	Vertical climber
Loaded carries	

For example, one HIIT protocol is 5 seconds of maximal activity followed by 45 seconds of rest for 10 rounds. On week 1 you could perform a kettlebell swing, week 2 a sled push, week 3 roundhouse kicks to a bag, and so on. Perform no single protocol more than three times in a row with the same exercise before substituting it for another option.

Unlike many books out there, in this chapter you won't see specific exercises programmed, such as 45 minutes of jogging on one day and 10 minutes of sprints on another. Instead, you'll see the recommended duration of activity for LISS and the work:rest ratio for HIIT. Choose the activities you like best and mix things up.

Sample Fat-Burning Programs

The following three 12-week resistance training plans consist of three resistance training sessions per week with 48 hours' rest between each session. Before each workout, perform a dynamic warm-up (see chapter 3) to prepare your body for exercise. The programs are Fat Burner 1 (FB1), Fat Burner 2 (FB2), and Fat Burner 3 (FB3). They are not arranged in any particular order and are all equally effective for burning fat. The purpose of three different plans is to give you a variety of choices based on your available equipment. Remember, when resistance training, train the right and left side of your body with equal volume. This means that whenever you see a one-limb version programmed (e.g., one-arm overhead press), start with your weaker side and then perform the *same* number of reps on the opposite side, even if you can do more. Rest as little as possible between the right and left side. Also, no progression is predetermined for any of the resistance training plans because it is very difficult to set new PRs when you're in a caloric deficit. So if you can increase the load or add an extra rep to a set or two, you're one of the lucky few.

You'll perform three LISS and two or three HIIT sessions each week. The LISS sessions are intended to be performed on the days you don't lift weights in order to burn fat, accelerate recovery, and reduce the likelihood of an interference effect.

If that doesn't fit your schedule, perform them earlier or later on the days you lift weights, or directly before or after those sessions. Perform two or three HIIT sessions each week. These are intended to be at the end of your workouts since they can create significant fatigue, which is also why it might be best to perform just two in a week. A caloric deficit can drain your energy and impair recovery. And just like the LISS sessions, you can put the HIIT sessions somewhere else in the week if it better suits your schedule.

There are distinctly different protocols for your LISS and HIIT sessions. You'll rotate between the three different protocols before repeating. The protocols are as follows:

LISS

Each week perform a 30-, 45-, or 60-minute session on three of your nonlifting days.

HIIT

Rotate between the following three protocols two or three times per week. If you do two sessions one week, perform the third at the start of the following week, and continue rotating between them:

- *5:45 protocol:* 5 seconds of maximal activity followed by 45 seconds of rest. Repeat for 10 rounds.
- *10:60 protocol:* 10 seconds of maximal activity followed by 60 seconds of rest; 10 seconds of maximal activity followed by 60 seconds of rest; 10 seconds of maximal activity followed by 2 minutes of rest. Repeat for three rounds.
- *15:45 protocol:* 15 seconds of maximal activity followed by 45 seconds of rest; 15 seconds of maximal activity followed by 2 minutes of rest. Repeat for four rounds.

Fat Burner 1 (FB1)

The FB1 plan is designed around a large selection of training equipment. It is intended for a commercial gym or an elaborate home gym.

EQUIPMENT NEEDED

Pull-up/dip station

Cable station with adjustable pulley

Long resistance band

Heavy and moderately heavy dumbbells or large selection of pairs of kettlebells

Trap bar

Adjustable bench

Chin/dip belt

Gymnastics rings

FB1 WORKOUT A

Exercise or *rest*	Reps	Page
1a. Overhand-grip pull-up or pull-down	3	152, 153
Rest 45 sec		
1b. One-arm overhead push press	6 each side	179
Rest 60 sec		
1c. Incline bench press	8	170
Rest 45 sec; perform exercises 1a-1c for 3 rounds		
2a. Straight-arm lat pull-down	12	158
Rest 30 sec		
2b. Romanian deadlift (RDL)	8	95
Rest 60 sec; perform exercises 2a-2b for 3 rounds		

FB1 WORKOUT B

Exercise or *rest*	Reps	Page
1a. Inverted row	AMRAP	142
Rest 45 sec		
1b. One-arm cable or band chest press	10 each side	171
Rest 45 sec		
1c. Reverse lunge	8 each side	82
Rest 60 sec; perform exercises 1a-1c for 3 rounds		
2a. Band lying leg raise	12	132
Rest 45 sec		
2b. Goblet squat	14	68
Rest 90 sec; perform exercises 2a-2b for 3 rounds		

AMRAP = as many repetitions as possible

FB1 WORKOUT C

Exercise or *rest*	Reps/time	Page
1a. Hammer-grip pull-up or pull-down	2	154, 155
Rest 45 sec		
1b. Staggered-stance hip thrust	6 each side	102
Rest 60 sec		
1c. Dip	6	173
Rest 45 sec; perform exercises 1a-1c for 3 rounds		
2a. Turkish get-up	2 each side	137
Rest 60 sec		
2b. Loaded carry (walk in figure-eight pattern)	30 sec	135
Rest 60 sec; perform exercises 2a-2b for 3 rounds		

FB1 WORKOUT A

Exercise or *rest*	Reps/time	Page
1a. Split-stance row	4	144
Rest 45 sec		
1b. One-arm overhead press	8 each side	178
Rest 30 sec		
1c. One-arm loaded carry (walk in figure-eight pattern)	20 sec each side	136
Rest 60 sec		
1d. Goblet squat	10	68
Rest 90 sec; perform exercises 1a-1d for 4 rounds		
2. One-leg calf raise	20 (AMRAP in rounds 2 and 3)	107
Rest 30 sec; perform exercise 2 for 2 more rounds, then repeat on the other side		

AMRAP = as many repetitions as possible

FB1 WORKOUT B

Exercise or *rest*	Reps/time	Page
1a. Hammer-grip pull-up or pull-down	4	154, 155
Rest 45 sec		
1b. Dumbbell or kettlebell bench press	12	168
Rest 30 sec		
1c. Half-kneeling Pallof press	30 sec each side	126
Rest 45 sec		
1d. Split squat	5 each side	78
Rest 60 sec; perform exercises 1a-1d for 4 rounds		
2. Lying triceps extension	20 (AMRAP in rounds 2 and 3)	192
Rest 30 sec; perform exercise 2 for 2 more rounds		

AMRAP = as many repetitions as possible

FB1 WORKOUT C

Exercise or *rest*	Reps	Page
1a. Face pull	18	148
Rest 45 sec		
1b. Dip	6	173
Rest 45 sec		
1c. Stir the pot	3 each direction, slow	124
Rest 30 sec		
1d. Trap bar deadlift	3	94
Rest 60 sec; perform exercises 1a-1d for 4 rounds		
2. Biceps curl	20 (AMRAP in rounds 2 and 3)	188
Rest 30 sec; perform exercise 2 for 2 more rounds		

AMRAP = as many repetitions as possible

FB1 WORKOUT A

Exercise or *rest*	Reps/time	Page
1a. Hammer-grip pull-up or pull-down	6	154, 155
Rest 45 sec		
1b. Stacked side plank	Max time each side	121
Rest 60 seconds		
1c. Belt squat	15	74
Rest 90 sec; perform exercises 1a-1c for 3 rounds		
2a. Face pull	12	148
Rest 30 sec		
2b. Dip	8	173
Rest 60 sec; perform exercises 2a-2b for 3 rounds		

FB1 WORKOUT B

Exercise or *rest*	Reps	Page
1a. One-arm row	12 each side	146
Rest 45 sec		
1b. One-arm cable or band chest press	12 each side	171
Rest 45 sec		
1c. Deficit reverse lunge	6 each side	83
Rest 60 sec; perform exercises 1a-1c for 3 rounds		
2a. Straight-arm lat pull-down	6	158
Rest 30 sec		
2b. Romanian deadlift (RDL)	4	95
Rest 60 sec; perform exercises 2a-2b for 3 rounds		

FB1 WORKOUT C

Exercise or *rest*	Reps	Page
1a. Turkish get-up	2 each side	137
Rest 60 sec		
1b. Staggered-stance hip thrust	6 each side	102
Rest 60 sec		
1c. Overhand-grip pull-up or pull-down	6	152, 153
Rest 60 sec; perform exercises 1a-1c for 3 rounds		
2a. Step-up	5 each side	88
Rest 60 sec		
2b. Hanging leg raise	AMRAP	133
Rest 45 sec; perform exercises 2a-2b for 3 rounds		

AMRAP = as many repetitions as possible

Fat Burner 2 (FB2)

This program combines a mix of old-school strength exercises, such as a Zercher squat and Ahrens press, with new-school movements such as the kettlebell high pull and hip thrust. You'll use straps for some body weight exercises and then fill in any remaining gaps with dumbbells. This program is aimed at lifters who want to focus on full-body strength while they get lean.

EQUIPMENT NEEDED

Barbell

Moderate to heavy dumbbells or kettlebells

Long resistance band

Suspension trainer straps

Adjustable bench

FB2 WORKOUT A

Exercise or *rest*	Reps	Page
1a. Split-stance row	5	144
Rest 45 sec		
1b. Hip thrust	5	101
Rest 45 sec		
1c. One-arm floor press	10 each side	172
Rest 45 sec		
1d. Step-up	5 each side	88
Rest 90 sec; perform exercises 1a-1d for 4 rounds		

FB2 WORKOUT B

Exercise or *rest*	Reps	Page
1a. One-arm overhead press	5 each side	178
Rest 45 sec		
1b. Straight-arm lat pull-down	8	158
Rest 30 sec		
1c. Sumo deadlift	5	93
Rest 60 sec		
1d. Split squat	7 each side	78
Rest 90 sec; perform exercises 1a-1d for 4 rounds		

FB2 WORKOUT C

Exercise or *rest*	Reps/time	Page
1a. Inverted row	AMRAP	142
Rest 45 sec		
1b. Rings or straps push-up	AMRAP	166
Rest 45 sec		
1c. Pallof press	20 sec each side	125
Rest 45 sec		
1d. Reverse lunge	6 each side	82
Rest 90 sec; perform exercises 1a-1d for 4 rounds		

AMRAP = as many repetitions as possible

FB2 WORKOUT A

Exercise or *rest*	Reps	Page
1a. Yates row	4	145
Rest 45 sec		
1b. Incline bench press	8	170
Rest 45 sec		
1c. Push-up	AMRAP	161
Rest 45 sec		
1d. One-leg Romanian deadlift	8 each side	97
Rest 90 sec; perform exercises 1a-1d for 4 rounds		

AMRAP = as many repetitions as possible

FB2 WORKOUT B

Exercise or *rest*	Reps/time	Page
1a. One-arm overhead push press	8 each side	179
Rest 45 sec		
1b. Hand walk push-up	AMRAP	165
Rest 45 sec		
1c. Side plank	20 sec each side	120
Rest 45 sec		
1d. Zercher squat	4	72
Rest 90 sec; perform exercises 1a-1d for 4 rounds		

AMRAP = as many repetitions as possible

FB2 WORKOUT C

Exercise or *rest*	Reps/time	Page
1a. One-arm row	8 each side	146
Rest 45 sec		
1b. Staggered-stance hip thrust	AMRAP each side	102
Rest 45 sec		
1c. Ahrens press	10	181
Rest 45 sec		
1d. Half-kneeling Pallof press	20 sec each side	126
Rest 45 sec		
1e. Forward lunge	5 each side	84
Rest 90 sec; perform exercises 1a-1e for 3 rounds		

AMRAP = as many repetitions as possible

FB2 WORKOUT A

Exercise or *rest*	Reps	Page
1a. Feet-elevated inverted row	AMRAP	143
Rest 45 sec		
1b. Hip thrust	6	101
Rest 45 sec		
1c. One-arm overhead press	8 each side	178
Rest 45 sec		
1d. Lateral lunge	4 each side	86
Rest 90 sec; perform exercises 1a-1d for 4 rounds		

AMRAP = as many repetitions as possible

FB2 WORKOUT B

Exercise or *rest*	Reps	Page
1a. Rings or straps inverted push-up	AMRAP	185
Rest 45 sec		
1b. Band lying leg raise	8, slow	132
Rest 45 sec		
1c. Deadlift	3	91
Rest 90 sec; perform exercises 1a-1c for 5 rounds		

AMRAP = as many repetitions as possible

FB2 WORKOUT C

Exercise or *rest*	Reps/time	Page
1a. Face pull	12	148
Rest 45 sec		
1b. Explosive push-up	3	164
Rest 45 sec		
1c. Stacked side plank	20 sec each side	121
Rest 45 sec		
1d. Step-through lunge	5 each side	85
Rest 90 sec; perform exercises 1a-1d for 4 rounds		

Fat Burner 3 (FB3)

The FB3 plan prioritizes your body weight for resistance. Additionally, you'll need a moderately heavy kettlebell, long resistance band, and Swiss ball to fill in the gaps. Since a range of loads isn't possible, most of the sets are performed for as many repetitions as possible (AMRAP). Stop each set one rep short of failure. On the last set you can push closer to exhaustion, as long as it doesn't compromise your form in any way.

Your full-body strength relies heavily on your core. Since it's common to lose strength while cutting calories, this program emphasizes making your midsection stronger. That's why your core exercises in this program are almost always performed first, when you have the most energy, instead of at the end of a workout when you're fatigued.

EQUIPMENT NEEDED

One moderately heavy kettlebell (or dumbbells)

Long resistance band

Swiss ball

Short box or step

FB3 WORKOUT A

Exercise or *rest*	Reps	Page
1a. Swiss ball rollout	AMRAP	117
Rest 45 sec		
1b. One-arm overhead push press	AMRAP each side	179
Rest 45 sec		
1c. One-arm row	AMRAP each side	146
Rest 45 sec		
1d. Reverse lunge	AMRAP each side	82
Rest 90 sec; perform exercises 1a-1d for 4 rounds		

AMRAP = as many repetitions as possible

FB3 WORKOUT B

Exercise or *rest*	Reps/time	Page
1a. Hardstyle plank	10 sec max effort	115
Rest 45 sec		
1b. Face pull	12	148
Rest 45 sec		
1c. One-arm floor press	AMRAP each side	172
Rest 45 sec		
1d. Step-up	AMRAP each side	88
Rest 90 sec; perform exercises 1a-1d for 4 rounds		

AMRAP = as many repetitions as possible

FB3 WORKOUT C

Exercise or *rest*	Reps/time	Page
1a. Pallof press	20 sec each side	125
Rest 45 sec		
1b. Feet-elevated push-up	AMRAP	162
Rest 45 sec		
1c. Straight-arm lat pull-down	12	158
Rest 30 seconds		
1d. Kettlebell swing	5	99
Rest 90 sec; perform exercises 1a-1d for 4 rounds		

AMRAP = as many repetitions as possible

FB3 WORKOUT A

Exercise or *rest*	Reps/time	Page
1a. One-leg hardstyle plank	5 sec max effort each side	116
Rest 45 sec		
1b. Face pull	16	148
Rest 45 sec		
1c. Explosive push-up	3	164
Rest 45 sec		
1d. Lateral lunge	AMRAP each side	86
Rest 90 sec; perform exercises 1a-1d for 4 rounds		

AMRAP = as many repetitions as possible

FB3 WORKOUT B

Exercise or *rest*	Reps/time	Page
1a. Half-kneeling Pallof press	20 sec each side	126
Rest 45 sec		
1b. Inverted push-up	AMRAP	182
Rest 45 sec		
1c. Stir the pot	3 each direction, slow	124
Rest 30 sec		
1d. Goblet squat	AMRAP	68
Rest 90 sec; perform exercises 1a-1d for 4 rounds		

AMRAP = as many repetitions as possible

FB3 WORKOUT C

Exercise or *rest*	Reps	Page
1a. Hand walkout	AMRAP	118
Rest 45 sec		
1b. One-arm row	AMRAP each side	146
Rest 45 sec		
1c. One-arm overhead press	AMRAP each side	178
Rest 45 sec		
1d. Forward lunge	AMRAP each side	84
Rest 90 sec; perform exercises 1a-1d for 4 rounds		

AMRAP = as many repetitions as possible

FB3 WORKOUT A

Exercise or *rest*	Reps/time	Page
1a. Tall-kneeling Pallof press	20 sec each side	127
Rest *45 sec*		
1b. Hand walk push-up	AMRAP	165
Rest *45 sec*		
1c. Straight-arm lat pull-down	16	158
Rest *30 sec*		
1d. Kettlebell swing	7	99
Rest *90 sec;* perform exercises 1a-1d for 4 rounds		

AMRAP = as many repetitions as possible

FB3 WORKOUT B

Exercise or *rest*	Reps/time	Page
1a. One-arm row	AMRAP each side	146
Rest *45 sec*		
1b. Turkish get-up	2 each side	137
Rest *45 sec*		
1c. One-arm plank	5 sec each side	129
Rest *45 sec*		
1d. Step-through lunge	AMRAP each side	85
Rest *90 sec;* perform exercises 1a-1d for 4 rounds		

AMRAP = as many repetitions as possible

FB3 WORKOUT C

Exercise or *rest*	Reps	Page
1a. Band lying leg raise	AMRAP	132
Rest *45 sec*		
1b. Face pull	20	148
Rest *45 sec*		
1c. Swiss ball push-up	AMRAP	167
Rest *45 sec*		
1d. One-leg Romanian deadlift	AMRAP each side	97
Rest *90 sec;* perform exercises 1a-1d for 4 rounds		

AMRAP = as many repetitions as possible

Final Thoughts

It's likely the resistance training programs in this chapter have longer rest periods than you've seen in many other fat-loss workouts. Complexes, for example, are often programmed with the intention of burning fat since they force you to transition between exercises without rest. Conversely, the resistance sessions covered have rest periods that allow for full recovery before repeating a lift. The goal is to stimulate muscle and strength gains with the lowest volume possible, even though it will be difficult to build either when you're in a caloric deficit. In other words, these resistance workouts are not intended to ramp up your heart rate to stimulate fat loss. That's what the LISS and HIIT sessions are for.

Finally, the resistance programs in this chapter are designed to equally stimulate all your major muscle groups with three workouts per week. For some of you, a higher frequency will be necessary for lagging muscle groups. So in the next chapter, we cover how you can train a body part or two more frequently, even when your primary goal is fat loss.

CHAPTER 10

Body Part–Specific Programs

Certain types of athletes can teach us a lot about muscle growth. All you have to do is look at the thighs of speed skaters, or the lats of swimmers, or the deltoids of boxers, or the biceps of gymnasts who specialize in the rings to see that frequently training a muscle group can result in tremendous development. In this chapter we cover the principles for targeting and stimulating growth in underdeveloped muscle groups using high frequency training (HFT) plans. If you're one of the lucky few who has proportional development from head to toe, this information might not be applicable to you. But for those who need to balance out their physique, the following HFT strategies are a terrific addition to your overall program.

The Genesis of HFT

By 2001 I'd been a full-time personal trainer for five years, with a long, diverse list of clients who'd successfully built muscle, increased strength, and improved performance. All of them used the same basic system of three full-body workouts a week. It was, I believed, the best starting point for any off-season athlete, CEO, or fitness enthusiast.

But some of those clients had muscle groups that simply didn't grow as fast as other areas. Those lagging, underdeveloped body parts were a problem for clients who were mainly focused on aesthetics. And if they had a problem, I had a problem, because my business depended on them getting all the muscle growth they were looking for, from head to toe.

I found the solution from two sources. One of them, to no one's surprise, was arguably the greatest bodybuilder of all time. The other was completely unexpected. Here's how it happened:

I heard about a Cirque du Soleil show called *Mystère*, which was playing in Las Vegas, a few hours up the road from Tucson, Arizona, where I lived in 2001. When the Alexis brothers took the stage for their part of the show, my first thought was, "Wow, I've never seen better physiques on two guys."

Then they began their routine. One brother would lift and lower the other in the most challenging ways you can imagine. I'd seen impressive feats of strength in the gym, including a triple body weight deadlift, but I'd never seen anything like this. Each part of the routine was more astonishing than the last. I couldn't believe they could do it without tearing a muscle. Not only that, they did it twice a day, five days a week, for months on end.

How was this possible? How could two guys develop such incredible physiques and put their mind-blowing strength on display 10 times a week? Nothing I'd learned in my exercise science courses could explain it, regardless of any pharmaceutical help they may or may not have had.

That show made me reevaluate my clients' training programs. I knew that training a muscle more often will lead to more muscle growth, but I also knew that growth requires sufficient recovery between training sessions (see figure 10.1). I thought three sessions a week was the highest training frequency you could use without compromising recovery. But if three sessions weren't enough to maximize growth in muscles like the biceps or calves, it made sense to have those clients target those muscles with a few sets outside of their full-body workouts.

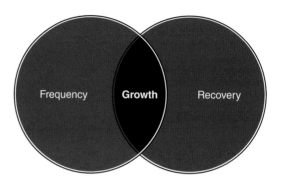

FIGURE 10.1 Optimal growth requires optimal overlap between training and recovery.

One thing became clear almost immediately: More was indeed better. The open question was how much more. That led to a lot of trial and error over the next few years as I searched for the right balance between extra training sessions and recovery. By 2012 I had accumulated enough data and experimentation to write *High Frequency Training*, followed by *High Frequency Training 2* in 2014.

What you'll find in this chapter is simpler and more effective than what I published in those books. In part those refinements come from the data and feedback I've accumulated from clients and patients since 2014. They're also based on a key element to faster muscle growth that I should have learned back in 2001. No, I'm not talking about the Alexis brothers. I'm talking about Arnold Schwarzenegger.

Back in 2001, when I saw the Alexis brothers perform, I was also reading Schwarzenegger's *New Encyclopedia of Modern Bodybuilding* (1987). This passage is especially relevant to what you'll see in the programming later in this chapter:

"My left arm used to be slightly smaller than my right arm. I noticed that whenever I was asked to show my biceps, I would automatically flex the right arm. So I consciously made an effort to flex my left arm as much or more than my right, to work that weak point instead of trying to ignore it, and eventually I was able to make my left biceps the equal of my right."

Back then, I used that quote to support the idea that training a muscle more frequently would lead to more growth. Today I have a different interpretation, and a more practical way to apply it. That's because I now know that simply squeezing a muscle three times each day will augment the results of a targeted HFT plan. The tension you achieve with an intense contraction can be similar to the levels you achieve with weights in the gym. That's why professional bodybuilders often report muscle soreness the day after practicing their posing routine.

That brings us to an essential point about any HFT plan to develop lagging body parts: You need to perform exercises that overload the muscles more than the joints. The barbell bench press might be a good exercise to build the pectorals, but it also places a lot of strain on the shoulder joints. But a one-arm fly with a resistance band targets the chest with minimal stress on the shoulders.

In this chapter we cover the ideal HFT exercises for each muscle group. These are the exercises that target muscles as directly as possible for maximal growth with minimal strain on your joints. Three other times throughout the day, you'll simply squeeze those muscles to peak contraction for 6 seconds. You can do these contractions anywhere, without any equipment, in whatever clothes you happen to be wearing, with no warm-up required.

These daily squeezes have significantly improved the muscle-building results of my HFT programs. I just wish I'd properly interpreted Schwarzenegger's quote years before I did.

Now it's time to show you what I'm talking about.

HFT Targeted Plans

In this section we cover the HFT plans that target specific muscle groups. Since you'll be performing three full-body workouts on top of these plans, choose no more than two muscle groups to attack at any given time. Any more than that will create excessive fatigue and compromise your overall recovery. For example, if you feel your calves and biceps are underdeveloped, add those plans to your program. Or maybe you just need to develop your triceps. In any case, continue with the plan until the muscle group has grown to the level that suits you. Later we'll cover what you can do to keep the gains you've made.

For the HFT targeted plans you will perform two sets on the scheduled days. When you're training a muscle twice a day, outside of your normal full-body workouts, the last thing you'll want to worry about is finding exercise equipment. That is why the recommended exercises for an HFT targeted plan are based on the minimum equipment possible. Ideally, all exercises could be performed with just your body weight, but that is not practical for targeting certain muscle groups. The good news is that the only exercises that require a weight are the lateral raise and wrist extension and flexion, and they often require nothing heavier than a 10-pound (4.5 kg) dumbbell. The other exercises are performed with your body weight or a resistance band. The ideal way to perform any HFT exercise is one limb at a time since it's likely you can produce more force than if you worked both limbs at the same time (Aune et al. 2013). There are three primary reasons why:

- You can better focus on the targeted muscle to improve motor unit recruitment.
- You can identify strength imbalances between the left and right side.
- Sometimes it's necessary to train only one limb, such as rehabilitation from surgery.

That being said, it's not always necessary to perform your HFT exercises one limb at a time. Sometimes you'll be short on time, or the exercise is well suited for working both limbs simultaneously, or the resistance band needs to be significantly stretched to produce enough tension to challenge you. In any of those cases, it might be more beneficial to train both limbs at the same time.

Variety is an important aspect of training to minimize joint stress when using heavy loads. That is why the full-body workouts in this book rotate between different exercises and repetitions. For targeted HFT plans, however, I've found that you can perform the same exercise for months at a time without impairing your results. These quick sets are simply intended to activate and fatigue the muscle so it will grow. Since all of the exercises we're about to cover accomplish that goal with minimal joint stress, no other variety is necessary. You will get all the variety you need by performing your sets in more challenging ways as you get stronger, which we cover later in this chapter. For now, the recommended exercises are shown in table 10.1.

TABLE 10.1   Recommended Exercises for HFT Targeted Plans

Targeted body part	HFT exercise	Page
Calves	One-leg calf raise	107
Quadriceps	Split squat	78
Hamstrings	Slider leg curl	103
Glutes	Standing fire hydrant	105
Pectoralis major	One-arm band fly	196
Latissimus dorsi (lats)	Straight one-arm lat pull-down	159
Upper back	One-arm band face pull	149
Middle deltoid	One-arm lateral raise	198
Upper trapezius	One-arm band shrug	199
Biceps	One-arm band biceps curl	191
Triceps	One-arm band triceps press-down	195
Forearms	One-arm wrist extension and flexion	200

Next, we cover strategies for getting the most out of your HFT sessions in minimal time. In the early days of my HFT protocols, I would have my clients train their lagging muscle groups each day, which I later discovered was unnecessary and, in some cases, impractical if any equipment was required. Since then, I've codified a simpler plan to help you grow where you need it most.

Frequency: three days on, one day off

For many years I had clients perform one set in the morning and evening hours, six days in a row, followed by a day of rest. After accumulating much data I've found that three days on and then resting every fourth day not only produces similar results but in some cases accelerates muscle growth. To be clear, your rest day from an HFT targeted plan might fall on a day you perform full-body training, so it won't necessarily be a complete rest day.

Timing of the sets: 8 to 12 hours apart

On the days of your HFT targeted plan you'll perform two sets, each one spaced 8 to 12 hours apart. Ideally, the sets will always be 12 hours apart, such as 8:00 a.m. and 8:00 p.m., since that allows for the most recovery, but that can be impractical at times. As long as you rest at least 8 hours between HFT sessions, you will reap the benefits, even if you perform a full-body workout during that break.

Most of my clients prefer to perform one of the HFT sets as part of their full-body workout, if it's scheduled that day. In that case, perform your HFT set at the beginning of your full-body workout when you have the most energy. In any case, as long as you rest 8 to 12 hours between sets of the HFT exercise, the timing of your full-body workout is irrelevant.

Intensity: every set taken to momentary muscular failure

Each set you perform is taken to momentary muscular failure. Any intensity lower than that will not create a stress that's large enough to optimize the hypertrophy response (Morton et al. 2019). The muscle group must be burning or pumped by the end of the set. The muscle pump, especially, might be a potent trigger for muscle growth (Schoenfeld and Contreras, 2014). If you fail to feel an intense muscle burn or a muscle pump, follow the strategies covered later in this section to make each set more challenging.

Repetitions or time: 30 repetitions or 30 seconds per set

Over the years I've experimented with a vast array of rep ranges for HFT plans, ranging anywhere from 20 to 100 per set. The sweet spot for almost everyone is 30 continuous repetitions. That number requires a load that is light enough to perform frequently but challenging enough to stimulate muscle growth (Lasevicius et al. 2019). Plus, it's quicker to perform 30 reps than 100, making it even easier to fit into a busy schedule. My patients find creative ways to fit the sets into their day, such as doing calf raises while putting gas in their car, or peak contraction squeezes of the glutes while waiting in line at the grocery store, which we cover shortly. The general tempo for each repetition is a controlled, moderate pace—basically, a count of "one-one thousand" on the way up and down. However, some of my patients prefer to perform the repetitions more explosively, while others prefer a slower tempo. Whichever tempo feels best to achieve tension and elicit a muscle pump is probably what's best for you.

Your brain's motor cortex has a very small area devoted to the glutes, which is one explanation why some people find it difficult to feel their glutes contract (Fischer et al. 2016). Therefore, the standing fire hydrant is performed as an isometric hold instead of repetitions. You will hold the muscle contraction for 30 seconds, and then progress to stronger bands as your strength increases in the weeks and months ahead.

Modifications: make sets more challenging

The goal of each set is to reach momentary muscular failure on the 30th repetition, give or take a repetition, without stopping any sooner. For the standing fire hydrants, you should feel an intense muscle burn in the glutes of your stance leg by 30 seconds. In either case, achieving that goal right from the start is both unlikely and unnecessary. Let's say you want to boost development of your calves, so you start on the HFT plan with the one-leg calf raise. You might not be able to perform 30 continuous repetitions through a full range of motion on day 1. As you experience fatigue on, say, repetition 18, start performing repetitions through a partial range of motion until you reach the 30th repetition. And if you reach momentary muscular failure before 30, rest for 15 seconds and continue until you hit the mark.

In this case, your first goal is to achieve 30 full range of motion repetitions, which might take weeks or months. Once you reach that goal, it's time to consider strategies to make the exercise more challenging because, as mentioned earlier, your calves must be burning or pumped when you reach failure on the 30th repetition. Once you can perform more than 30 full range of motion one-leg calf raises, or any other HFT exercise, do one of the following:

- Squeeze the peak contraction of the last 10 repetitions for 1 to 3 seconds.
- Perform a 10- to 30-second negative on the last one or two repetitions.
- Perform a 5- to 10-second peak contraction squeeze at the beginning or end of the set, or both.

You can use any combination of the aforementioned strategies to increase the intensity of a set. Finally, it's important to understand that strength gains are not linear. Much like a stock can fluctuate day to day, what matters is that the overall trend is upward. Some days you'll need the aforementioned strategies to reach muscle failure on the 30th repetition; other times you'll just need to blast through the repetitions and hope to reach 30. But your overall performance will drastically improve over the weeks and months, just like any good investment.

Peak Contraction Squeezes

Peak contraction squeezes (PCSs) are relatively new to my HFT plans. These intense isometric contractions have augmented my patients' results ever since I implemented them. In this section we cover how to get the most out of this simple addition to your plan that you can do anywhere, anytime.

When performing a PCS, you squeeze an intense peak contraction of the targeted muscle group for 6 seconds, three times per day. This improves your mind–muscle connection by improving neural drive through the cortical motor pathway (Fisher et al. 2016). That carries over to your ability to recruit more motor units, and thereby stimulate more growth, in your sets of 30 repetitions. Furthermore, professional bodybuilders extol the virtues of intense contractions during their posing routines to improve muscle hardness and overall definition.

As is the case with sets of the HFT exercises, it's ideal to spread the three PCS exercises as evenly as possible throughout the day. For example, if your two sets of the HFT exercise are performed at 8:00 a.m. and 8:00 p.m., you could do the three PCSs at, say, 11:00 a.m., 2:00 p.m. and 5:00 p.m., or any interval around that time frame. The key is to just spread out the three squeezes and do them six days per week. You should always have one day of complete rest, meaning no HFT exercise, no PCSs, and no full-body training.

Also, perform the PCSs one limb at a time: 6 seconds on the right, then 6 seconds on the left, or just one side if that's all you need to target (e.g., rehabilitation after surgery). Squeeze and hold the PCS with around 8 out of 10 effort. A 10 out of 10 effort usually results in excessive tension elsewhere in the body, which is not recommended.

Most guys already know how to intensely squeeze their biceps. They've been doing it ever since puberty. Other muscle groups, such as the latissimus dorsi (lats) or hamstrings, might not be so easy for someone without a background in competitive bodybuilding. Therefore, we finish out this chapter by covering guidelines for the PCS exercises.

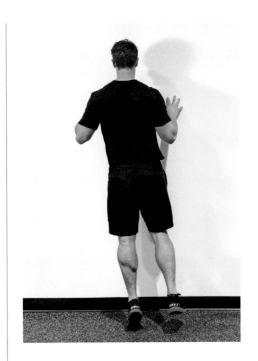

Calves PCS

Stand facing a wall or secure object for balance support. Place the fingertips of one or both hands on the wall, stand on your left leg, and perform a one-leg calf raise. Squeeze the peak contraction of your left calf for 6 seconds. Repeat on the opposite side.

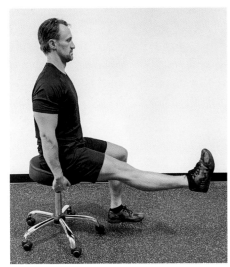

Quadriceps PCS

Sit tall in a chair, knees bent and feet flat on the floor. Fully extend your right leg. Squeeze the peak contraction of your right quadriceps for 6 seconds. Repeat on the opposite side.

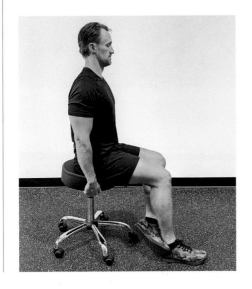

Hamstrings PCS

Sit tall in a chair, knees bent and feet flat on the floor. Place your left ankle behind your right heel. Pull your right heel back against the resistance from your left leg. No actual movement should occur at the knee once you achieve the peak contraction of the right hamstrings. Squeeze the peak contraction of your right hamstrings for 6 seconds. Repeat on the opposite side.

Glutes PCS

Stand tall with your feet shoulder-width apart. Slightly flex your right knee and place the ball of your right foot approximately 6 inches (15 cm) behind you. Fully extend your right hip. Squeeze the peak contraction of your right glutes for 6 seconds. Repeat on the opposite side.

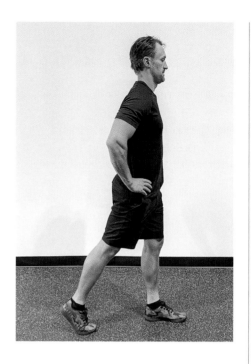

Pectoralis Major PCS

Stand approximately 18 inches (45 cm) in front of a wall's corner or secure object, with your feet slightly wider than shoulder width. Place your left palm over your navel as a tactile cue to brace your abdomen. Place the palm of your right hand against the wall, with your arm parallel to the ground. Your right palm should be directly in line with the center of your right pectoralis. Pull your right palm against the resistance of the wall. Squeeze the peak contraction of your right pectoralis for 6 seconds. Repeat on the opposite side.

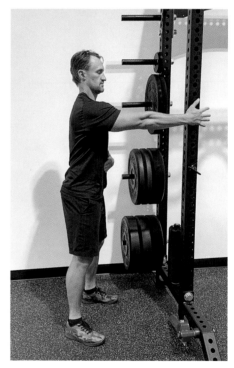

Latissimus Dorsi PCS

Stand tall with your feet slightly wider than shoulder width. Place your left palm over your navel as a tactile cue to brace your abdomen. Flex your right elbow to 90 degrees, and make a fist with your right hand. Brace your midsection, and then pull your right elbow against the side of your torso. Squeeze the peak contraction of your right latissimus dorsi for 6 seconds. Repeat on the opposite side.

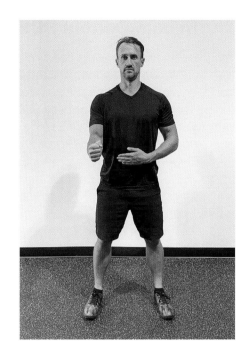

Upper Back PCS

Stand tall with your feet slightly wider than shoulder width. Place your left palm over your navel as a tactile cue to brace your abdomen. Lift your right arm 45 degrees away from the side of your torso. Fully flex your right elbow, with your palm facing forward. Brace your midsection, then pull your right elbow as far behind you as possible. Squeeze the peak contraction of your right upper back muscles for 6 seconds. Repeat on the opposite side.

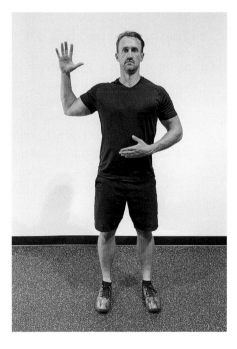

Middle Deltoid PCS

Technically, the following position is not the middle deltoid's peak contraction; however, it's the position that is often ideal for performing your squeezes. Stand tall with the corner of a wall or secure object approximately 12 inches (30 cm) to your right. Place your left palm over your navel as a tactile cue to brace your abdomen. Flex your right elbow to 90 degrees, make a fist, and then elevate your forearm until it touches the wall. Your right upper arm should be approximately 45 degrees away from the side of your torso. Push your right forearm into the resistance of the wall without shrugging your right shoulder. Squeeze the peak contraction of your right middle deltoid for 6 seconds. Repeat on the opposite side.

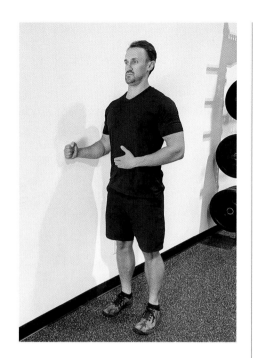

Upper Trapezius PCS

Be sure to have a physician or physical therapist clear you for this exercise if you have a history of neck problems. This exercise is not appropriate for everyone. Get in a split stance, with your left leg in front and feet shoulder-width apart. Place your left palm over your navel as a tactile cue to brace your abdomen. Shift your trunk slightly forward, make a fist with your right hand, and then shrug your right shoulder as high as possible toward the back of your right ear. Squeeze the peak contraction of your right upper trapezius for 6 seconds. Repeat on the opposite side.

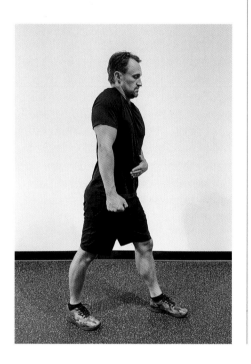

Biceps PCS

Stand tall with your feet slightly wider than shoulder width. Place your left palm over your navel as a tactile cue to brace your abdomen. Abduct your right arm to parallel, make a fist, and then maximally flex your elbow and wrist. Squeeze the peak contraction of your right biceps for 6 seconds. Repeat on the opposite side.

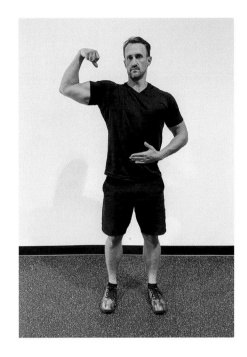

Triceps PCS

Get in a split stance, with your left leg in front and feet shoulder-width apart, and shift your trunk slightly forward. Place your left palm over your navel as a tactile cue to brace your abdomen. With your right arm hanging down at your side, make a fist with your right hand, and turn your palm so it faces behind you. Fully extend your right elbow. Squeeze the peak contraction of your right triceps for 6 seconds. Repeat on the opposite side.

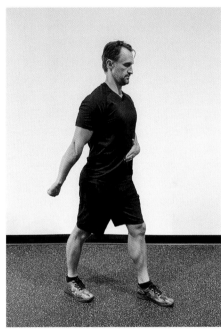

How to Maintain Your Gains

Since I wrote *High Frequency Training* in 2012, the most common question I get asked is, How can I maintain the gains I made from the HFT plans? The answer is relatively straightforward and consists of three key points:

- Keep training that muscle group three times per week as part of your full-body workouts.

- Perform one set to failure at the beginning of your workout. This is the time when you'll have the most energy, and not surprisingly, it has been shown to elicit the best results (Spineti et al. 2010).

- The single set should be as challenging as possible, based on the modifications covered earlier. Most of my patients have found that starting the set with a 10-second peak contraction squeeze and ending it with a slow negative, such as 30 seconds, is sufficient to maintain the HFT gains.

Forearm PCS

This consists of two squeezes on each side: one for the wrist extensors and one for the wrist flexors. Sit tall in a chair, knees bent and feet flat on the floor. Rest the inside of your right forearm, palm facing down, on the top of your right thigh. Make a fist with your right hand, and then pull your right knuckles as high as possible (i.e., wrist extension). Place your left palm over your right knuckles to provide resistance. Pull your right knuckles against the resistance of your left palm. Squeeze the peak contraction of your right wrist extensors for 6 seconds. Next, place the top of your right forearm, palm facing up, on your right thigh. Make a fist with your right hand and pull your knuckles as high as possible (i.e., wrist flexion). Pull your right knuckles against the resistance of your left palm. Squeeze the peak contraction of your right wrist flexors for 6 seconds. Repeat on the opposite side.

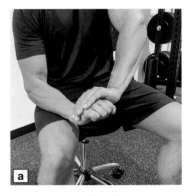

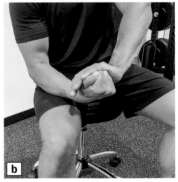

Final Thoughts

As we close out this chapter, it is worth mentioning there's a lack of research devoted to training a muscle group with any frequency higher than three times per week. However, it's thought that more frequent training results in more frequent boosts in muscle protein synthesis, which can accelerate growth over the weeks and months (Dankel et al. 2017). My anecdotal evidence definitely supports that hypothesis, and I hope you'll achieve results like my patients have.

PART IV

MUSCLE MAINTENANCE

CHAPTER 11

Nutrition for Muscle Growth or Fat Loss

I'm not a registered dietitian, nor do I have an advanced degree in nutrition. But I learned early in my coaching career that I couldn't help my clients reach their performance or physique goals without focusing as much on nutrition as I do on training and recovery.

It's a surprisingly complex topic. For example, if you want to lose fat, you should eat less. The math is pretty simple, right? But the more aggressively you cut calories, the harder it will be to continue training with enough volume and intensity to achieve the physique you want. You'll compromise your recovery between workouts and probably disrupt the quality of your sleep as well. You can still lose fat, if you tough it out long enough. But it's a miserable way to reach your goals, and it makes your new lower body fat percentage nearly impossible to sustain.

Or let's say you want to gain muscle. Again, the math is pretty simple: The more you eat, the more muscle you can pack on. But there are good and bad ways to do it. Without a smart nutrition plan, the muscle you gain will come with more fat than you anticipated, and it may take years to lose it. No matter your goals—muscle gain, fat loss, or physique maintenance—you need to get two things right: total calories per day and protein intake.

In this chapter we cover the elements of your nutrition plan that apply to muscle growth, fat loss, and recovery. We first discuss the importance of getting your calories and protein intake dialed in. We also outline healthy sources of carbohydrate, fat, and protein, as well as guidelines for workout nutrition and hydration. Intermittent fasting is discussed along with simple guidelines to clean up any diet. By the end of this chapter you'll have all the nutrition strategies you need to accelerate fat loss and muscle growth in sensible, sustainable ways, allowing for full recovery and optimal health to maximize your nutrition for any goal.

Dialing in Your Calories and Protein

Losing fat requires an energy deficit, meaning you need to eat fewer calories per day than your body needs for maintenance. Gaining muscle requires an energy surplus. For that, it doesn't help to increase your protein intake beyond 1.6 grams per kilogram of body weight, the recommended amount of protein we discussed in chapter 3. Protein is highly satiating, which means it helps reduce your appetite. That's why increasing protein can contribute to fat loss; even if you don't deliberately cut calories, you'll probably eat less simply because you aren't as hungry, thanks to the excess protein. But when you're trying to eat more, the last thing you want to do is overconsume a macronutrient that suppresses your desire to eat.

This may seem counterintuitive to you. After all, if muscle tissue is made of protein, and muscle growth requires a positive protein balance, why wouldn't higher protein intake contribute to bigger muscles? Think of it in terms of your energy balance—the number of calories required to maintain your current body weight. If you eat fewer calories than your body expends, you lose weight. If you eat more, you gain weight. All of this is in constant flux. Your body is very good at downregulating your metabolism in response to an energy deficit, which is one reason it's so difficult to lose weight in a steady, predictable way. You move less, and you burn fewer calories when you do. That's another reason why increasing your protein intake helps with fat loss. Protein has a higher thermic effect than the other macronutrients, which means your body burns more calories processing it (Halton and Hu 2004).

Given the importance of getting your calories right, you might be surprised to know that I almost never have my patients count them. Even if you carried around a nutrition almanac, the likelihood of being accurate is very low, not to mention frustrating and time consuming. And frankly, it's usually unnecessary. In the early stages, all you need to keep track of is your protein intake. From there, it's often best (and easiest) to consume the other foods we cover later in this chapter and not worry about how many calories they contain. By nature, most of the recommended foods are high in nutrients and relatively low in calories. This makes them both satisfying and difficult to eat too much of.

If you are someone who wants to count calories, a good starting point for daily calories for a nonobese person follows. We'll use a 200-pound (91 kg) person as an example:

- *Lose fat:* 10 × body weight in pounds (2,000 calories/day)
- *Maintain current weight:* 12 × body weight in pounds (2,400 calories/day)
- *Gain muscle:* 14 × body weight in pounds (2,800 calories/day)

Importantly, these are just estimates and can be greatly affected by age, activity levels, and metabolic health. For example, an in-season 200-pound football player would likely lose weight if he consumed 2,800 calories per day. Conversely, if you're obese the aforementioned calculation for fat loss might be much higher than what's optimal. In that case, you should consult with a registered dietitian to determine your recommended daily calories, which will likely be based on your fat free mass. In any case, use an abdomen measurement, mirror, and scale as your guide to determine if you need to increase or decrease your calories. If you need to increase your calories, choose healthy sources of carbohydrate and fat that we cover later.

Maximizing Your Macronutrients

In this section we cover the three types of macronutrients: protein, fat, and carbohydrate. These nutrients provide the calories your body needs for energy, growth, and repair. When you choose the right sources of macronutrients, you'll also optimize your intake of micronutrients, which are the vitamins and minerals necessary for optimal health and performance. The following information will help you design a nutrition plan that pleases your body as well as your taste buds.

Protein

Sufficient protein intake is the same for someone trying to build muscle with a calorie surplus or maintain it during a caloric deficit (Martin-Rincon et al. 2019):

1.6 grams × weight in kilograms = minimum daily protein requirement

Let's say you weigh 200 pounds. Divide the weight in pounds by 2.2 to determine the weight in kilograms (200/2.2 = 91). Then multiply that number by 1.6 (91 × 1.6 = 146). So a 200-pound person needs 146 grams of protein each day.

On the days you lift weights, consume approximately 25 grams within an hour before and another 25 within an hour after you train. Most people prefer a high-quality protein powder for pre- and postworkout nutrition since it's easier to digest, but whole food sources work just as well. In either case, it covers 50 grams' worth of your daily needs. Spread the remaining 96 grams across three meals per day, which equates to around 32 grams at each meal. You could also spread it across four meals if you prefer more frequent feedings.

Protein intake should remain constant at least six days per week. There is some evidence that short periods of low protein intake, such as one day, might provide benefits to your metabolic health (Avruch et al. 2009; Levine and Kroemer 2008). Dave Asprey, author of *The Bulletproof Diet*, recommends eating 15 grams of protein one day per week to promote autophagy, a process your body goes through to clean out damaged cells and regenerate new ones (Parzych and Klionsky 2014). The majority of your calories that day come from healthy fats and carbohydrate. Check with your physician to determine if that is right for you.

There is also some evidence that more protein can accelerate fat loss when you're dieting (Jäger et al. 2017). But in my experience, it's best to start with the aforementioned amount for four weeks. Then, if you're disappointed by your rate of fat loss, you can increase it to 2.0 grams per kilogram of body weight. If that works, and you see steady decreases in your waist circumference, you can stick with higher protein for the rest of your dieting phase. If it doesn't improve fat loss, it's probably better to focus on the other factors you can manipulate— decreasing your total calorie intake or increasing your metabolic work, as covered in chapter 9.

Recommended Sources of Protein

All proteins are not created equal since they can be either complete or incomplete in nature. A complete protein contains all the 20 amino acids a human requires. Of those 20 amino acids, nine are essential and must be consumed from foods. Beans and tofu, for example, are incomplete proteins since they lack some of the essential amino acids. So are egg whites. They have been stripped of many of the key amino acids, vitamins, and minerals found in their yolk. In fact, the yolk arguably contains the healthiest part of the egg (Xiao et al. 2020). An ideal protein source is one that contains all 20 amino acids and has sufficient amounts of branched-chain amino acids (BCAAs), which have been shown to improve protein synthesis and possibly ward off certain diseases (Neinast, Murashige, and Arany 2019). Animal proteins and dairy are recommended protein sources since they provide all the amino acids, including BCAAs, your body needs

Creatine: More Muscle but Less Hair?

Powdered creatine was first introduced to the world back in the mid-1990s. Within a few years, creatine arguably gained more popularity, and at a faster rate, than any other performance-boosting supplement. It became a global sensation that generated many millions of dollars, and it still does to this day.

If you're reading this book you're probably a lot like me: a middle-aged guy who wants to use every natural advantage possible to safely build more muscle. And if you're like me, you also don't want to lose any hair in the process. I've never met a guy who looked forward to having less hair on his head. This is where things get tricky with creatine.

Although creatine supplementation is associated with an increase in dihydrotestosterone (DHT), a hormone that can contribute to hair loss, no substantial body of research shows that creatine can accelerate balding. Back in 2009, one small study of 20 college-aged rugby players demonstrated an increase in DHT levels after they added creatine to their diets (van der Merwe, Brooks, and Myburgh 2009). Since the study didn't directly measure for hair loss, it's not enough to hang your hat on—no pun intended. However, you only need to do a quick internet search to find loads of anecdotal evidence that supplementing with creatine may indeed cause hair loss. This is a classic case where research doesn't support or refute the claim. We just don't know yet.

Alan Bauman, founder of Bauman Medical Hair Transplant and Hair Loss Treatment Center, considers creatine supplementation to be "risky for those susceptible to hair loss." Given the tens of thousands of patients he's treated, that seems to be a pretty strong warning for those who are trying to keep their domes covered.

for growth, repair, and metabolic health. The quality of the proteins you eat is essential for keeping inflammation at bay, so whenever possible, consume the following protein sources:

- Grass-finished or 100% grass-fed beef (This means the animal was fed grass through its entire life)
- Organic chicken breast
- Organic turkey breast
- Pasture-raised organic whole eggs (not egg whites)
- Organic dairy
- Wild fish and shellfish

Whey protein powder contains a high level of leucine, one of the three BCAAs. Leucine increases protein synthesis and energy metabolism (Duan et al. 2016). This is one reason whey is a popular choice for pre- and postworkout consumption (Churchward-Venne et al. 2012). Casein is another good option, as well as a mix of whey and casein (Traylor et al. 2019). Supplementing with protein powders, although not necessary, has been shown to improve muscle and strength (Morton et al. 2020). Most of my patients prefer an unflavored whey protein concentrate that has been cold processed to keep key nutrients intact. Others prefer to drink organic milk before and after training. In any case, use the version that feels best in your gut.

Another advantage of a protein powder, or dairy product, is that you can read the label to determine how much protein you're getting. With food, you'll need to do a little guesswork since it's virtually impossible to determine exactly how much protein is in a piece of meat or fish or an egg. As a general rule, expect one ounce of animal protein and one large egg to contain 7 grams of protein. So in our previous example of 32 grams of protein at each meal, you could consume five ounces of grass-finished beef, or five whole eggs, or three ounces of beef plus two eggs, all of them equally somewhere around 35 grams. Sure, it's not exactly 32 grams, but it gets the job done without measuring fractions of ounces or consuming part of an egg.

Fat

Concern about the amounts and types of fat in our diets first took root in the 1950s. Heart disease was the leading cause of death in the United States, killing half a million Americans each year, twice as many as all cancers combined. Ancel Keys, the country's most respected nutrition scientist (he invented K rations, which fed millions of American soldiers in World War II), set out to prove it was caused by saturated fat consumption (Keys, Anderson, and Grande 1965).

Keys was right about a few things. Postwar prosperity allowed Americans to stuff themselves, and he was among the first to sound the alarm on the emerging obesity epidemic. He also raised awareness of the connection between high blood cholesterol levels and heart disease risk. Finally, he was the first to promote what he called a Mediterranean diet, with lots of plant-based foods (fruits, vegetables, grains, olive oil) and very little meat.

The problem wasn't the theory. It was the application. Once the government got behind the idea that saturated fat was the dietary equivalent of communism, the solutions were catastrophic. Food manufacturers replaced animal fats with oils made from corn, soybeans, and cottonseed, which were previously unknown in the human diet and pro-inflammatory (Ng et al. 2014). The production of another substitute, palm oil, is considered both an environmental and human rights disaster (Kadandale, Marten, and Smith 2019).

The availability of all these new fats, combined with cheap sweeteners made from corn, made convenience foods cheaper and more ubiquitous than ever, leading to massive overconsumption. The rise in obesity was apparent by the mid-1980s (Hales et al. 2018). Although many factors beyond the food on your plate contribute to obesity, there's little doubt that the campaign to reduce and replace saturated fat in the diet backfired.

Recommended Sources of Fat

Earlier we talked about how not all proteins are created equal. Neither are fats—not by a long shot. Some types of fat can contribute to heart disease; other types can reduce it. The same is true for chronic inflammation, a significant problem that contributes to heart disease and makes it hard to reduce belly fat (Golia et al. 2014; Monteiro and Azevedo 2010).

All the protein sources we covered earlier—grass-finished beef, wild fish, organic eggs, and so on—contain healthy forms of fat.

Those fats contribute to your health in a number of ways, by

- providing satiety, leaving you less hungry between meals;
- supplying the building blocks of cellular membranes;

- slowing the release of glucose into the blood; and
- giving you a steady source of energy.

Polyunsaturated fats, such as omega-3s, should be part of your daily fat intake to reduce inflammation and promote cardiovascular health (Calder 2017; Shahidi and Ambigaipalan 2018). Excellent sources of omega-3s are wild salmon, mackerel, and other fatty fish or seafood. But virtually no other foods contain enough omega-3s to derive substantial health benefits. So if you're not a fan of fish or seafood, consider a high-quality fish oil supplement. Other forms of healthy polyunsaturated fats are found in walnuts, sunflower seeds, and flax seeds. Eating these foods has been shown to improve heart health (Liu et al. 2017).

Monounsaturated fats finish our list of healthy fats to add to your nutrition plan. The superstar is extra virgin olive oil, which has shown to have a positive impact on virtually every aspect of aging (Fernández del Río et al. 2016). That is why it should be used as your cooking oil and drizzled on your salads and vegetables. Organic avocados and nuts are an excellent source as well.

To recap, high-quality protein sources contain a significant amount of healthy fats, but they're not enough to derive all the potential health and performance benefits from your daily fat consumption. Therefore, add one or more of the following to your nutrition plan each day:

- Extra virgin olive oil
- Organic avocado
- Organic nuts
- Organic seeds
- Fish oil (if you don't consume fish at least twice per week)

Carbohydrate

Carbohydrate is the focus of more online arguments among fitness enthusiasts than the other two macronutrients combined. At one extreme, advocates of ketogenic and carnivore diets say carbohydrate isn't an essential macronutrient. Humans can live perfectly well on fat and protein. It's accurate enough, although it's an odd argument to make. You can also survive without indoor plumbing. But why would you want to?

Among nutrition scientists, there's hardly any debate at all. We know beyond any reasonable doubt that carbohydrate-rich fruits, vegetables, whole grains, legumes, nuts, and seeds are all correlated with health and longevity (Herforth et al. 2019). Plant-based foods are the only dietary source of fiber and the best source of vitamin C and other crucial antioxidants. By contrast, animal foods are the only dietary source of vitamin B_{12} and creatine. Most other nutrients in meat, eggs, fish, and dairy can also be found in plants.

In addition, plant foods often provide a lot more than carbohydrate. Legumes are relatively high in protein, while avocados, nuts, and seeds are great sources of healthy fats. (Dairy is the only animal-based source of carbohydrate.)

Notice we're talking about whole or minimally processed foods here. Processing removes most of the fiber and many of the vitamins and minerals, leaving a more concentrated source of energy that's easy to overconsume. Consider potatoes, for example. A single baked potato, including the skin, includes four grams of fiber and five grams of surprisingly high-quality protein. That's in addition to much of your daily requirement for vitamins C and B$_6$ and a long list of minerals, including potassium and magnesium. They're also one of the most satiating foods you can eat.

But simply peeling the potatoes removes all the fiber and much of the mineral content. Frying the skinless potatoes adds calories. Turning them into chips and other highly palatable snack foods makes them a weapon of mass consumption. A one-ounce serving of potato chips—about 15 chips—is typically 160 calories, or more than 10 calories per chip. It's no big deal if you can stop yourself after the first handful of chips. But if you can't, or if you dip them in sour cream or guacamole, you're looking at hundreds of calories with little nutritional value and extremely low satiety.

Nutrients aside, when we talk about carbohydrate, the most important questions are how much energy you need, and when you need it. Your body converts the carbohydrate you eat to glucose, which it can either use for immediate energy or store as glycogen in your muscles and liver. (When needed, it can also convert protein to glucose.)

Most of the time, a healthy body burns a higher percentage of fat for energy. Your brain, which accounts for about 20 percent of your total energy needs, gets 100 percent of its fuel from glucose, while your muscles and organs use a mix of fat and carbohydrate (Mergenthaler et al. 2013). That changes when you exercise. The harder you work, the higher the percentage of glucose your body uses (De Feo et al. 2003). Your muscle contractions when you lift are almost entirely fueled by glucose. Therefore, it's recommended to consume carbohydrate in your preworkout nutrition. One fast-acting and easy-to-digest source is tart cherry juice, which has been shown to improve recovery after a workout (Vitale, Hueglin, and Broad 2017). Research demonstrates that consuming 8 to 12 ounces (240-360 ml) per day can decrease inflammation, oxidative stress, and blood pressure (Chai et al. 2019). Another great option is pomegranate juice, which has been shown to decrease oxidative stress after resistance training, help protect your neurons, and lower blood pressure (Ammar et al. 2017; Kujawska et al. 2019; Sahebkar et al. 2017). If tart cherry or pomegranate juice isn't an option, grape juice is a good choice. As is the case with any food, always choose the organic version of tart cherry, pomegranate, or grape juice since it has more nutrients and fewer pesticides than its nonorganic counterpart (Crinnion 2010; Worthington 2001).

Recommended Sources of Carbohydrate

If you eat before you work out, stick to easily digested carbohydrate like bananas, rice, or potatoes. High-fiber carbohydrate sources take longer to digest and could leave you with stomach discomfort while you train. In any case, consume 30 to 40 grams of carbohydrate in your preworkout nutrition. Here are some options that work well within an hour before you lift weights:

- One cup of organic tart cherry juice in 8 ounces (240 ml) of water
- One-half cup of organic pomegranate juice in 16 ounces (480 ml) of water
- One-half cup of organic grape juice in 16 ounces (480 ml) of water
- One banana

- Three-quarters of a cup of cooked rice
- One large baked potato
- One large sweet potato

After a workout, your body quickly reverts to burning a higher percentage of fat. The carbohydrate you eat is likely to be used to replace glycogen in your muscles and liver. It doesn't really matter how soon you eat that carbohydrate. As long as you aren't starving yourself, 24 hours is plenty of time to refuel your muscles for the next workout.

Carbohydrate foods are tricky for fat loss. Since they're not essential, it's easiest to just minimize them to keep your overall calories down and better manage insulin. In most cases, my patients who are trying to lose fat limit their carbohydrate intake to preworkout nutrition. The other meals consist of healthy protein, fat, and cruciferous vegetables. Berries work well for fat loss since they're high in nutrients and low in carbohydrate. One cup of raspberries has 5 grams of carbohydrate compared with one cup of banana or pineapple, which has 24 and 20 grams, respectively. For gaining muscle, carbohydrate helps a lot. The following sources add high-quality calories that provide additional nutrients to support growth and repair:

- Organic white or brown rice
- Organic white or sweet potato or yam
- Any organic whole fruits (not juices)
- Organic oatmeal
- Organic quinoa
- Organic Ezekiel bread
- Any organic berries (usually for a fat-loss plan)

It is likely that people who are significantly overweight or have difficulty losing weight have insulin resistance or leptin resistance. Insulin resistance is very similar to type II diabetes (Petersen and Shulman 2018). You have too much blood glucose and too much insulin at the same time, causing chronic inflammation and a resistance to fat loss (Wu and Ballantyne 2017). Leptin resistance means your body is telling you it's starving when it's really not, which causes excessive food intake that worsens the problem even more (Liu et al. 2018). Following a low-carbohydrate diet is an effective strategy for overcoming insulin resistance, and maybe it will help with leptin resistance as well (Liu et al. 2018; Westman et al. 2018). That is why the nutrition plan for fat loss in this book consists of around 50 grams of carbohydrate per day. But for muscle gain, there are many benefits to increasing your carbohydrate intake well beyond that. For decades professional bodybuilders have consumed up to 60 percent of their calories from carbohydrate to build muscle with minimal fat gain. The tricky part of that plan is keeping your fat to 10 percent of calories per day since the other 30 percent should be protein.

Finally, avoid consuming fruit juices of any kind, even tart cherry juice, outside of your preworkout nutrition. Fruit juices have been stripped of many of their nutrients, including fiber, which drastically increases their rate of absorption, elevating your blood glucose too quickly.

Time to Veg Your Bets?

Of all the debates about which foods you should or shouldn't eat, everyone seems to agree on one thing: vegetables. All of us should be eating more plant-based foods in general, and more vegetables specifically.

And for good reason: Vegetables are low in calories and high in nutrients. One cup of broccoli and one cup of white rice might feel like the same amount of food when you're eating them. But the rice has 200 calories while the broccoli has just 30, along with 2.5 grams of fiber and 135 percent of the daily recommended value of vitamin C. That cup of rice, meanwhile, has just 0.5 gram of fiber and negligible amounts of vitamins or minerals.

To be clear, I'm not saying rice is always a poor nutrition choice. Its lack of fiber makes it a good source of preworkout fuel if you need it, or to replenish your glycogen afterwards. But when your goal is fat loss, cruciferous vegetables are pretty much free food. A large bowl of steamed veggies with a bit of olive oil is an excellent way to fill your stomach with relatively few calories.

That said, not everyone agrees on the value of a plant-heavy diet. Paul Saladino, author of *The Carnivore Code*, has gone as far as saying that plants are generally toxic. He's not entirely wrong. If you were stranded in a forest and had to forage for every meal, there's a much greater chance you'd get sick, and perhaps even die, from eating a living plant than a dead animal (as long as the animal hasn't been dead too long).

Plants produce a long list of toxins—phytoalexins, oxalates, and lectins, to name just a few—to protect themselves from hungry animals. The only animals that live long enough to reproduce are the ones that avoid poisonous plants. They in turn teach their offspring to avoid them.

To be sure, the dose makes the poison, as the adage goes. Some plants aren't safe in any amount, while others are harmless no matter how much you eat. Fruits, for example, evolved to be eaten.

The organic plants in your grocery store, the potatoes and vegetables and herbs, are generally low in natural defense chemicals, which is why we eat them. The biggest risk comes from eating something that upsets your GI tract. Stick to the veggies that feel best in your gut, and avoid the ones that give you indigestion or make you feel bloated, no matter what you read about their health benefits.

Water and Electrolytes

Approximately 60 percent of the human body is water, maybe a little higher than that depending on your source. If we stick to the lower end, that means a 200-pound (91 kg) person has about 120 pounds (54 kg) of water. This is a very large pool for the body to pull from during exercise, during extreme heat, or when you're not drinking enough water. Indeed, it's common for an athlete to lose 6 or 8 pounds (2.7-3.6) of water when exercising in high heat. Research indicates that losing as little as 2 percent of your body weight, or 4 pounds (1.8 kg) for a 200-pound person, causes dehydration that significantly impairs your performance (Magee, Gallagher, and McCormack 2017). That lack of water can also stress your kidneys (Lippi et al. 2008).

As a general rule, aim to consume at least 0.5 ounce (15 ml) of water per pound of body weight per day (i.e., 100 ounces [3 liters] for a 200-pound person). The majority of that water should be consumed during the fasting phase. Your urine should always be clear. If it's not, you need more water. You can consume unsweetened tea or black coffee as part of any nutrition plan.

An essential aspect of your overall hydration and performance is linked to the balance of your sodium, potassium, magnesium, and chloride (Shirreffs and Sawka 2011). These electrolytes regulate the amount of water that goes in and out of your cells, driving important metabolic processes and muscle contractions (Chenevey 1987).

One excellent source of most electrolytes is fresh coconut water. The only thing it's missing is sodium, which is easily solved by adding a few pinches of salt. For those who want to avoid carbohydrates, an electrolyte supplement is recommended. There are many powder and liquid forms on the market with zero or near zero carbohydrate. Mix it in a large glass of water to dilute the metallic taste, and consume once or twice each day when you're exercising in high temperatures. Electrolytes are also recommended during a fasting phase, which we cover shortly.

Finally, exercise can quickly drain your body of water, especially when you're sweating a lot. That is why every expert recommends consuming water while exercising. However, what you're consuming might not be enough. One simple way to determine how much water you need is to weigh yourself before and after a long, intense workout and then replace the difference with electrolyte-rich water. For example, if you lost two pounds (0.9 kg), drink 32 ounces (960 ml). Ensure you are fully hydrated before the workout weigh in.

At this point we've covered all the key elements to design your nutrition plan. First, calculate how many grams of protein you need each day. Second, determine if your goal is to lose fat or gain muscle. For fat loss, get the remainder of your calories from healthy fats and veggies. For muscle gain, add healthy carbohydrate foods to one or more meals. In other words, the only difference between a nutrition plan for fat loss and muscle gain is the carbohydrate you add for the latter. You still need healthy fats and veggies for either plan. Third, try to consume pre- and postworkout nutrition; for most people, it's an easy way to help meet your daily protein requirement. Importantly, workout nutrition applies only to resistance training, not cardio sessions. Fourth, spread your food over three or more meals per day. Table 11.1 shows a sample nutrition plan for fat loss or muscle gain for a 200-pound (91 kg) person.

TABLE 11.1   Sample Nutrition Plan for Fat Loss or Muscle Gain

Time	Fat loss	Muscle gain
8:00 a.m.	5 eggs + veggies + berries	5 eggs + veggies + 1 banana
12:30 p.m.	5 oz (150 g) fish + veggies	5 oz (150 g) fish + veggies + rice
5:00 p.m.	Preworkout: whey + juice	Preworkout: whey + juice
5:30-6:30 p.m.	Resistance training	Resistance training
6:45 p.m.	Postworkout: whey in water	Postworkout: whey in water
8:00 p.m.	5 oz (150 g) chicken + avocado	5 oz (150 g) chicken + avocado + potato

These plans are appropriate for a 200-pound (91 kg) person who trains at 5:30 p.m.

A Tale of Two Nutrients

A number of vitamins and minerals play important roles in your body. But the ones we focus on tend to change with the seasons. Consider vitamin D and magnesium. Although both are crucial for health and performance, you've probably heard a lot more about the former than the latter in recent years (Erem, Atfi, and Razzaque 2019).

It's not as if vitamin D went out and hired a better PR agency. Research over the past 10 years shows how importance it is for a wide range of immune, health, and performance benefits. We now know there are genuine consequences to your health and performance if you're deficient. Low levels can increase your risk of cancer and type 2 diabetes, among many other problems (Holcik et al. 2011). Here's how it all breaks down:

- *Deficiency:* <20 ng/mL
- *Insufficiency:* <25 ng/mL
- *Sufficient:* >30 ng/mL

Recent estimates suggest a billion people have vitamin D deficiency or insufficiency (Holick 2017). That's about 13 percent of the global population at the time. If your blood test indicates a level of vitamin D below 30 ng/mL, you should probably consider taking a supplement (Rondanelli et al. 2020). Or you could spend more time in the sun, if that's an option. Sunlight is a cheaper and more efficient way to get more vitamin D in your system (Nair and Maseeh 2012).

Magnesium gets much less attention in the media than vitamin D, but it deserves at least as much. It's involved in hundreds of metabolic processes and plays essential roles in cell proliferation, growth, and survival. Magnesium deficiency can cause chronic inflammation, fatigue, muscle weakness, and even heart failure (de Baaij, Hoenderop, and Bindels 2015; DiNicolantonio, O'Keefe, and Wilson 2018). It can worsen insulin resistance, which makes it nearly impossible to lose fat, and can contribute to depression (Kostov 2019; Serefko et al. 2013). And if trying to wrap your mind around all this gives you a migraine, you should know that, too, might be caused by low magnesium (Volpe 2013).

Fifty years ago, most people got sufficient magnesium from the foods they ate. But depleted soil means your food has less magnesium, and much of that is stripped by food processing (Rosanoff, Weaver, and Rude 2012; Worthington 2001). Current estimates suggest about 60 percent of adults don't consume the recommended 320 to 420 milligrams a day of magnesium, and 45 percent are deficient (Workinger, Doyle, and Bortz 2018).

Unlike vitamin D levels, which can be measured with a simple blood test during your annual checkup, it's hard to determine your magnesium level if your doctor suspects you're deficient. It typically requires a blood test combined with a 24-hour urine sample (Workinger, Doyle, and Bortz 2018). To avoid that possibility, you can get your daily magnesium from leafy greens, pumpkin seeds, and avocados. Dark chocolate with at least 88 percent cocoa can be another good source, although you have to watch out for added sugar (Garcia et al. 2018).

Finally, vitamin D and magnesium affect each other. Trying to overcome a vitamin D deficiency by taking high doses of supplements, such as 20,000 IUs or more in one day, can lead to a magnesium deficiency and possibly toxicity (Reddy and Edwards 2019). Consult with your physician to make sure you don't create more problems than you fix.

Using Intermittent Fasting to Your Advantage

Now that we've covered the key principles for building a nutrition plan, let's cover one modification that can work well when your goal is fat loss: intermittent fasting (IF). This style of eating also works well for people who don't like to eat much during the day because of a busy schedule.

One of the simplest ways I've found to help my patients lose weight and improve overall health is with restricted periods of eating, or IF. The practical application of IF is simple: Restrict the vast majority of your calories to 4 hours in each 24-hour period. One caveat: The 20:4 ratio takes some mettle to work up to, as discussed shortly. The other 20 hours should consist of plenty of water as well as some unsweetened tea or coffee for those who need a caffeine boost. Caffeine might help curb hunger, so it works especially well when you can't eat (Schubert et al. 2018).

There isn't a lot of research on IF, but there's enough evidence to suggest that restricting your eating to, say, 4 hours each day could have a positive effect on cardiovascular health, obesity, and diabetes (Dong et al. 2020). Put another way, IF might be good for your heart, blood sugar control, and fat loss. There are three steps for making IF work for you.

Step 1: Determine the time of your feeding phase.

When you follow IF, each 24-hour period consists of two phases: fasting and feeding. During the fasting phase you'll either consume no calories or limit your calories to two servings of an easily digestible protein powder such as whey or a blend of whey and casein, making it a pseudo-fasting phase. Most of my patients prefer to consume protein powder during the fasting phase for two reasons. First, it helps curb hunger and maintain energy. Second, it's easier to meet your daily protein requirements. Consuming 1.6 grams of protein per kilogram of body weight is not easy to accomplish, nor recommended, during a 4-hour period. Morbidly obese people might be better served to spend the fasting phase avoiding any calories, including protein powders, since it might have a more positive impact on weight loss and health (Fernando et al. 2019; Santos and Macedo 2018). In either case, determine when a 4-hour feeding phase best fits into your schedule.

Let's say it's 4:00 p.m. to 8:00 p.m. each day. This window should remain constant because if you move it, the time you eat the next day will be affected. The goal is to have 20 hours between finishing your last meal and the start of your feeding phase the next day. The trick here is to fit your lifting sessions into the feeding phase since you'll be consuming calories pre- and postworkout.

The ideal structure is to start your feeding phase with your preworkout nutrition, train, have your postworkout nutrition immediately after, and then start your feeding phase. This works especially well for people who like to consume food for pre- and postworkout nutrition. If you consume protein powder during those times, as well as two servings during your fasting phase, it comes to four servings of protein powder per day. That is neither enjoyable nor sustainable for most people. Table 11.2 shows an example of a 20:4 IF plan for a 200-pound (91 kg) person, requiring around 146 grams of protein. This plan can be adjusted in any way to fit your schedule. All that matters is you fast for 20 hours in any 24-hour period and keep that basic plan consistent.

TABLE 11.2   Sample 20:4 IF Plan for a 200-Pound Person

Phase	Time	Eat, sleep, or train
Fast	8:00 p.m.	End of final meal
	11:00 p.m.-7:00 a.m.	Sleep
	8:00 a.m.	25 g protein powder in water
	12:00 p.m.	25 g protein powder in water
Feed	4:00 p.m.	Preworkout: 5 oz (150 g) chicken + 1 banana
	4:30-5:30 p.m.	Train
	6:00 p.m.	Postworkout: 4 oz (120 g) fish + veggies
	7:45 p.m.	5 oz (150g) beef + veggies + avocado

Step 2: Work up to a 20-hour fast or at least 18 hours.

It's likely you consume breakfast, lunch, and dinner on a relatively set schedule. So you probably have a good idea how much time you already fast between your last meal at night and breakfast the following day. Let's say it's typically 12 hours. Increase that duration by 2 hours for two days (i.e., 14 hours). Then add another hour the third day, followed by another hour the fourth day. At this point your IF lasts 16 hours. Keep adding 1 or 2 hours each day, or every other day, until you reach 20. There is no perfect way to do this as long as you don't add more than 2 hours on any given day. Give your body time to adjust as you work up to 20 hours.

For you, only 4 hours of eating each day might not be enough time. Either you can't consume all your food in such a limited window or you just don't like being that tightly restricted. In that case, follow an 18:6 structure, which expands your feeding phase to 6 hours. Any duration longer than 6 hours hasn't shown to be enough of a time restriction on eating to get the fat-burning results my patients were happy with.

Step 3: Avoid dehydration and electrolyte imbalances.

When you're not eating for a long period of time, it's easy to get dehydrated. This can cause people who are new to IF to get light-headed or dizzy. Be sure to drink plenty of water, as covered earlier, during the fasting phase, and take electrolytes to maintain physiological health.

If all the aforementioned information seems too daunting to tackle right now, there is a simple strategy that might help you lose fat, gain energy, and improve recovery between workouts. As mentioned earlier, chronic inflammation is associated with belly fat, disease, and poor performance. The simplest way to improve your nutrition plan and health is to eliminate foods that cause the high levels of inflammation (Giugliano, Ceriello, and Esposito 2006; Myles 2014; Ng et al. 2014). Those foods are as follows:

- Vegetable oils
- Refined sugars
- Refined grains

Put another way, eat nothing but fruits, veggies, and healthy protein sources. That single change might give you all the results you want. And if you'd like to progress a bit beyond those guidelines, follow the Healthy Eating Index, which has been shown to reduce all causes of mortality, including heart disease and cancer (Onvani et al. 2017).

Final Thoughts

All of this brings us to the final point I want to make in this chapter: Fat loss and muscle gain are different goals requiring different strategies. Someone who's new to resistance training, or returning to it after a layoff, might be able to gain some muscle while losing some fat, resulting in an improvement in body composition even without a change in scale weight. But the longer you train, the less likely that is to happen. That's why you have to focus on one goal or the other:

- Eat more to gain muscle, with the understanding that you'll probably gain some fat in the process.
- Eat less to lose fat, knowing you'll probably lose a little muscle.

Weight gain and weight loss are never 100 percent one thing or the other. Throughout this chapter I discuss ways to minimize fat gain during a calorie surplus and to minimize muscle loss during a calorie deficit. But the idea that an experienced and fit lifter can lose fat and gain muscle simultaneously is akin to trying to drive north and south at the same time.

CHAPTER 12

Strong and Lean for Life

Most books about resistance training are written for two types of lifters: (1) new or relatively inexperienced lifters, or enthusiasts who're ready to get serious for the first time, and (2) trained lifters who want to reach their peak for strength, size, or aesthetics. Some books focus on one or the other. Others, including this one, offer guidance for both new and advanced lifters. But what about the lifters who began in their teens or 20s and have now been training for decades?

Many of them tell a familiar story: They started working out in their garage or basement with nothing but a barbell and bench, focusing mostly on the bench press and curls. Or they played sports or were in the military and did hundreds of push-ups and dozens of pull-ups a week while pounding their joints on the field or obstacle course. They eventually found a home away from home in the weight room, where they pushed themselves to squat, press, and deadlift heavy weights, year in and year out, rarely taking breaks until forced to by injury or illness. Now, in middle age, they still want to be strong, lean, and muscular, but they can't do it the way they used to. Most have one or more compromised joints—shoulders, lower back, hips, knees—thanks to the usual suspects: too much load and volume, poor form, and unfortunate program design.

If this describes you, the information in this chapter will help you train both seriously and sustainably. You'll learn to protect your most vulnerable joints instead of inflicting more damage, and we'll address a hard truth: It is not wise for older lifters to train the way they did in their 20s. The aging lifter has to battle more inflammation, joint problems, and muscle loss than his younger peers. Not to mention poorer balance and a nagging injury or two. The good news is we cover practical strategies to keep you in the iron game so you can remain strong and lean for life. And if you're not yet in that "wounded weightlifter" demographic, you'll learn to adjust your workouts now to avoid dealing with these things down the road.

How Your Body Changes With Age

Everything you want to accomplish in your training program occurs during recovery. That's when your body repairs and rebuilds your muscles and connective tissues, making them bigger and stronger. Ask a group of 50-year-olds who are lifelong gym-goers and they'll tell you that everything vital to recovery slows down with age.

Protein synthesis is less efficient, which means it takes more protein to build new tissue (Burd, Gorissen, and van Loon, 2013). But because of your slowing metabolism, it's harder to consume enough protein from food without gaining excessive body fat. Fat, in turn, triggers inflammation, which can be either good or bad for a lifter. Acute inflammation after a workout is an important part of the recovery process, sending chemical signals that trigger muscle hypertrophy (Chazaud 2020). But an aging body is more likely to have some degree of chronic inflammation, which impairs muscle growth and repair (Furman et al. 2019). Furthermore, this inflammation is associated with increased levels of abdominal fat (Cabral et al. 2019). Sleep is also important to recovery for a number of reasons we discuss in chapter 3. And, yes, both sleep duration and quality decline as you get older (Dzierzewski, Dautovich, and Ravyts 2018).

Biomechanically, there's a price to pay for years of lifting hard and heavy. The small aches and pains you gladly tolerated in your 20s and 30s, when your body had unrestricted range of motion and little inflammation, were a warning of bigger problems to come. By ignoring them, you wore down cartilage in your shoulders, knees, and hips. Once it's gone, it's gone. Most areas of cartilage have an extremely low blood supply, which inhibits regeneration (Hardingham, Tew, Murdoch 2002). As a doctor of physical therapy, I assure you there's no way to replace it, and probably won't be for a long time. Without cartilage, your bones begin to grind against each other, or the tendons attaching muscles to bones become inflamed. And that age-related chronic inflammation we discussed earlier might negatively affect your cartilage as well (Berenbaum 2013).

Structurally, some bodies simply aren't designed for the most popular lifts. Some of us, for example, have deep hip sockets that aren't suited for deep squats. If you have deep hip sockets and force yourself to squat below parallel, two things will probably happen:

1. You'll wear down the cartilage in your hip joints that allows smooth movement and provides a cushion between your femur and pelvis.
2. You'll shift your lumbar spine out of the neutral position to achieve the range of motion, wearing down the tissues protecting the discs in your lower back and irritating the nerves (McGill 2015).

Extending from the shoulder blade is a bony structure called the acromion process. In about 40 percent of us, this bony protuberance is shaped like a hook (Shah, Bayliss, and Malcolm 2001) that literally digs into your tissues as you lift overhead. This causes damage that can, with enough time and volume, make it painful to lift your arms above parallel to the floor (Nyffeler and Meyer 2017). And that's just one of the many ways your training can irritate, inflame, or injure the tangle of muscles, connective tissues, and bones that make up your shoulder joints.

The lower back, similarly, shows a range of structural and functional variations that can affect your lifting form and be affected by it. Larger lumbar vertebrae can provide a strong base for heavy squats and deadlifts but also make the spinal discs more vulnerable to injury from twisting movements in anything from core training to yoga to golf (McGill 2015). Conversely, someone whose lumbar spine more naturally accommodates rotational movements might be at higher risk when an exercise requires high tension to stabilize the core.

Skateboard Your Way to Better Health and Performance

As a kid, you spent your days running, jumping, climbing, and chasing your sibling who stole your favorite toy. Now that you're older, you spend most of your day sitting or walking to your car or standing in line at the grocery store. So it doesn't take a neuroscientist to understand why your older self has poorer balance: You don't train it.

If you're over 25 years old, it's almost certain your brain has reached full maturity. After that age, scientists long believed that any significant changes within the brain were no longer possible. Sure, you could learn a new language or memorize a list of random facts at any age. But the formation of new neurons that we experienced early in life was thought to be science fiction.

Around 2002, that thinking started to shift (Shors et al. 2002). Today scientists know that neurogenesis, the process of creating new neurons, can occur in your hippocampus throughout life. But it won't happen on its own: You need to give it a good reason. Social interactions, exercise, and learning a new skill are three such reasons (Curlik and Shors 2013; Opendak, Briones, and Gould 2016; Sun, Sun, and Qi 2017).

It's not a shock that as adults age, they lose their balance more easily (Khow and Visvanathan 2017). That's why I like to have my patients promote neurogenesis each day through skill training that challenges their balance. You can start with a simple task, such as standing on one leg with your eyes closed, and work to double or triple your time. Then move on to a more challenging activity such as martial arts or tai chi. From there, if you have the drive, work to more youthful challenges such as learning to surf or skateboard. The key is to constantly try to learn new skills to keep your brain healthy and strong throughout life.

Practical Strategies for Older Lifters

Let's make one thing clear up front: You don't have to stop doing everything you enjoy in the weight room and switch to an "over 50" training program. An older lifter is still a lifter. But to continue lifting safely and successfully, you need to acknowledge your body is different from a young lifter's.

That's not really bad news. Your experience has made you smarter. You know what works for your body, and you probably do it with better form than the crazy dudes whose workouts would leave you with crippling pain. (I say "dudes" because we rarely see young women lifting near-maximal weights with poor form.) Here are some simple ways to take advantage of your hard-earned knowledge.

Volume

All the program design principles in chapters 8 and 9 are still in play for an older lifter, except one: volume. More is rarely better. For you, less can sometimes be more. But getting more done with fewer sets requires more focus on each one. You aren't just grinding out repetitions. You're *feeling* each rep, especially as you get near the end of a set. Make sure the targeted muscles are doing the work and achieving the optimal level of fatigue. Get it right on the second or third set and there's no need to do a fourth, fifth, or sixth.

Frequency

Different bodies recover at different rates, and different muscles within each body also recover at different rates. Thus, there's no single standard of ideal workout frequency for all lifters in their 40s or 50s or beyond. They will most certainly tell you that the older you get, the longer it takes for *your* body and *your* muscles to recover. They won't care if research can't confirm it (Deschenes et al. 2019; Fell and Williams 2008).

Even if your schedule allows you to do long, challenging workouts five or six days a week, as you did with great success in your 20s or 30s, that's almost certainly too much for you in middle age. Forget the idea that if you train chest

Hip Impingement and Squat Depth

Your hip is a ball-and-socket joint. The ball is the head of your femur, and the socket is the acetabulum in your pelvis. The acetabulum is a concave, dome-like structure that can be either relatively flat to create a shallow hip socket or relatively deep to create— you guessed it—a deep hip socket (see figure 12.1).

If you aspire to achieve the squat depth necessary to excel at Olympic lifting, you will need shallow hip sockets and sufficient elasticity of the hip joint capsule. If you weren't born that

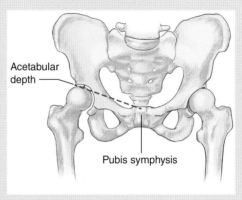

FIGURE 12.1   Hip joint.

way, surgery is the only way to change it, and no reputable surgeon would recommend such an invasive procedure to improve your squat.

Aging and excessive exercise can also limit your squat depth. One common hip problem is femoroacetabular impingement, or FAI. Basically speaking, FAI is due to excessive bone growth from aging or too much loading stress on the hip. Let's briefly cover each type of impingement:

- *Cam impingement:* Growth on the head or neck of the femur causes a bony protrusion that pushes into cartilage within the joint space.
- *Pincher impingement:* Either the hip socket is too deep or there's excessive bone growth on the acetabulum that limits range of motion.
- *Combined impingement:* Both of the problems previously mentioned are present; this is the most common type of impingement.

In any of the aforementioned cases, a deep squat will cause a pinching pain in the hip socket. Over time, that pinching causes microtears and degeneration of the hip's cartilage, which can lead to osteoarthritis. When this happens, a common course of intervention is hip arthroscopy, a minimally invasive procedure that removes any excess bone growth as well as damage to the cartilage. The best course of action, either to prevent FAI or minimize further damage, is to have a reputable physical therapist help you determine your optimal squat depth based on the structure of your hips.

one day and back the next day, you aren't working the same body parts two days in a row. You are.

Your pecs, lats, biceps, triceps, and deltoids all act on the shoulder joints. If there's a weighted object in your hands, your forearm muscles are involved. You can't avoid using your elbows if you're pushing or pulling those weights. Your traps work to move or stabilize your shoulder blades in almost any exercise worth doing. Same with your core muscles.

Older lifters typically do well with three full-body training sessions a week, alternating two workouts that focus on different movement patterns. Here's an example:

Workout A: horizontal push, horizontal pull, knee-emphasis movement (squat, lunge, or leg press)

Workout B: vertical push, vertical pull, hip-emphasis movement (deadlift variation)

If you have the time and ambition to work out more often, try some low-impact cardio—walking, cycling, swimming. Those activities speed up recovery without beating up your muscles or joints and have been shown to elicit an anti-aging effect on your arteries (Seals 2014).

Exercise Selection

Older lifters often want to cling to their youth by continuing to push their bench press, squat, and deadlift, no matter how much their bodies protest. It's the weight-room equivalent of buying a new Harley. But if a barbell bench press makes your right shoulder ache, or a back squat causes radiating pain down to your pelvis, or a traditional deadlift from the floor tweaks your lower back, you have to stop doing them and seek council from a reputable physical therapist who can determine which pains can be fixed. If you don't get help from a qualified professional, those exercises will likely never become less painful, and the pain you feel may actually understate the damage you're doing to those joints.

I've already mentioned how structural differences in your shoulders and hips can make some exercises easier or harder for individual lifters. But it's actually more complicated than that. Human bodies aren't perfectly symmetrical. The same person can have significant differences in the shape and positioning of their hip joints. Your shoulders may be wider on one side, and your arms may have more or less internal or external rotation. Ignoring those anomalies sets you up for injury, especially when you're training with a barbell that forces each side of your body to work exactly the same way.

Here are some joint-friendly alternatives to three powerlifts:

- *Barbell bench press:* My favorite alternative is the standing one-arm chest press with a cable, band, or tubing. Besides working your chest and shoulders, it's one of the best core exercises you can do. Mix those with dumbbell bench presses with one or both arms, and experiment with different degrees of incline or decline. Generally, a slightly declined bench is less stressful on the shoulders.

- *Barbell squat:* You can get results with goblet squats with a dumbbell or kettlebell or front squats with two kettlebells. These variations allow you to adjust the exercise to your anatomy and achieve a full range of motion with less strain on your lower back. The most back-friendly variation of all is a belt squat, which is terrific for building lower body strength while sparing your lower back.

- *Barbell deadlift from the floor:* Very few lifters have the long arms and short legs that make them ideally proportioned for traditional deadlifts from the floor. Many will do well if they elevate the weights a few inches off the floor, using weight plates, boxes, or the supports on a squat rack. And almost everyone can deadlift successfully by using the high handles of a hex bar. You can also elevate the hex bar on one or two weight plates to further shorten the range of motion and make it a little more back friendly.

Can a Cobra Save Your Low Back?

It's almost certain that you've experienced low back pain at some point in your life. (And if you haven't, know you're one of the lucky few.) Without a doubt, low back pain is a significant problem around the globe, even if hard numbers across different populations are difficult to determine (Trompeter, Fett, and Platen 2017).

Two of the most common causes of low back pain are disc herniations (i.e., bulging discs) and spinal stenosis, which is a narrowing of the spinal canal. Herniated discs can be especially painful when the bulge presses against a spinal nerve. When that occurs, it is often beneficial to perform a movement that extends the spine (Alhakami et al. 2019). One of the most popular extension-based movements goes by three different names: McKenzie extension, sloppy push-up, or cobra. We'll refer to it here as a cobra since it sounds the coolest of the three options.

I prescribe the cobra for both rehabilitation and prehabilitation purposes. After a disc herniation, the cobra can be a great rehabilitation exercise to restore range of motion and reduce pain. Importantly, if you have low back pain you must first see a licensed physical therapist or orthopedic doctor to diagnose the underlying problem, which might not be a disc problem. Don't try to self-diagnose because your source of pain might actually worsen with a cobra, which is usually the case when you have spinal stenosis.

If you're currently not suffering from low back pain, use the cobra as a prehabilitation exercise to keep your discs healthy. I often program 10 to 15 repetitions of a cobra after each set of an exercise that stresses the low back, such as a deadlift or barbell back squat. It is also a great exercise to perform after you've been sitting for long periods of time. That's because sitting causes the following problems: shortening of hip flexors, shortening of abdominals, loss of spinal extension, and increased pressure on the discs. The cobra reverses those ill effects through one simple move:

1. Lie on your abdomen on the floor. Place your hands directly below your shoulders, or wherever feels most comfortable (see figure 12.2a).

2. Push your chest as far away from the floor as possible by straightening your arms (see figure 12.2b). Lower to the starting position. Keep your hips and legs relaxed throughout the movement.

3. Perform 10 to 15 repetitions after each set of an exercise that challenges your low back, and every hour while sitting.

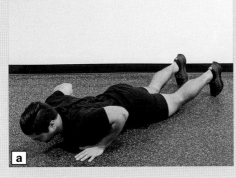
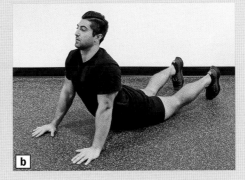

FIGURE 12.2   Cobra.

Training to Failure and Pursuing PRs

Pushing yourself to momentary muscular failure is a technique you want to use sparingly. It works best with body weight or single-joint exercises. Most of the time, you want to stop a set a few reps short of failure, and before you need to change your form to achieve a repetition.

As for PRs, you can still pursue them, with two caveats:

1. If you just turned 40, think of every set you do as a new PR for you in your 40s. Same if you just turned 50 or 60. There's no point comparing your current lifts against what you did in your 20s or 30s.

2. Don't think of them as a one-repetition max. Establish a 5RM on a joint-friendly exercise like the dumbbell bench press or hex-bar deadlift. Push yourself to surpass it once or twice a year, but back away if it feels uncomfortable or if you have to change your form to go heavier.

Rest

This is the most important rule of all. If you feel like you need an extra day between workouts, you do. Same for those days when you get to the gym and realize everything feels a little "off." Spend that workout doing light cardio, or go home and give your body the rest it needs. The gym will still be there tomorrow or the next day or the next week.

Understanding your body's signals is one of the biggest benefits of the aging process. You've earned these insights the hard way, with thousands of workouts and perhaps dozens of injuries. If you listen to your body at the right moments, you'll enjoy thousands more workouts with minimal risk of inflicting new aches and pains.

Final Thoughts

Now that we've reached the end of the book, there are a few key things to keep in mind. First, be patient. Making significant improvements in muscle mass or fat loss takes months, not weeks. Sure, you should see some visual changes in the mirror every few weeks, as we covered back in chapter 1, but for most of you, the body and performance you seek most will require many months of hard work and dedication. Second, take a few days off or decrease the volume of your workouts when you're feeling run down. If you've been training intensely and haven't missed any workouts for many weeks straight, often five to seven days off actually increases your strength and muscle mass. Third, if your fat loss comes to a halt, the culprit is almost always your nutrition plan. Adhere to the guidelines for fat loss covered in chapter 11.

REFERENCES

Chapter 1

Agrawal Y, Carey JP, Hoffman HJ, Sklare DA, Schubert MC. The modified Romberg balance test: Normative data in U.S. adults. *Otol Neurotol.* 2011;32(8):1309-1311.

Butcher SJ, Rusin JS. Core strength and functionality with loaded carries. *NSCA Coach.* 2016;4(3).

Butryn ML, Phelan S, Hill JO, Wing RR. Consistent self-monitoring of weight: A key component of successful weight loss maintenance. *Obesity.* 2007;15(12):3091-3096.

Castro-Piñero J, Ortega FB, Artero EG, et al. Assessing muscular strength in youth: Usefulness of standing long jump as a general index of muscular fitness. *J Strength Cond Res.* 2010;24(7):1810-1817.

Cools AM, Johansson FR, Borms D, Maenhout A. Prevention of shoulder injuries in overhead athletes: A science-based approach. *Braz J Phys Ther.* 2015;19(5):331-339.

Cooper KH. A means of assessing maximal oxygen intake: Correlation between field and treadmill testing. *J Am Med Assoc.* 1968; 203:201-204.

Duren DL, Sherwood RJ, Czerwinski SA, et al. Body composition methods: Comparisons and interpretation. *J Diabetes Sci Technol.* 2008;2(6):1139-1146.

Golec de Zavala A, Lantos D, Bowden D. Yoga poses increase subjective energy and state self-esteem in comparison to 'power poses.' *Front Psychol.* 2017;8:752.

Helander EE, Vuorinen A-L, Wansink B, Korhonen IKJ. Are breaks in daily self-weighing associated with weight gain? *PLoS ONE.* 2014;9(11):e113164.

Hester GM, Ha PL, Dalton BE, et al. Rate of force development as a predictor of mobility in older adults. *J Geriatr Phys Ther.* 2020 Jan 6.

Kandel ER, Schwartz JH, Jessell TM, et al. *Principles of Neural Science.* 5th ed. McGraw-Hill Medical; 2013.

Kim SH, Kwon OY, Park KN, Jeon IC, Weon JH. Lower extremity strength and the range of motion in relation to squat depth. *J Hum Kinet.* 2015;45:59-69.

Komi PV. *Strength and Power in Sport.* 2nd ed. Blackwell Science; 2003.

Loprinzi PD, Brosky JA Jr. Objectively measured physical activity and balance among U.S. adults. *J Strength Cond Res.* 2014;28(8):2290-2296.

Lunsford BR, Perry J. The standing heel-rise test for ankle plantar flexion: Criterion for normal. *Phys Ther.* 1995;75(8):694-698.

Macht JW, Abel MG, Mullineaux DR, Yates JW. Development of 1RM prediction equations for bench press in moderately trained men. *J Strength Cond Res.* 2016;30(10):2901-2906.

Madigan CD, Daley AJ, Lewis AL, Aveyard P, Jolly K. Is self-weighing an effective tool for weight loss: A systematic literature review and meta-analysis. [published correction] *Int J Behav Nutr Phys Act.* 2016;13:42.

Markovic G, Dizdar D, Jukic I, Cardinale M. Reliability and factorial validity of squat and countermovement jump tests. *J Strength Cond Res.* 2004;18(3):551-555.

Masharawi Y, Haj A, Weisman A. Lumbar axial rotation kinematics in an upright sitting and with forward bending positions in men with nonspecific chronic low back pain. *Spine (Phila Pa 1976).* 2020;45(5):e244-e251.

Mayorga-Vega D, Bocanegra-Parrilla R, Ornelas M, Viciana J. Criterion-related validity of the distance- and time-based walk/run field tests for estimating cardiorespiratory fitness: A systematic review and meta-analysis. *PLoS One.* 2016;11(3):e0151671.

Mazur LJ, Yetman RJ, Risser WL. Weight-training injuries: Common injuries and preventative methods. *Sports Med.* 1993;16(1):57-63.

Miller JR, Van Hooren B, Bishop C, Buckley JD, Willy RW, Fuller JT. A systematic review and meta-analysis of crossover studies comparing physiological, perceptual and performance measures between treadmill and overground running. *Sports Med.* 2019;49(5):763-782.

Page P. Shoulder muscle imbalance and subacromial impingement syndrome in overhead athletes. *Int J Sports Phys Ther.* 2011;6(1):51-58.

Peterson MD, Alvar BA, Rhea MR. The contribution of maximal force production to explosive movement among young collegiate athletes. *J Strength Cond Res.* 2006;20(4):867-873.

Reynolds JM, Gordon TJ, Roberts RA. Prediction of one repetition maximum strength from multiple repetition maximum testing and anthropometry. *J Strength Cond Res.* 2006;20(3):584-592.

Richens B, Cleather DJ. The relationship between the number of repetitions performed at given intensities is different in endurance and strength trained athletes. *Biol Sport.* 2014;31(2):157-161.

Riemann B. Is there a link between chronic ankle instability and postural instability. *J Athl Train.* 2002;37(4):386-393.

Roach SM, San Juan JG, Suprak DN, Lyda M, Bies AJ, Boydston CR. Passive hip range of motion is reduced in active subjects with chronic low back pain compared to controls. *Int J Sports Phys Ther.* 2015;10(1):13-20.

Rose G. *TPI Level 1 Seminar Manual.* Version 2.5. TPI Nevada Star I LP; 2019.

Rothman KJ. BMI-related errors in the measurement of obesity. *Int J Obes.* 2008;32(Suppl 3):S56-S59.

Shumway-Cook A, Horak FB. Assessing the influence of sensory interaction of balance: Suggestion from the field. *Phys Ther.* 1986;66(10):1548-1550.

Stastny P, Lehnert M, Zaatar AM, Svoboda Z, Xaverova Z. Does the dumbbell-carrying position change the muscle activity in split squats and walking lunges? *J Strength Cond Res.* 2015;29(11):3177-3187.

U.S. Department of Health and Human Services. Physical Activity Guidelines for Americans, 2nd edition. Washington, DC: U.S. Department of Health and Human Services; 2018.

Weiglein L, Herrick J, Kirk S, Kirk EP. The 1-mile walk test is a valid predictor of VO(2max) and is a reliable alternative fitness test to the 1.5-mile run in U.S. Air Force males. *Mil Med.* 2011;176(6):669-673.

Wells JC, Fewtrell MS. Measuring body composition. *Arch Dis Child.* 2006;91(7):612-617.

Whitehead PN, Schilling BK, Peterson DD, Weiss LW. Possible new modalities for the Navy Physical Readiness Test. *Mil Med.* 2012;177(11):1417-1425.

Yang L, Cao C, Kantor ED, et al. Trends in sedentary behavior among the US population, 2001-2016. *JAMA.* 2019;321(16):1587-1597.

Yang J, Christophi CA, Farioli A, et al. Association between push-up exercise capacity and future cardiovascular events among active adult men. *JAMA Netw Open.* 2019;2(2):e188341.

Chapter 2

Aragon AA, Schoenfeld BJ, Wildman R, et al. International Society of Sports Nutrition position stand: Diets and body composition. *J Int Soc Sports Nutr.* 2017;14:16.

Cava E, Yeat NC, Mittendorfer B. Preserving healthy muscle during weight loss. *Adv Nutr.* 2017;8(3):511-519.

Clamp LD, Hume DJ, Lambert EV, Kroff J. Enhanced insulin sensitivity in successful, long-term weight loss maintainers compared with matched controls with no weight loss history. *Nutr Diabetes.* 2017;7(6):e282.

Hubal MJ, Gordish-Dressman H, Thompson PD, et al. Variability in muscle size and strength gain after unilateral resistance training. *Med Sci Sports Exerc.* 2005;37(6):964-972.

Huovinen HT, Hulmi JJ, Isolehto J, et al. Body composition and power performance improved after weight reduction in male athletes without hampering hormonal balance. *J Strength Cond Res.* 2015;29(1):29-36.

Institute of Medicine (US) Subcommittee on Military Weight Management. *Weight Management: State of the Science and Opportunities for Military Programs.* National Academies Press; 2004.

Pedersen BK, Febbraio MA. Muscles, exercise and obesity: Skeletal muscle as a secretory organ. *Nat Rev Endocrinol.* 2012;8(8):457-465.

Pion CH, Barbat-Artigas S, St-Jean-Pelletier F, et al. Muscle strength and force development in high- and low-functioning elderly men: Influence of muscular and neural factors. *Exp Gerontol.* 2017;96:19-28.

Schoenfeld BJ, Alto A, Grgic J, et al. Alterations in body composition, resting metabolic rate, muscular strength, and eating behavior in response to natural bodybuilding competition preparation: A case study. *J Strength Cond Res.* 2020;34(11):3124-3138.

Schoenfeld BJ, Contreras B, Krieger J, et al. Resistance training volume enhances muscle hypertrophy but not strength in trained men. *Med Sci Sports Exerc.* 2019;51(1):94-103.

Tsametis CP, Isidori AM. Testosterone replacement therapy: For whom, when and how? *Metabolism.* 2018;86:69-78.

Chapter 3

Campbell BI, Aguilar D, Conlin L, et al. Effects of high versus low protein intake on body composition and maximal strength in aspiring female physique athletes engaging in an 8-week resistance training program. *Int J Sport Nutr Exerc Metab.* 2018;28(6):580-585.

Chennaoui M, Arnal PJ, Drogou C, Sauvet F, Gomez-Merino D. Sleep extension increases IGF-I concentrations before and during sleep deprivation in healthy young men. *Appl Physiol Nutr Metab.* 2016;41:963-970.

Dankel SJ, Mattocks KT, Jessee MB, et al. Frequency: The overlooked resistance training variable for inducing muscle hypertrophy? *Sports Med.* 2017;47(5):799-805.

Goodwin ML, Harris JE, Hernández A, Gladden LB. Blood lactate measurements and analysis during exercise: A guide for clinicians. *J Diabetes Sci Technol.* 2007;1(4):558-569.

Grgic J, Schoenfeld BJ, Davies TB, Lazinica B, Krieger JW, Pedisic Z. Effect of resistance training frequency on gains in muscular strength: A systematic review and meta-analysis. *Sports Med.* 2018;48(5):1207-1220.

Hayashi M, Motoyoshi N, Hori T. Recuperative power of a short daytime nap with or without stage 2 sleep. *Sleep.* 2005;28:829-836.

Helms ER, Zinn C, Rowlands DS, Brown SR. A systematic review of dietary protein during caloric restriction in resistance trained lean athletes: A case for higher intakes. *Int J Sport Nutr Exerc Metab.* 2014;24(2):127-138.

Henneman E. Relation between size of neurons and their susceptibility to discharge. *Science.* 1957;126(3287):1345-1347.

Hostler D, Crill MT, Hagerman FC, et al. The effectiveness of 0.5-lb increments in progressive resistance exercise. *J Strength Cond Res.* 2001;15(1):86-91.

Kandel ER, Schwartz JH, Jessell TM, et al. *Principles of Neural Science.* 5th ed. McGraw-Hill Medical; 2013.

Killgore WD. Effects of sleep deprivation on cognition. *Prog Brain Res.* 2010;185:105-129.

Liebenson C. *Functional Training Handbook.* Lippincott Williams & Wilkins; 2014.

Lim JJ, Kong PW. Effects of isometric and dynamic postactivation potentiation protocols on maximal sprint performance. *J Strength Cond Res.* 2013;27(10):2730-2736.

McBride JM, Nimphius S, Erickson TM. The acute effects of heavy-load squats and loaded countermovement jumps on sprint performance. *J Strength Cond Res.* 2005;19(4):893-897.

McCrary JM, Ackermann BJ, Halaki M. A systematic review of the effects of upper body warm-up on performance and injury. *Br J Sports Med.* 2015;49(14):935-942.

Moro T, Ebert SM, Adams CM, Rasmussen BB. Amino acid sensing in skeletal muscle. *Trends Endocrinol Metab.* 2016;27(11):796-806.

Mougin F, Bourdin H, Simon-Rigaud ML, Nguyen Nhu U, Kantelip JP, Davenne D. Hormonal responses to exercise after partial sleep deprivation and after hypnotic drug-induced sleep. *J Sports Sci.* 2001;19:89-97.

Mukherjee S, Patel SR, Kales SN, et al. American thoracic society ad hoc committee on healthy sleep. An official American Thoracic Society statement: The importance of healthy sleep. Recommendations and future priorities. *Am J Respir Crit Care Med.* 2015;191:1450-1458.

Osmond AD, Directo DJ, Elam ML, et al. The effects of leucine-enriched branched-chain amino acid supplementation on recovery after high-intensity resistance exercise. *Int J Sports Physiol Perform.* 2019;14(8):1081-1088.

Patel SR, Malhotra A, White DP, Gottlieb DJ, Hu FB. Association between reduced sleep and weight gain in women. *Am J Epidemiol.* 2006;164:947-954.

Reilly T, Deykin T. Effects of partial sleep loss on subjective states, psychomotor and physical performance tests. *J Hum Mov Stud.* 1983;9:157-170.

Reilly T, Piercy M. The effect of partial sleep deprivation on weight-lifting performance. *Ergonomics.* 1994;37:107-115.

Reyner LA, Horne JA. Sleep restriction and serving accuracy in performance tennis players, and effects of caffeine. *Physiol Behav.* 2013;120:93-96.

Rixon KP, Lamont HS, Bemben MG. Influence of type of muscle contraction, gender, and lifting experience on postactivation potentiation performance. *J Strength Cond Res.* 2007;21(2):500-505.

Sanchez-Sanchez J, Rodriguez A, Petisco C, Ramirez-Campillo R, Martínez C, Nakamura FY. Effects of different post-activation potentiation warm-ups on repeated sprint ability in soccer players from different competitive levels. *J Hum Kinet.* 2018;61:189-197.

Schoenfeld BJ. The mechanisms of muscle hypertrophy and their application to resistance training. *J Strength Cond Res.* 2010;24(10):2857-2872.

Schoenfeld BJ, Aragon AA. How much protein can the body use in a single meal for muscle-building? Implications for daily protein distribution. *J Int Soc Sports Nutr.* 2018;15:10.

Schoenfeld BJ, Contreras B, Krieger J, et al. Resistance training volume enhances muscle hypertrophy but not strength in trained men. *Med Sci Sports Exerc.* 2019;51(1):94-103.

Schoenfeld BJ, Grgic J, Krieger J. How many times per week should a muscle be trained to maximize muscle hypertrophy? A systematic review and meta-analysis of studies examining the effects of resistance training frequency. *J Sports Sci.* 2019;37(11):1286-1295.

Schoenfeld BJ, Ogborn D, Krieger JW. Effects of resistance training frequency on measures of muscle hypertrophy: A systematic review and meta-analysis. *Sports Med.* 2016;46(11):1689-1697.

Schoenfeld BJ, Ogborn D, Krieger JW. Dose-response relationship between weekly resistance training volume and increases in muscle mass: A systematic review and meta-analysis. *J Sports Sci.* 2017;35(11):1073-1082.

Seitz LB, Haff GG. Factors modulating post-activation potentiation of jump, sprint, throw, and upper-body ballistic performances: A systematic review with meta-analysis. *Sports Med.* 2016;46(2):231-240.

Souissi N, Chtourou H, Aloui A, et al. Effects of time-of-day and partial sleep deprivation on short-term maximal performances of judo competitors. *J Strength Cond Res.* 2013;27:2473-2480.

Todd JS, Shurley JP, Todd TC. Thomas L. DeLorme and the science of progressive resistance exercise. *J Strength Cond Res.* 2012;26(11):2913-2923.

UCSD Center for Pulmonary and Sleep Medicine. Sleep hygiene patient information handout [Brochure]. University of California San Diego; 2017.

Wallace BJ, Shapiro R, Wallace KL, Abel MG, Symons TB. Muscular and neural contributions to postactivation potentiation. *J Strength Cond Res.* 2019;33(3):615-625.

Waterhouse J, Atkinson G, Edwards B, Reilly T. The role of a short post-lunch nap in improving cognitive, motor, and sprint performance in participants with partial sleep deprivation. *J Sports Sci.* 2007;25:1557-1566.

Zatsiorsky VM. Intensity of strength training facts and theory: Russian and Eastern European approach. *Natl Strength Cond Assoc J.* 1992;14(5):46-57.

Chapter 4

Alcaraz PE, Sanchez-Lorente J, Blazevich AJ. Physical performance and cardiovascular responses to an acute bout of heavy resistance circuit training versus traditional strength training. *J Strength Cond Res.* 2008;22(3):667-671.

Burd NA, West DW, Staples AW, et al. Low-load high volume resistance exercise stimulates muscle protein synthesis more than high-load low volume resistance exercise in young men. *PLoS One.* 2010;5(8):e12033.

Cermak NM, Res PT, de Groot LC, Saris WH, van Loon LJ. Protein supplementation augments the adaptive response of skeletal muscle to resistance-type exercise training: A meta-analysis. *Am J Clin Nutr.* 2012;96:1454-1464.

Eftestøl E, Egner IM, Lunde IG, et al. Increased hypertrophic response with increased mechanical load in skeletal muscles receiving identical activity patterns. *Am J Physiol Cell Physiol.* 2016;311(4):C616-C629.

Egner IM, Bruusgaard JC, Gundersen K. Satellite cell depletion prevents fiber hypertrophy in skeletal muscle. *Development.* 2016;143(16):2898-2906.

Fry AC, Kraemer WJ. Resistance exercise overtraining and overreaching: Neuroendocrine responses. *Sports Med.* 1997;23:106-129.

Greer BK, Sirithienthad P, Moffatt RJ, Marcello RT, Panton LB. EPOC comparison between isocaloric bouts of steady-state aerobic, intermittent aerobic, and resistance training. *Res Q Exerc Sport.* 2015;86(2):190-195.

Haun CT, Vann CG, Osburn SC, et al. Muscle fiber hypertrophy in response to 6 weeks of high-volume resistance training in trained young men is largely attributed to sarcoplasmic hypertrophy. *PLoS One.* 2019;14(6):e0215267.

Hay N, Sonenberg N. Upstream and downstream of mTOR. *Genes Dev.* 2004;18(16):1926-1945.

Jenkins ND, Housh TJ, Buckner SL, et al. Neuromuscular adaptations after 2 and 4 weeks of 80% versus 30% 1 repetition maximum resistance training to failure. *J Strength Cond Res.* 2016;30(8):2174-2185.

Jorgenson KW, Phillips SM, Hornberger TA. Identifying the structural adaptations that drive the mechanical load-induced growth of skeletal muscle: A scoping review. *Cells.* 2020;9(7):1658.

Mitchell CJ, Churchward-Venne TA, West DW, et al. Resistance exercise load does not determine training-mediated hypertrophic gains in young men. *J Appl Physiol (1985).* 2012;113(1):71-77.

Phillips SM, Tipton KD, Aarsland A, Wolf SE, Wolfe RR. Mixed muscle protein synthesis and breakdown after resistance exercise in humans. *Am J Physiol Endocrinol Metab.* 1997;273:e99-e107.

Roberts MD, Haun CT, Vann CG, Osburn SC, Young KC. Sarcoplasmic hypertrophy in skeletal muscle: A scientific "unicorn" or resistance training adaptation? *Front Physiol.* 2020;11:816.

Schoenfeld B. The mechanisms of muscle hypertrophy and their application to resistance training. *J Strength Cond Res.* 2010;24(10):2857-2872.

Schoenfeld BJ, Alto A, Grgic J, et al. Alterations in body composition, resting metabolic rate, muscular strength, and eating behavior in response to natural bodybuilding competition preparation: A case study. *J Strength Cond Res.* 2020;34(11):3124-3138.

Thomas G, Hall MN. TOR signaling and control of cell growth. *Curr Opin Cell Biol.* 1997;9:782-787.

Tokunaga C, Yoshino K, Yonezawa K. mTOR integrates amino acid- and energy-sensing pathways. *Biochem Biophys Res Commun.* 2004;313(2):443-446.

Toigo M, Boutellier U. New fundamental resistance exercise determinants of molecular and cellular muscle adaptations. *Eur J Appl Physiol.* 2006;97:643-663.

Vierck J, O'Reilly B, Hossner K, et al. Satellite cell regulation following myotrauma caused by resistance exercise. *Cell Biol Int.* 2000;24:263-272.

West DW, Baehr LM, Marcotte GR, et al. Acute resistance exercise activates rapamycin- sensitive and -insensitive mechanisms that control translational activity and capacity in skeletal muscle. *J Physiol.* 2016;594:453-468.

Williams CB, Zelt JG, Castellani LN, et al. Changes in mechanisms proposed to mediate fat loss following an acute bout of high-intensity interval and endurance exercise. *Appl Physiol Nutr Metab.* 2013;38(12):1236-1244.

Chapter 6

Bautista D, Durke D, Cotter JA, Escobar KA, Schick EE. A comparison of muscle activation among the front squat, overhead squat, back extension and plank. *Int J Exerc Sci.* 2020;13(1):714-722.

Butcher SJ, Rusin JS. Core strength and functionality with loaded carries. *NSCA Coach.* 2016;4(3).

Desmoulin GT, Pradhan V, Milner TE. Mechanical aspects of intervertebral disc injury and implications on biomechanics. *Spine (Phila Pa 1976).* 2020;45(8):e457-e464.

Hewit JK, Jaffe DA, Crowder T. A comparison of muscle activation during the pull-up and three alternative pulling exercises. *J Phy Fit Treatment & Sports.* 2018;5(4):555669.

McGill S. *Low Back Disorders.* 3rd ed. Human Kinetics; 2015.

Sanchis-Moysi J, Serrano-Sánchez JA, González-Henríquez JJ, Calbet JAL, Dorado C. Greater reduction in abdominal than in upper arms subcutaneous fat in 10- to 12-year-old tennis players: A volumetric MRI study. *Front Pediatr.* 2019;7:345.

Vagner M, Malecek J, Tomšovský L, Kubový P, Levitova A, Stastny P. Isokinetic strength of rotators, flexors and hip extensors is strongly related to front kick dynamics in military professionals. *J Hum Kinet.* 2019;68:145-155.

Chapter 8

Alcaraz PE, Perez-Gomez J, Chavarrias M, Blazevich AJ. Similarity in adaptations to high-resistance circuit vs. traditional strength training in resistance-trained men. *J Strength Cond Res.* 2011;25(9):2519-2527.

Colquhoun RJ, Gai CM, Walters J, et al. Comparison of powerlifting performance in trained men using traditional and flexible daily undulating periodization [published correction appears in *J Strength Cond Res.* 2017;31(4):e70]. *J Strength Cond Res.* 2017;31(2):283-291.

Fink J, Schoenfeld BJ, Kikuchi N, Nakazato K. Effects of drop set resistance training on acute stress indicators and long-term muscle hypertrophy and strength. *J Sports Med Phys Fitness.* 2018;58(5):597-605.

Fry AC, Kraemer WJ. Resistance exercise overtraining and overreaching: Neuroendocrine responses. *Sports Med.* 1997;23:106-129.

Helms ER, Fitschen PJ, Aragon AA, Cronin J, Schoenfeld BJ. Recommendations for natural bodybuilding contest preparation: Resistance and cardiovascular training. *J Sports Med Phys Fitness.* 2015;55(3):164-178.

Hornberger TA, Chien S. Mechanical stimuli and nutrients regulate rapamycin-sensitive signaling through distinct mechanisms in skeletal muscle. *J Cell Biochem.* 2006;97:1207-1216.

Izquierdo M, Ibañez J, González-Badillo JJ, et al. Differential effects of strength training leading to failure versus not to failure on hormonal responses, strength, and muscle power gains. *J Appl Physiol (1985).* 2006;100(5):1647-1656.

Krieger JW. Single vs. multiple sets of resistance exercise for muscle hypertrophy: A meta-analysis. *J Strength Cond Res.* 2010;24(4):1150-1159.

McGill S. *Low Back Disorders.* 3rd ed. Human Kinetics; 2015.

Miranda FS, Simao R, Rhea MR, et al. Effects of linear vs. daily undulating periodized resistance training on maximal and submaximal strength gains. *J Strength Cond Res.* 2011;25:1824-1830.

Mitchell CJ, Churchward-Venne TA, West DW, et al. Resistance exercise load does not determine training-mediated hypertrophic gains in young men. *J Appl Physiol (1985).* 2012;113(1):71-77.

Morton RW, Oikawa SY, Wavell CG, et al. Neither load nor systemic hormones determine resistance training-mediated hypertrophy or strength gains in resistance-trained young men. *J Appl Physiol (1985).* 2016;121(1):129-138.

Muñoz-Martínez FA, Rubio-Arias JÁ, Ramos-Campo DJ, Alcaraz PE. Effectiveness of resistance circuit-based training for maximum oxygen uptake and upper-body one-repetition maximum improvements: A systematic review and meta-analysis. *Sports Med.* 2017;47(12):2553-2568.

Patterson SD, Hughes L, Warmington S, et al. Blood flow restriction exercise: Considerations of methodology, application, and safety. *Front Physiol.* 2019;10:533.

Schoenfeld, B. The mechanisms of muscle hypertrophy and their application to resistance training. *J Strength Cond Res.* 2010;24(10):2857-2872.

Schoenfeld BJ, Contreras B, Krieger J, et al. Resistance training volume enhances muscle hypertrophy but not strength in trained men. *Med Sci Sports Exerc.* 2019;51(1):94-103.

Schoenfeld BJ, Grgic J, Ogborn D, Krieger JW. Strength and hypertrophy adaptations between low- vs. high-load resistance training: A systematic review and meta-analysis. *J Strength Cond Res.* 2017;31(12):3508-3523.

Schoenfeld BJ, Ogborn D, Krieger JW. Dose-response relationship between weekly resistance training volume and increases in muscle mass: A systematic review and meta-analysis. *J Sports Sci.* 2017;35(11):1073-1082.

Schoenfeld BJ, Ogborn D, Krieger JW. Effects of resistance training frequency on measures of muscle hypertrophy: A systematic review and meta-analysis. *Sports Med.* 2016;46(11):1689-1697.

Schoenfeld BJ, Pope ZK, Benik FM, et al. Longer interset rest periods enhance muscle strength and hypertrophy in resistance-trained men. *J Strength Cond Res.* 2016;30(7):1805-1812.

Simao RS, Spineti J, de Salles BF, et al. Comparison between nonlinear and linear periodized resistance training: Hypertrophy and strength effects. *J Strength Cond Res.* 2012;26:1389-1395.

Takada S, Okita K, Suga T, et al. Blood flow restriction exercise in sprinters and endurance runners. *Med Sci Sports Exerc.* 2012;44(3):413-419.

Vierck J, O'Reilly B, Hossner K, et al. Satellite cell regulation following myotrauma caused by resistance exercise. *Cell Biol Int.* 2000;24:263-272.

Chapter 9

Hellsten Y, Nyberg M. Cardiovascular adaptations to exercise training. *Compr Physiol.* 2015;6(1):1-32.

Hickson RC. Interference of strength development by simultaneously training for strength and endurance. *Eur J Appl Physiol Occup Physiol.* 1980;45(2-3):255-263.

Ismail I, Keating SE, Baker MK, Johnson NA. A systematic review and meta-analysis of the effect of aerobic vs. resistance exercise training on visceral fat. *Obes Rev.* 2012;13(1):68-91.

Maffetone P. *The Big Book of Endurance Training and Racing.* Skyhorse Publishing; 2010.

Murawska-Cialowicz E, Wolanski P, Zuwala-Jagiello J, et al. Effect of HIIT with tabata protocol on serum irisin, physical performance, and body composition in men. *Int J Environ Res Public Health.* 2020;17(10):3589.

Petré H, Löfving P, Psilander N. The effect of two different concurrent training programs on strength and power gains in highly-trained individuals. *J Sports Sci Med.* 2018;17(2):167-173.

Qaisar R, Bhaskaran S, Van Remmen H. Muscle fiber type diversification during exercise and regeneration. *Free Radic Biol Med.* 2016;98:56-67.

Tabata I, Nishimura K, Kouzaki M, et al. Effects of moderate-intensity endurance and high-intensity intermittent training on anaerobic capacity and VO2max. *Med Sci Sports Exerc.* 1996;28(10):1327-1330.

Tabata I. Tabata training: One of the most energetically effective high-intensity intermittent training methods. *J Physiol Sci.* 2019;69(4):559-572.

Tsatsouline P. *Strong Endurance.* 2nd ed. Power by Pavel;2018.

Volek JS, Noakes T, Phinney SD. Rethinking fat as a fuel for endurance exercise. *Eur J Sport Sci.* 2015;15(1):13-20.

Chapter 10

Aune TK, Aune MA, Ettema G, Vereijken B. Comparison of bilateral force deficit in proximal and distal joints in upper extremities. *Hum Mov Sci.* 2013;32(3):436-444.

Dankel SJ, Mattocks KT, Jessee MB, et al. Frequency: The overlooked resistance training variable for inducing muscle hypertrophy? *Sports Med.* 2017;47(5):799-805.

Fisher BE, Southam AC, Kuo YL, Lee YY, Powers CM. Evidence of altered corticomotor excitability following targeted activation of gluteus maximus training in healthy individuals. *Neuroreport.* 2016;27(6):415-421.

Lasevicius T, Schoenfeld BJ, Silva-Batista C, et al. Muscle failure promotes greater muscle hypertrophy in low-load but not in high-load resistance training [published online ahead of print, 2019 Dec 27]. *J Strength Cond Res.* 2019;10.

Morton RW, Sonne MW, Farias Zuniga A, et al. Muscle fibre activation is unaffected by load and repetition duration when resistance exercise is performed to task failure. *J Physiol.* 2019;597(17):4601-4613.

Schoenfeld BJ, Contreras B. The muscle pump: Potential mechanisms and applications for enhancing hypertrophic adaptations. *Strength Cond J.* 2014;36(3):21-25.

Schwarzenegger A. *The New Encyclopedia of Modern Bodybuilding.* Simon & Schuster; 1987.

Spineti J, de Salles BF, Rhea MR, et al. Influence of exercise order on maximum strength and muscle volume in nonlinear periodized resistance training. *J Strength Cond Res.* 2010;24(11):2962-2969.

Chapter 11

Ammar A, Turki M, Hammouda O, et al. Effects of pomegranate juice supplementation on oxidative stress biomarkers following weightlifting exercise. *Nutrients.* 2017;9(8):819.

Avruch J, Long X, Ortiz-Vega S, Rapley J, Papageorgiou A, Dai N. Amino acid regulation of TOR complex 1. *Am J Physiol Endocrinol Metab.* 2009;296(4):e592-e602.

Calder PC. Omega-3 fatty acids and inflammatory processes: From molecules to man. *Biochem Soc Trans.* 2017;45(5):1105-1115.

Chai SC, Jerusik J, Davis K, Wright RS, Zhang Z. Effect of Montmorency tart cherry juice on cognitive performance in older adults: A randomized controlled trial. *Food Funct.* 2019;10(7):4423-4431.

Chenevey B. Overview of fluids and electrolytes. *Nurs Clin North Am.* 1987;22(4):749-759.

Churchward-Venne TA, Burd NA, Mitchell CJ, et al. Supplementation of a suboptimal protein dose with leucine or essential amino acids: Effects on myofibrillar protein synthesis at rest and following resistance exercise in men. *J Physiol.* 2012;590(11):2751-2765.

Crinnion WJ. Organic foods contain higher levels of certain nutrients, lower levels of pesticides, and may provide health benefits for the consumer. *Altern Med Rev.* 2010;15(1):4-12.

de Baaij JH, Hoenderop JG, Bindels RJ. Magnesium in man: Implications for health and disease. *Physiol Rev.* 2015;95(1):1-46.

De Feo P, Di Loreto C, Lucidi P, et al. Metabolic response to exercise. *J Endocrinol Invest.* 2003;26(9):851-854.

DiNicolantonio JJ, O'Keefe JH, Wilson W. Subclinical magnesium deficiency: A principal driver of cardiovascular disease and a public health crisis [published correction appears in *Open Heart.* 2018;5(1):e000668corr1]. *Open Heart.* 2018;5(1):e000668.

Dong TA, Sandesara PB, Dhindsa DS, et al. Intermittent fasting: A heart healthy dietary pattern? *Am J Med.* 2020;133(8):901-907.

Duan Y, Li F, Li Y, et al. The role of leucine and its metabolites in protein and energy metabolism. *Amino Acids.* 2016;48(1):41-51.

Erem S, Atfi A, Razzaque MS. Anabolic effects of vitamin D and magnesium in aging bone. *J Steroid Biochem Mol Biol.* 2019;193:105400.

Fernández del Río L, Gutiérrez-Casado E, Varela-López A, Villalba JM. Olive oil and the hallmarks of aging. *Molecules.* 2016;21(2):163.

Fernando HA, Zibellini J, Harris RA, Seimon RV, Sainsbury A. Effect of Ramadan fasting on weight and body composition in healthy non-athlete adults: A systematic review and meta-analysis. *Nutrients.* 2019;11(2):478.

Garcia JP, Santana A, Baruqui DL, Suraci N. The cardiovascular effects of chocolate. *Rev Cardiovasc Med.* 2018;19(4):123-127.

Giugliano D, Ceriello A, Esposito K. The effects of diet on inflammation: Emphasis on the metabolic syndrome. *J Am Coll Cardiol.* 2006;48(4):677-685.

Golia E, Limongelli G, Natale F, et al. Inflammation and cardiovascular disease: From pathogenesis to therapeutic target. *Curr Atheroscler Rep.* 2014;16(9):435.

Hales CM, Fryar CD, Carroll MD, Freedman DS, Ogden CL. Trends in obesity and severe obesity prevalence in US youth and adults by sex and age, 2007-2008 to 2015-2016. *JAMA.* 2018;319(16):1723-1725.

Halton TL, Hu FB. The effects of high protein diets on thermogenesis, satiety and weight loss: A critical review. *J Am Coll Nutr.* 2004;23(5):373-385.

Herforth A, Arimond M, Álvarez-Sánchez C, Coates J, Christianson K, Muehlhoff E. A global review of food-based dietary guidelines [published correction appears in *Adv Nutr.* 2019;10(4):730]. *Adv Nutr.* 2019;10(4):590-605.

Holick MF. The vitamin D deficiency pandemic: Approaches for diagnosis, treatment and prevention. *Rev Endocr Metab Disord.* 2017;18(2):153-165.

Holick MF, Binkley NC, Bischoff-Ferrari HA, et al. Evaluation, treatment, and prevention of vitamin D deficiency: An Endocrine Society clinical practice guideline [published correction appears in *J Clin Endocrinol Metab.* 2011;96(12):3908]. *J Clin Endocrinol Metab.* 2011;96(7):1911-1930.

Jäger R, Kerksick CM, Campbell BI, et al. International Society of Sports Nutrition position stand: Protein and exercise. *J Int Soc Sports Nutr*. 2017;14:20.

Kadandale S, Marten R, Smith R. The palm oil industry and noncommunicable diseases. *Bull World Health Organ*. 2019;97(2):118-128.

Keys A, Anderson JT, Grande F. Serum cholesterol response to changes in the diet: IV. Particular saturated fatty acids in the diet. *Metabolism*. 1965;14(7):776-787.

Kostov K. Effects of magnesium deficiency on mechanisms of insulin resistance in type 2 diabetes: Focusing on the processes of insulin secretion and signaling. *Int J Mol Sci*. 2019;20(6):1351.

Kujawska M, Jourdes M, Kurpik M, et al. Neuroprotective effects of pomegranate juice against Parkinson's disease and presence of ellagitannins-derived metabolite—urolithin A—in the brain. *Int J Mol Sci*. 2019;21(1):202.

Levine B, Kroemer G. Autophagy in the pathogenesis of disease. *Cell*. 2008;132(1):27-42.

Lippi G, Schena F, Salvagno GL, et al. Acute variation of estimated glomerular filtration rate following a half-marathon run. *Int J Sports Med*. 2008;29(12):948-951.

Liu AG, Ford NA, Hu FB, Zelman KM, Mozaffarian D, Kris-Etherton PM. A healthy approach to dietary fats: Understanding the science and taking action to reduce consumer confusion. *Nutr J*. 2017;16(1):53.

Liu J, Yang X, Yu S, Zheng R. The leptin resistance. *Adv Exp Med Biol*. 2018;1090:145-163.

Magee PJ, Gallagher AM, McCormack JM. High prevalence of dehydration and inadequate nutritional knowledge among university and club level athletes. *Int J Sport Nutr Exerc Metab*. 2017;27(2):158-168.

Martin-Rincon M, Perez-Suarez I, Pérez-López A, et al. Protein synthesis signaling in skeletal muscle is refractory to whey protein ingestion during a severe energy deficit evoked by prolonged exercise and caloric restriction. *Int J Obes (Lond)*. 2019;43(4):872-882.

Mergenthaler P, Lindauer U, Dienel GA, Meisel A. Sugar for the brain: The role of glucose in physiological and pathological brain function. *Trends Neurosci*. 2013;36(10):587-597.

Monteiro R, Azevedo I. Chronic inflammation in obesity and the metabolic syndrome. *Mediators Inflamm*. 2010;2010:289645.

Morton RW, Murphy KT, McKellar SR, et al. A systematic review, meta-analysis and meta-regression of the effect of protein supplementation on resistance training-induced gains in muscle mass and strength in healthy adults [published correction appears in *Br J Sports Med*. 2020;54(19):e7]. *Br J Sports Med*. 2018;52(6):376-384.

Myles IA. Fast food fever: Reviewing the impacts of the Western diet on immunity. *Nutr J*. 2014;13:61.

Nair R, Maseeh A. Vitamin D: The "sunshine" vitamin. *J Pharmacol Pharmacother*. 2012;3(2):118-126.

Neinast M, Murashige D, Arany Z. Branched chain amino acids. *Annu Rev Physiol*. 2019;81:139-164.

Ng CY, Leong XF, Masbah N, Adam SK, Kamisah Y, Jaarin K. Heated vegetable oils and cardiovascular disease risk factors. *Vascul Pharmacol*. 2014;61(1):1-9.

Onvani S, Haghighatdoost F, Surkan PJ, Larijani B, Azadbakht L. Adherence to the Healthy Eating Index and Alternative Healthy Eating Index dietary patterns and mortality from all causes, cardiovascular disease and cancer: A meta-analysis of observational studies. *J Hum Nutr Diet*. 2017;30(2):216-226.

Parzych KR, Klionsky DJ. An overview of autophagy: Morphology, mechanism, and regulation. *Antioxid Redox Signal*. 2014;20(3):460-473.

Petersen MC, Shulman GI. Mechanisms of insulin action and insulin resistance. *Physiol Rev*. 2018;98(4):2133-2223.

Reddy P, Edwards LR. Magnesium supplementation in vitamin D deficiency. *Am J Ther*. 2019;26(1):e124-e132.

Rondanelli M, Faliva MA, Gasparri C, et al. Current opinion on dietary advice in order to preserve fat-free mass during a low-calorie diet. *Nutrition*. 2020;72:110667.

Rosanoff A, Weaver CM, Rude RK. Suboptimal magnesium status in the United States: Are the health consequences underestimated? *Nutr Rev*. 2012;70(3):153-164.

Sahebkar A, Ferri C, Giorgini P, Bo S, Nachtigal P, Grassi D. Effects of pomegranate juice on blood pressure: A systematic review and meta-analysis of randomized controlled trials. *Pharmacol Res*. 2017;115:149-161.

Santos HO, Macedo RCO. Impact of intermittent fasting on the lipid profile: Assessment associated with diet and weight loss. *Clin Nutr ESPEN*. 2018;24:14-21.

Schubert MM, Irwin C, Seay RF, Clarke HE, Allegro D, Desbrow B. Caffeine, coffee, and appetite control: A review. *Int J Food Sci Nutr*. 2017;68(8):901-912.

Serefko A, Szopa A, Wlaź P, et al. Magnesium in depression. *Pharmacol Rep*. 2013;65(3):547-554.

Shahidi F, Ambigaipalan P. Omega-3 polyunsaturated fatty acids and their health benefits. *Annu Rev Food Sci Technol*. 2018;9:345-381.

Shirreffs SM, Sawka MN. Fluid and electrolyte needs for training, competition, and recovery. *J Sports Sci*. 2011;29(Suppl 1):S39-S46.

Traylor DA, Gorissen SHM, Hopper H, Prior T, McGlory C, Phillips SM. Aminoacidemia following ingestion of native whey protein, micellar casein, and a whey-casein blend in young men. *Appl Physiol Nutr Metab*. 2019;44(1):103-106.

van der Merwe J, Brooks NE, Myburgh KH. Three weeks of creatine monohydrate supplementation affects dihydrotestosterone to testosterone ratio in college-aged rugby players. *Clin J Sport Med*. 2009;19(5):399-404.

Vitale KC, Hueglin S, Broad E. Tart cherry juice in athletes: A literature review and commentary. *Curr Sports Med Rep*. 2017;16(4):230-239.

Volpe SL. Magnesium in disease prevention and overall health. *Adv Nutr.* 2013;4(3):378S-83S.

Westman EC, Tondt J, Maguire E, Yancy WS Jr. Implementing a low-carbohydrate, ketogenic diet to manage type 2 diabetes mellitus. *Expert Rev Endocrinol Metab.* 2018;13(5):263-272.

Workinger JL, Doyle RP, Bortz J. Challenges in the diagnosis of magnesium status. *Nutrients.* 2018;10(9):1202.

Worthington V. Nutritional quality of organic versus conventional fruits, vegetables, and grains. *J Altern Complement Med.* 2001;7(2):161-173.

Wu H, Ballantyne CM. Skeletal muscle inflammation and insulin resistance in obesity. *J Clin Invest.* 2017;127(1):43-54.

Xiao N, Zhao Y, Yao Y, et al. Biological activities of egg yolk lipids: A review. *J Agric Food Chem.* 2020;68(7):1948-1957.

Chapter 12

Alhakami AM, Davis S, Qasheesh M, Shaphe A, Chahal A. Effects of McKenzie and stabilization exercises in reducing pain intensity and functional disability in individuals with nonspecific chronic low back pain: A systematic review. *J Phys Ther Sci.* 2019;31(7):590-597.

Berenbaum F. Osteoarthritis as an inflammatory disease (osteoarthritis is not osteoarthrosis!). *Osteoarthritis Cartilage.* 2013;21(1):16-21.

Burd NA, Gorissen SH, van Loon LJ. Anabolic resistance of muscle protein synthesis with aging. *Exerc Sport Sci Rev.* 2013;41(3):169-173.

Cabral M, Bangdiwala SI, Severo M, Guimarães JT, Nogueira L, Ramos E. Central and peripheral body fat distribution: Different associations with low-grade inflammation in young adults? *Nutr Metab Cardiovasc Dis.* 2019;29(9):931-938.

Chazaud B. Inflammation and skeletal muscle regeneration: Leave it to the macrophages! *Trends Immunol.* 2020;41(6):481-492.

Curlik DM 2nd, Shors TJ. Training your brain: Do mental and physical (MAP) training enhance cognition through the process of neurogenesis in the hippocampus? *Neuropharmacology.* 2013;64(1):506-514.

Deschenes MR, Tufts HL, Noronha AL, Li S. Both aging and exercise training alter the rate of recovery of neuromuscular performance of male soleus muscles. *Biogerontology.* 2019;20(2):213-223.

Dzierzewski JM, Dautovich N, Ravyts S. Sleep and cognition in older adults. *Sleep Med Clin.* 2018;13(1):93-106.

Fell J, Williams D. The effect of aging on skeletal-muscle recovery from exercise: Possible implications for aging athletes. *J Aging Phys Act.* 2008;16(1):97-115.

Furman D, Campisi J, Verdin E, et al. Chronic inflammation in the etiology of disease across the life span. *Nat Med.* 2019;25(12):1822-1832.

Hardingham T, Tew S, Murdoch A. Tissue engineering: Chondrocytes and cartilage. *Arthritis Res.* 2002;4(Suppl 3):S63-S68.

Khow KSF, Visvanathan R. Falls in the aging population. *Clin Geriatr Med.* 2017;33(3):357-368.

McGill S. *Low Back Disorders.* 3rd ed. Human Kinetics; 2015.

Nyffeler RW, Meyer DC. Acromion and glenoid shape: Why are they important predictive factors for the future of our shoulders? *EFORT Open Rev.* 2017;2(5):141-150.

Opendak M, Briones BA, Gould E. Social behavior, hormones and adult neurogenesis. *Front Neuroendocrinol.* 2016;41:71-86.

Seals DR. Edward F. Adolph Distinguished Lecture: The remarkable anti-aging effects of aerobic exercise on systemic arteries. *J Appl Physiol (1985).* 2014;117(5):425-439.

Shah NN, Bayliss NC, Malcolm A. Shape of the acromion: Congenital or acquired—a macroscopic, radiographic, and microscopic study of acromion. *J Shoulder Elbow Surg.* 2001;10(4):309-316.

Shors TJ, Townsend DA, Zhao M, Kozorovitskiy Y, Gould E. Neurogenesis may relate to some but not all types of hippocampal-dependent learning. *Hippocampus.* 2002;12(5):578-584.

Sun L, Sun Q, Qi J. Adult hippocampal neurogenesis: An important target associated with antidepressant effects of exercise. *Rev Neurosci.* 2017;28(7):693-703.

Trompeter K, Fett D, Platen P. Prevalence of back pain in sports: A systematic review of the literature. *Sports Med.* 2017;47(6):1183-1207.

ABOUT THE AUTHOR

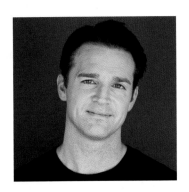

Chad Waterbury, PT, DPT, MS, graduated from the nation's top ranked doctor of physical therapy (DPT) program at the University of Southern California (USC), where he currently teaches the course Resistance Training Techniques for High-Performance Athletes for the master's degree in sports science program. He is the owner of Chad Waterbury LLC and author of *Huge in a Hurry* from Rodale Publishing. Waterbury has lectured for fitness organizations such as the National Strength and Conditioning Association (NSCA) and Perform Better. He has a master's degree in physiology from the University of Arizona, where his focus on the neurophysiology of human movement and performance led him to make radical changes in the way he trains competitive athletes as well as nonathletic clients. His workouts are now shorter and faster, producing superior results in strength, power, and muscular development, while at the same time inducing less fatigue and allowing for shorter recovery periods between workouts.

You read the book—now complete the companion CE exam to earn continuing education credit!

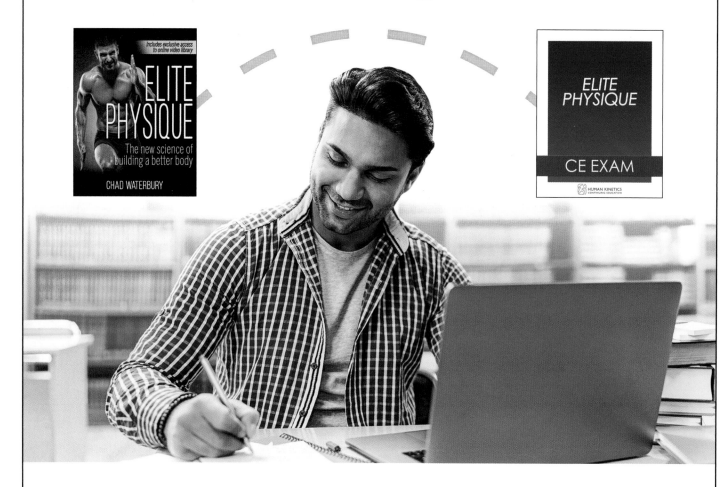

Find and purchase the companion CE exam here:
US.HumanKinetics.com/collections/CE-Exam
Canada.HumanKinetics.com/collections/CE-Exam

50% off the companion CE exam with this code

EP2022

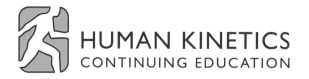